PEDIATRIC LIVER DISEASE

HEPATOLOGY
Research and Clinical Issues

Volume 1 • Viral Hepatitis
Edited by M. M. Fisher and J. W. Steiner
Canadian Medical Association Journal
(Vol. 106, Special Issue, pp. 417 – 528, 1972)

Volume 2 • Jaundice
Edited by C. A. Goresky and M. M. Fisher

Volume 3 • Alcohol and the Liver
Edited by M. M. Fisher and J. G. Rankin

Volume 4 • Gall Stones
Edited by M. M. Fisher, C. A. Goresky,
E. A. Shaffer, and S. M. Strasberg

Volume 5 • Pediatric Liver Disease
Edited by M. M. Fisher and C. C. Roy

PEDIATRIC LIVER DISEASE

Edited by

M. M. FISHER
University of Toronto
Toronto, Ontario, Canada

and

C. C. ROY
Université de Montréal
Montréal, Québec, Canada

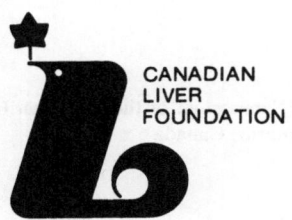

CANADIAN
LIVER
FOUNDATION

PLENUM PRESS · NEW YORK AND LONDON

Library of Congress Cataloging in Publication Data

Canadian Liver Foundation. International Symposium (5th: 1980: Toronto, Ont.)
  Pediatric liver disease.

  (Hepatology: research and clinical issues; v. 5)
  "Proceedings of the Fifth International Symposium of the Canadian Liver Founda-
tion held May 23-24, 1980, in Toronto, Ontario, Canada" — T.p. verso.
  Includes bibliographical references and index.
  1. Liver — Diseases — Congresses. 2. Pediatric gastroenterology — Congresses. I.
Fisher, M. M. (Murray M.), 1934–   . II. Roy, Claude C., 1928–   . III. Title. IV.
Series: Hepatology; v. 5. [DNLM: 2. Liver diseases — In infancy and childhood — Con-
gresses. W1 HE913 v.5/WS 310 P3715 1980]
  RJ456.L5C36 1980   618.92′362   82-18046

ISBN 978-1-4684-4387-5   ISBN 978-1-4684-4385-1 (eBook)
DOI 10.1007/978-1-4684-4385-1

Proceedings of the Fifth International Symposium of the Canadian Liver Foundation
held May 23-24, 1980, in Toronto, Ontario, Canada

© 1983 Plenum Press, New York
Softcover reprint of the hardcover 1st edition 1983
A Division of Plenum Publishing Corporation
233 Spring Street, New York, N.Y. 10013

PREFACE

    This was an important Symposium in a rapidly developing field of interest. It was designed to draw attention to areas which have been neglected in standard hepatology textbooks and to review areas of controversy. It was also meant to help bridge the communication gap between hepatologists caring for children and adults as well as between some areas of clinical and basic research.

    The Symposium was a substantial success. Unfortunately two of the twenty participants did not deliver a manuscript. The result is a publication which is late and which is not as complete as it should be. For this lateness and incompleteness the editors apologize most sincerely--especially to those participants who delivered their manuscripts on time but even to those who delivered their manuscripts late.

    Perhaps the most noteworthy feature of this publication is the fact that material presented in May 1980 is by no means out of date. Apart from the section on Viral Hepatitis, one of the most rapidly evolving fields of medicine, the context of the Symposium remains disturbingly current. The neglect continues, the controversies remain.

    We hope that this publication will help draw investigators into liver research, provide a useful point of reference for those in the field and stand as a monument to editors past, present and future, who have chased, are chasing and will chase manuscripts in vain.

M.M. Fisher
C.C. Roy

ACKNOWLEDGEMENTS

The Canadian Liver Foundation gratefully acknowledges the support of the Hospital for Sick Children Foundation which awarded a grant towards the expenses of the meeting and the cost of preparing the proceedings for publication.

CONTENTS

CONTENTS

EARLY DEVELOPMENT OF THE LIVER: A REVIEW

Robert L. Peters

Professor of Pathology, University of Southern
California School of Medicine
Los Angeles, California

INDUCTIVE PROCESS (LESS THAN 2.5 mm)

The earliest sign of liver formation in the developing human
embryo antedates any recognizable morphologic anlage.   At a
developmental time less than 21 post ovulatory days, when the
embryo is less than 2.5 mm long, the embryo is a convex caterpillar-
like structure, broadly connected to the yolk sac.   The infolding
that produces the head process, has brought the cardiac mesoderm
in close juxtaposition to the broad stalk of the yolk sac.   This
stalk forms the upright of a T with the horizontal arms making up
the fore and hind guts, at this stage.

Extrapolating from work performed in the chick (1,2) even in
the presomatic stages, stages corresponding to less than 20 post
ovulatory days in man, markers can be placed to allow identification
of "presumptive hepatic" areas.   However the mesodermal and endodermal areas so identified are not capable of forming liver by
self differentiation.   The liver develops from the endomesodermal
tissues that lie between the pericardium and the stalk of the yolk
sac.   However, the cardiac mesoderm is the inductive source and
is required for hepatic differentiation.   By about 21 days, (between
4 and 7 somites development), the endomesodermal tissue from which
the hepatic anlage is anticipated, can often, if transplanted to
chorioallantoic membrane, develop into hepatic parenchyma.   However
at 21 days if the mesodermal component is removed by trypsinization,
the residual endoderm will not differentiate into hepatoblasts, but
will retain the appearance of primative endodermal gut.   At 23 days
(2.5 mm) the foregut and the pericardial cavity are encased in
continuous mesenchyme(3,4).   A spongy transformation begins to
develop in the mesenchymal tissue of the transverse septum area

1

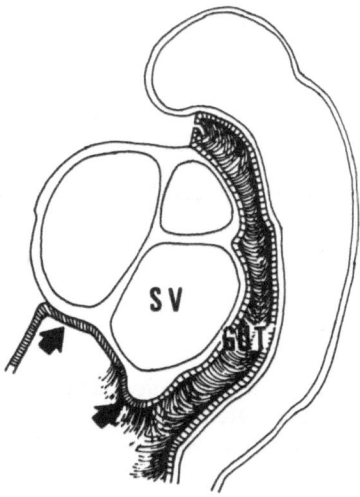

Fig. 1   *Diagram of human embryo at 23 days (2.5 mm).   Note that*
         the foregut opens to yolk sac.   The pericardial sac is
         separated from the gut by mesenchymal tissue that makes
         up the septum transversum.   Arrows demarcate the area
         of future hepatic diverticulum.   SV = sinus venosus.

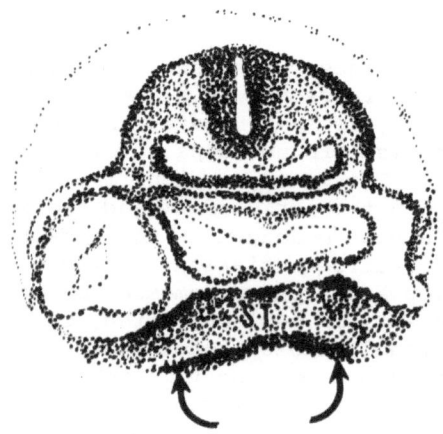

Fig. 2   *Thickening of gut wall preparatory to eventration of the*
         ductus choledochus.   Arrows enclose area of future
         hepatic diverticulum.   ST = septum transversum.

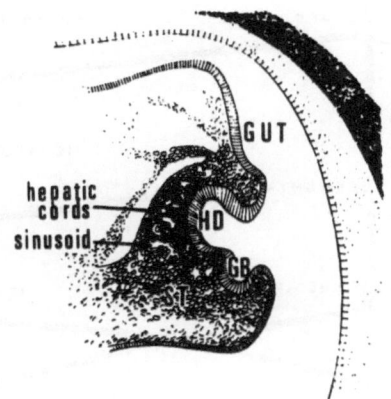

*Fig. 3   As the ductus choledochus invaginates the septum transversum,
          epithelial cells begin to bud off from the ductus tip.   By
          5 mm the epithelial buds and vascular spaces interdigitate.
          HD = hepatic diverticulum, GB = gallbladder, ST = septum
          transversum.*

that lies between pericardium and the gut wall, and the prehepatic
endodermal cells become enlongated (Figures 1,2).

PARENCHYMAL-MESENCHYMAL INTERACTION, 3 to 5 mm

     At about 25 days when the fetus is 3 mm long, the prehepatic
endodermal area begins to evaginate into the spongy splanchnic
mesoderm forming a diverticulum (Figure 3).   As the diverticulum
grows into the splanchnic mesoderm, epithelial cells with characteristics of hepatoblasts begin to proliferate from the tip of the
diverticulum.   At the same time, sinusoidal spaces develop in the
mesenchyme of the transverse septum.   The epithelial cells interdigitate with the developing vascular structures to form an hepatic
cord-sinusoid relationship.   As the foregut recedes from the septum
transversum, and the yolk-sac stalk shrinks while the elongating
gut retracts into the body cavity, mesoderm that surrounds the
hepatic diverticulum thins and becomes the hepatoduodenal ligament
dorsal to the liver, and the falciform ligament ventrally.

VASCULAR DEVELOPMENT, 3 to 5 mm

     All of the vascular spaces in the mesenchyme of the septum
transversum become filled very rapidly with blood islands consisting
principally of primitive hemacytoblasts.   The formation of vascular
spaces within the pre-hepatic mesenchyme is self differentiating,
requiring neither cardiac mesoderm nor the differentiating hepatoblasts for induction (1).   Instead, the sinusoids act as a template
for hepatic cord growth.   However, the hematopoietic potential of

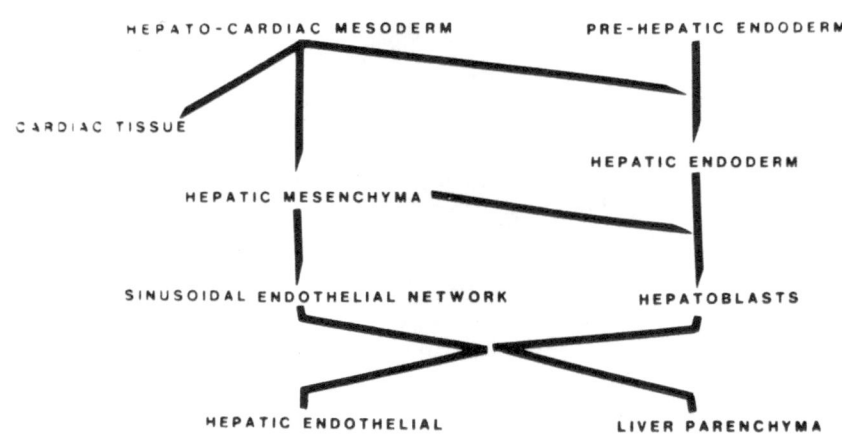

Fig. 4   *Chart showing interrelated inductive activity*

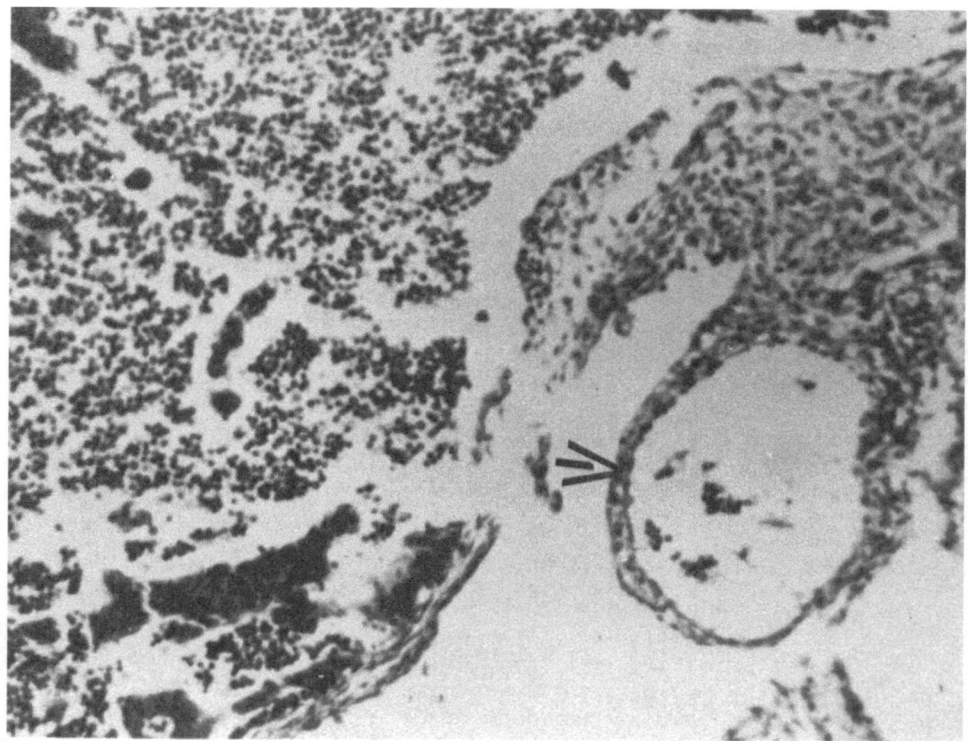

Fig. 5   *Liver with extensive erythropoiesis encroaching upon the*
         vitelline vein (arrow).   (H & E x 80)

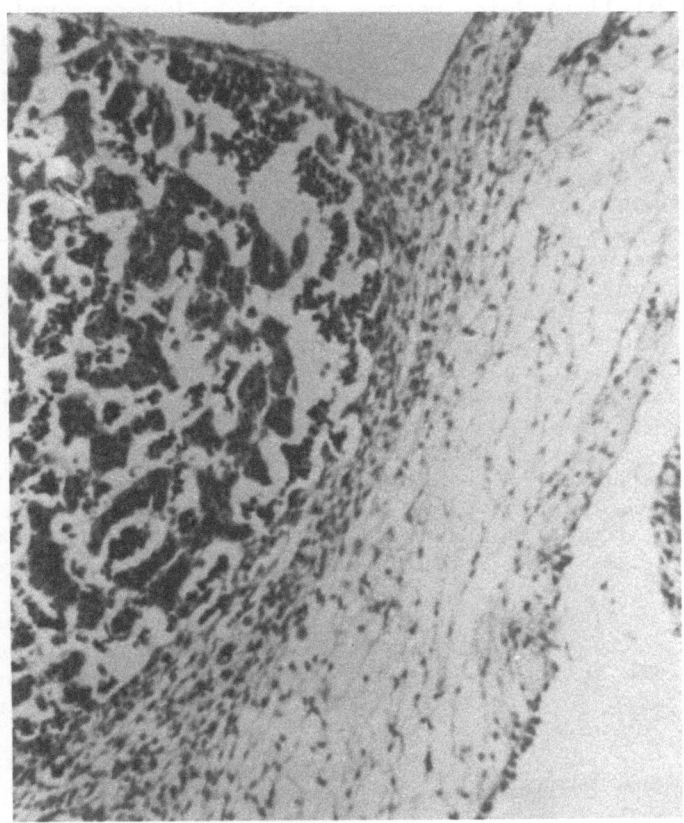

*Fig. 6   The vitelline vein has been invaded and the liver extends
across the abdominal cavity at 5 mm. (H & E x 100)*

the hepatic mesenchyme apparently requires the hepatoblasts for
induction.   Thus part of the hepatic mesoderm (the sinusoid lining)
is self inducing, the other part (hematopoietic) requires induction
by the endodermal portion (Figure 4).   The sinusoidal channels
become confluent so that by the time the vitelline and umbilical
veins are invaded, the sinusoidal bed is already complete.

The vitelline veins are situated laterally along the yolk sac,
draining that structure and passing on up to the heart.   As the
combined endomesodermal mass of hepatic anlage begins to grow, it
receives a rich blood supply from the vitelline veins, which may be
responsible for the liver's rapid growth.   By the 5 mm embryo size,
the liver extends all the way across the abdomen from the right
vitelline vein system to the left (Figure 5).

As the liver extends to the lateral margins of the abdominal cavity, the vitelline veins become completely incorporated into the hepatic mass so that the veins empty directly into the developing hepatic sinusoidal bed.   The blood egresses through the distal residua of the vitelline vein system that terminates in the right atrium of the developing heart (Figure 6).   The subhepatic section of the vitelline veins becomes the portal vein.   The more distal tributaries of the vitelline veins, originally ramifying over the yolk sac, become part of the mesenteric vein system, ultimately the splanchnic vasculature and the portal vein tributaries.   In a similar fashion to the vitelline veins, the left umbilical vein is first surrounded, then invaded by the growing endomesodermal mass.

At the five millimeter stage, the liver endodermal component forms a loose network of thin tubular structures.   The tubular parenchyma is interdigitated with dilated sinusoids.   From their onset the tubular parenchymal cells resemble hepatic epithelial cells and not duct structures.   Intrahepatic veins, both efferent and afferent branches of the vitelline and of the umbilical veins, become recognizable.   At 6 mm, the ductus venosus develops, reestablishing direct flow from the left umbilical vein to the inferior vena cava.   At 7 mm, the right umbilical vein atrophies.

The umbilical vein as it enters the ductus venosus, has sphincter activity that allows control of blood returning to the heart (5).   The sphincter control is presumed to offer protection against excessive fetal cardiac filling when maternal uterine contractions increase venous return.

LOBULAR (ACINAR) FORMATION

Until about 7.5 mm, the liver still consists of just one lobe made up of one lobule.   Since the entire liver is so small, vascular supply is adequate for total perfusion in spite of the single lobule configuration.   But as the liver mass grows in the caudal-cephalad plane, the portal vein structures and the hepatic vein structures become more widely separated, and the lobule begins to divide.   Ultimately the liver mass gets large enough to form separate lobules, two separate lobules by about 7.5 mm fetal length, 6 lobules by 11 mm length, and of course thousands by the time the infant is born.   It would appear as though hepatic vein prolifera- tion occurs earlier than does portal vein proliferation, and throughout the whole fetal development, more hepatic vein structures than portal veins can be found, usually two hepatic veins per portal vein.   Perhaps the proliferating hepatic vein system is either directly or indirectly stimulatory for division of the portal vein. Conversely, the portal vein may be slower to respond to the stimulus that affects both portal and hepatic veins.

The earliest intrahepatic portal veins (afferent vitelline

veins) moving into the liver substance are not associated with
connective tissue.   Soon however, the mesenchyme at the hilum of
the liver migrates in around the portal veins.   At first there is
only connective tissue and the vein itself.   Occasional portal
areas have a small interlobular bile duct.   This duct, most
investigators believe, is formed by a conversion from the adjacent
hepatic cords (6), induced by the invading mesenchyme.   The
lobular portal areas have no arterioles in early fetal life, only
large portal vein structures.

LYMPHATICS

       Little seems to have been written about the development of the
intrahepatic lymphatics.   There are many thin wall structures in
the developing portal areas, as there are in adult livers.
Structures that might represent lymphatics can be seen, but it is
difficult to prove histologically that any particular endothelialized
structure is a lymphatic.

ARTERIOLAR DEVELOPMENT

       In the first trimester arteriolar structures are sparse and
only in larger portal spaces (Figure 7).

       By the time the fetus has reached the third trimester of
intrauterine development, the lobular arterioles are plentiful but
are quite small relative to the size of the portal vein (Figure 8).
This probably reflects a lesser blood flow through the arteries,
just as in different animal species the relative size of intrahepatic arteries and portal veins seems to reflect the relative
blood flow in each.   The liver doesn't require much in the way of
hepatic arterial blood at this stage in its development, particularly
since arterial blood has no greater nutritive or oxygen carrying
capacity than the umbilical vein.

INTERLOBULAR DUCTS

       In the third trimester fetus, lobular bile ductules are still
deficient, but in fairly large portal areas, liver cords are
beginning to be incorporated by collagen at the margins, stimulating
conversion of cords into duct structures (6) (Figure 9).   In
Progressive Familial Cholestasis, the earliest biopsies show
unusually small portal areas.   The disease is characterized by
intrinsic impairment to bile flow.   Could some of these diseases
have their onset as a result of a deficiency or late development
of the sheath of connective tissue that induces duct formation?

       The portal area is highly vascularized around the bile ducts,
presumably the hepatic arteries branch around the duct in a
spiralling fashion.   Theoretically, damage or deficiency of hepatic

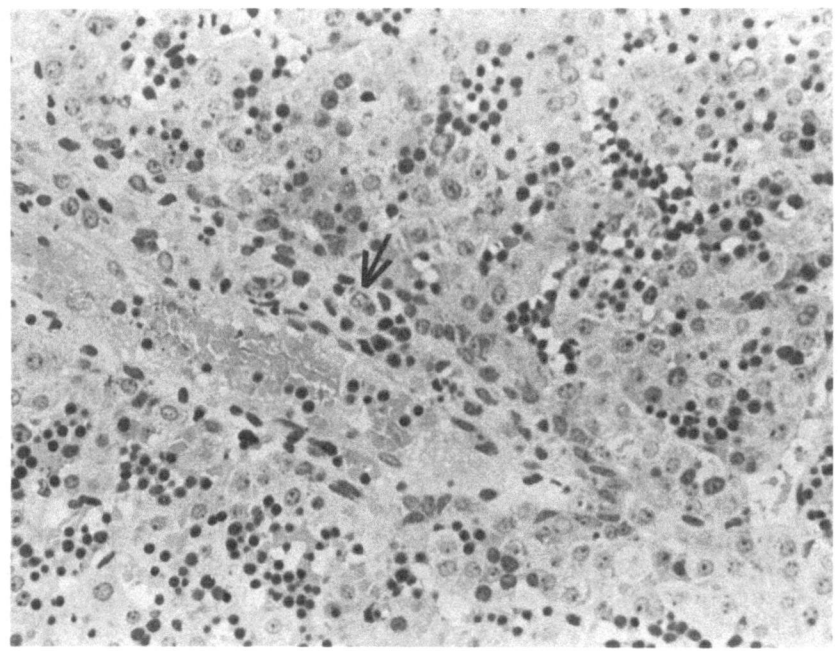

*Fig. 7 Portal area of first trimester fetus.   Note small
          arteriole (arrow).   (H & E x 180)*

arterial branches could cause some deficiency or abnormality of
ducts.   It is quite possible that arterioles in themselves may
play some role in the dissolution or the lack of development of
bile ducts, but the effect of arterial deficiency would probably
only begin to develop post-natally.

     At even very early stages of development of a duct, the lumen
is visible, even though duct epithelial cells are still quite
primitive, supporting again what some investigators have shown
about the early appearance of bile acids and bile pigments, not
only in the gut but in the gallbladder and elsewhere at 5 months
fetal age.

     The development of ducts in portal areas is still incomplete
into the newborn period.   In the smallest portal areas at birth,
ducts are still rather poorly developed as compared with those in
adult livers.   Lobule development is not complete at birth, and
there is continual growth of portal structures out into the lobule
and ongoing transformation of some of the cord structures into ducts.

     The liver cord, as it develops, has a canaliculus right from
its onset.   The canalicular wall simply represents the wall of the

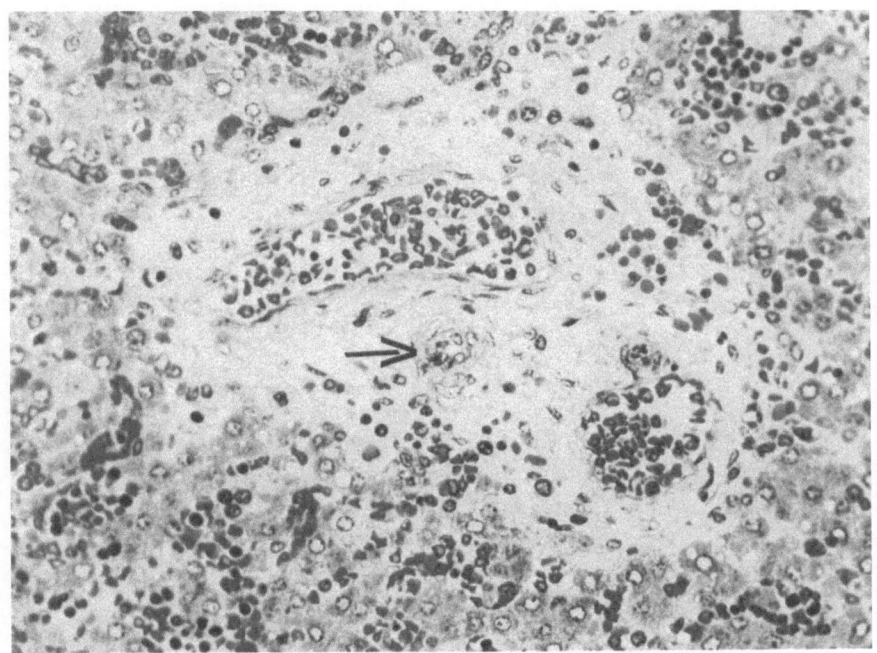

*Fig. 8 Portal area in 3rd trimester fetus.   Note small
        arteriole (arrow)   (H & E x 180)*

hepatocyte, but is more obvious than it is in the adult.   Only in
an abnormal hepatic condition will one identify a canaliculus in
adult liver cords that is as prominent as those normally seen in
the newborn (Figure 10).

ERYTHROPOIESIS

     Erythropoiesis is an important activity of the fetal liver.
At about two months it becomes quite striking and continues as a
major source of blood production until about seven months fetal
age.   There is some erythropoiesis continuing until birth, in many
hepatic pathologic conditions of the newborn one sees more erythropoiesis than in a normal newborn.   Term or near term infants dying
of pulmonary hyaline membrane disease at eight hours after birth
have increased hepatic erythropoiesis, even though one cannot
attribute the erythropoiesis to the brief anoxia.

     The islands of erythroid tissue develop, not in the sinusoids
but in subendothelial spaces, and within the liver cords in the
human, sometimes in the intercellular space invaginating into
hepatocytes (Figure 11).   Erythroid tissue constitutes a considerable

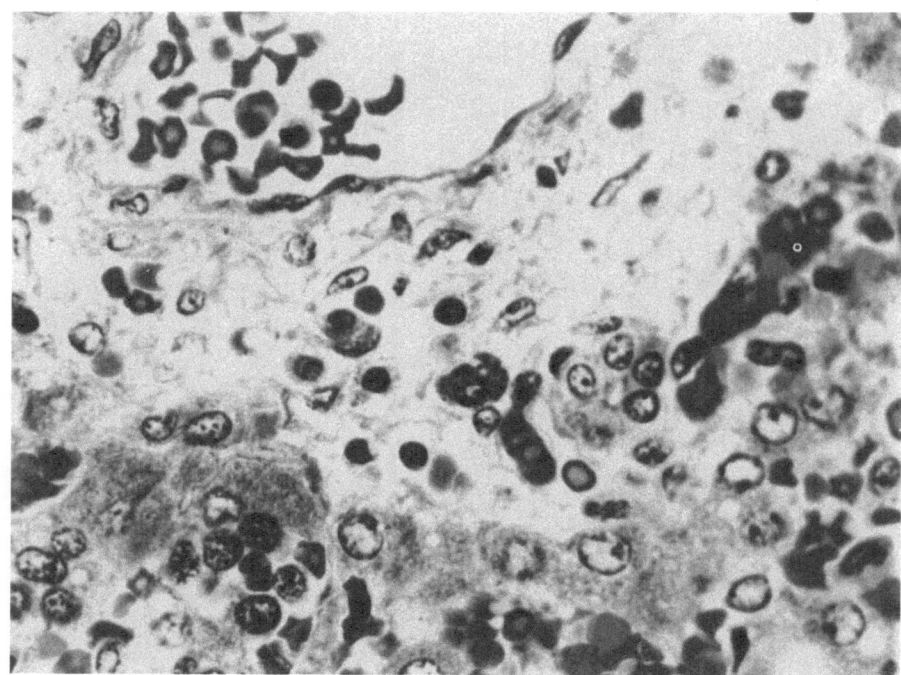

*Fig. 9 Portal area of 12 week fetus showing developing ductule
(large arrow). Note the patent lumen (small arrow).
(H & E x 900)*

portion of the mass of the liver. The erythroid tissue may resemble
confluent giant-cells. Erythropoiesis seems to be much more
prominent than myelopoiesis or megakaryocytopoiesis. One does
not see very many adult (nonnucleated) erythrocytes formed in the
liver until fetal age has nearly reached the point for hepatic
erythropoiesis to have stopped entirely. Then one can find an
occasional erythrocyte actually having lost its nucleus, extruding
its way out from the space of Disse, apparently trying to squeeze
into the sinusoid (Figure 12).

LYMPHOID TISSUE

The portal areas, which seem to be a site of some normal
lymphopoiesis in the adult, do not have abundant lymphoid tissue
in the fetus or the newborn, but there apparently are precursor
cells. The precursors to T cells have been demonstrated in liver
from 12 to 17 weeks of embryonic age (7). It is rather difficult
to identify some of the cells in portal areas; they are primitive
and since the primitive cells are still present in the newborn

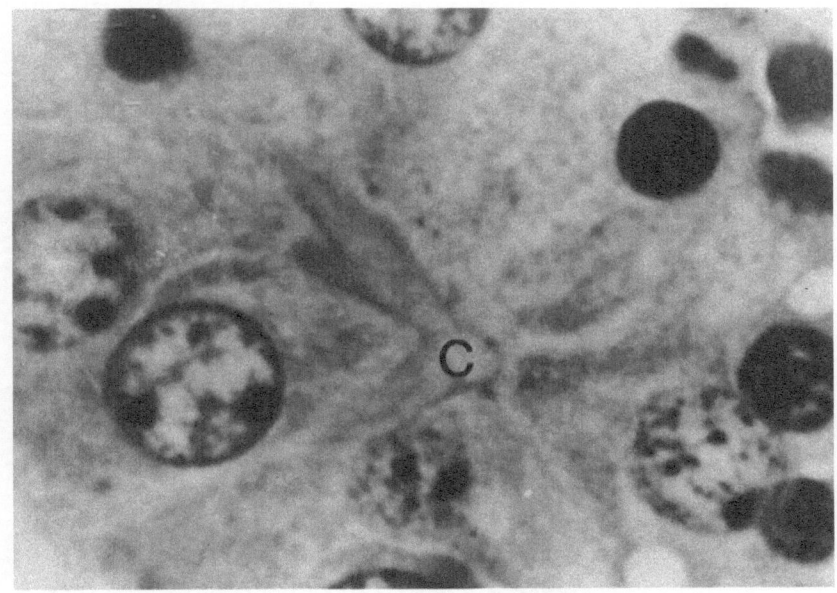

Fig. 10   Prominent canaliculus in fetal liver (C). (H & E x 2250)

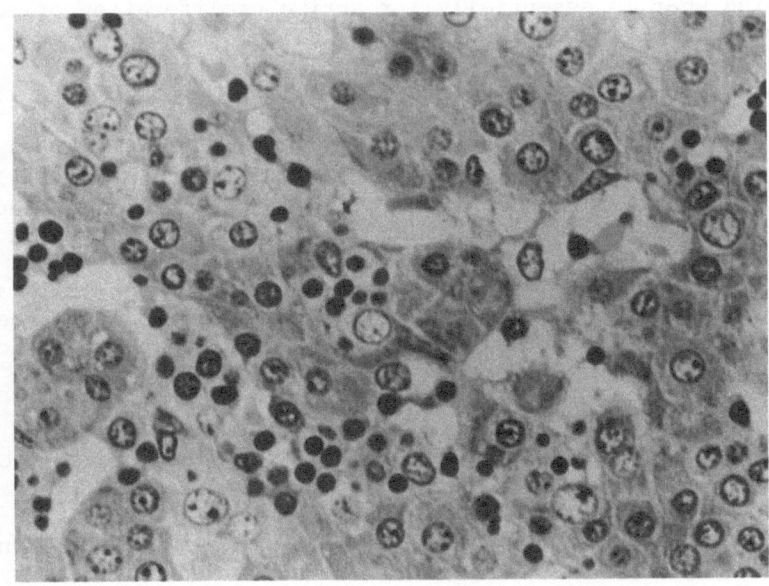

Fig. 11   Hemacytoblasts in liver cord.   (H & E x 450)

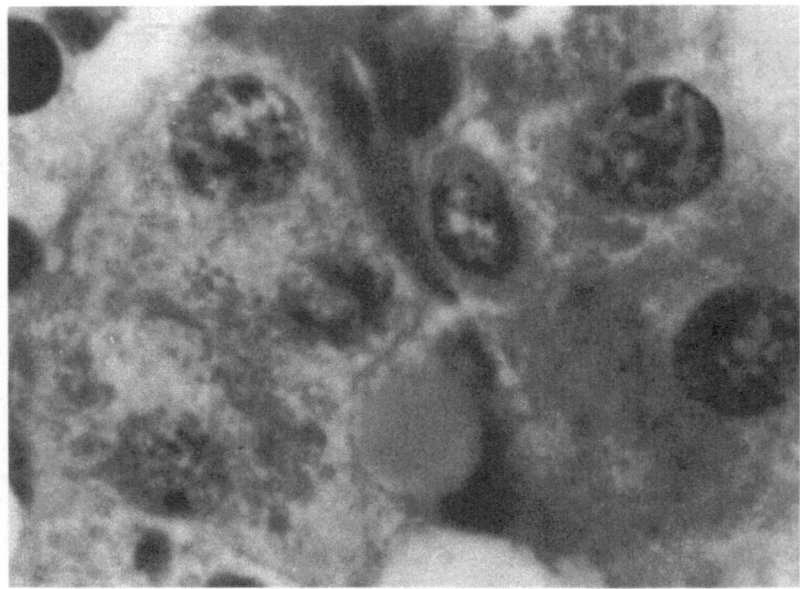

Fig. 12   Erythrocyte in the space of Disse (H & E x 2250)

period, it is easy to see how it might be quite difficult to
distinguish what is essentially a reactive proliferation of many
of the more primitive cells from true inflammation.

TRACE ELEMENTS

There are additional components of fetal and infant liver that
are not normally found in the adult liver.   Iron deposition is
common (although not visible in most late fetal periportal hepatocytes) even in the hepatocytes that are undergoing conversion into
duct epithelium.   This may be related to an increased amount of
iron entering the liver without a mechanism to dispose of it after
erythropoiesis has ceased.   The excess iron absorbed from the
gastrointestinal system is deposited mainly in hepatocytes, not in
the reticuloendothelial system.

Copper is deposited in the hepatocytes at most stages of fetal
development, and when one stains for copper binding protein, one
can see it even in the 950 g fetus.   Deposition is in the same
sites that one sees copper deposited in diseases in adults in which
there is chronic impairment of bile excretion.   One might wonder
whether or not copper fails to be excreted through the biliary tree
in the infant and if it may even act as some additional stimulus
for further developmental stages.

PROTEIN SYNTHESIS

    Specific protein production starts early in the liver.
Because of its occurrence as an onco-fetal antigen, alpha-fetoprotein
(AFP) has been studied extensively.   Fetal liver at 3-4 months
produces AFP which becomes the major fetal serum protein (8).   It
may be related to tissue immunity.   Experimentally induced absence
of AFP in the fetus results in multiple deformities (9).

    Fetal hepatic enzymes develop at variable stages of development.
Glycogen deposits are detectable by the 3rd or 4th intrauterine
month (5) and glycogen deposits increase to a level 2-4 times the
adult level by birth.   By 2 hours post-natally, liver cell glycogen
has fallen to 1/20 the level at birth.   Bile pigment production
starts at 4 months.   Many other cellular functions are well
developed by birth, others are not.   Most enzyme systems concerned
with detoxification develop after birth, some, such as glucuronyl
transferase, appearing only shortly before birth.

    There are many factors we do not understand about the relation-
ships of structural components to each other.   Function is very
difficult to establish in relationship to the morphological changes.
What association the inter-relationships between function and
structure may have to disease or to lack of disease in early childhood still needs further exploration.

SUMMARY

1)   The presumptive hepatic tissues respond to the inductive
qualities of cardiac mesoderm when the embryo is less than 2.5 mm
long, before hepatic tissue is recognizable.

2)   Transverse septal mesenchyme begins to develop a spongy sinusoidal character as the gut diverticulum (hepatic endoderm) evaginates
towards it.

3)   The transverse septal mesenchyme (hepatic mesoderm) is not
dependent upon the hepatic endoderm for induction.

4)   The tip of the hepatic diverticulum "sheds" tubularly arranged
hepatoblasts to interdigitate with the developing sinusoids.   The
hepatic endoderm is dependent upon the hepatic mesoderm for the
differentiation into hepatoblasts.

5)   The vitelline vein system and the left umbilical vein are
incorporated into the hepatic mass to form the portal vein and
umbilical vein respectively.

6)   Connective tissue from the primitive liver capsule grows into

the liver around the portal vein radicals.   The connective tissues induce the development of intrahepatic ducts.

7)   Bile formation is demonstrable by 4 months ovulatory fetal age, and bile passes into the gut by 5 months.

8)   Erythropoiesis, an important fetal hepatic function, persists into the post-natal period.

9)   Enzymatic activities, fetal and adult type protein production, glycogen production and excretory mechanisms are evident during the last half of fetal life.

10)   The inducing factors for the many diverse functions still remain largely unknown.

ACKNOWLEDGEMENT

     This investigation was supported in part by Account 6001 of the John Wesley Hospital Attending Staff Association.

REFERENCES

1.   LEDOUARIN NM: An experimental analysis of liver development.
       Med Biol 53:   427-455, 1975.

2.   CROISILLE Y, LEDOUARIN NM: Development and regeneration of the
       liver. In Organogenesis, DeHaan RL and Ursprung H (eds).
       Holt, Rinehart and Winston, 1965. Chapter 17.

3.   AREY LB: Developmental Anatomy. W.B. Saunders, 1974.
       pp. 255-259.

4.   SEVERN CG: A morphological study of the development of the
       human liver. II. Establishment of liver parenchyma,
       extrahepatic ducts and associated venous channels. Am J
       Anat 133: 85-107, 1972.

5.   HAMILTON WJ, BOYD JD, MOSSMAN HW: Alimentary and respiratory
       systems, pleural and peritoneal cavities. In Human
       Embryology, Hamilton WJ and Mossman HW (eds). Williams
       and Wilkins Co., 1972, Chapter 11.

6.   BLOOM W: The embryogenesis of human bile capillaries and
       ducts. Am J Anat 36: 451-465, 1926.

7. PYKE KW et al: Detection of T-precursor cells in human bone
        marrow and foetal liver.   Differentiation 5 (2-3):
        189-191, 1976.

8. SHYLTZE HE, HEREMANS JF: Plasma protein syntehsis in the
        fetus.   In Molecular Biology of Human Proteins, Shultze HE
        and Heremans JF (eds). Elsevier Publishing C., 1966,
        Chapter 3.

9. SMITH JA: Alpha-fetoprotein: A possible factor necessary for
        normal development of the embryo. Lancet 1: 851, 1972.

DEVELOPMENTAL ASPECTS OF THE HEPATIC CIRCULATION

Ian M. Taylor

Department of Anatomy, Faculty of Medicine
University of Toronto, Toronto, Ontario

The human embryo at the beginning of Horizon XI (13 somites, 24 days) has a midline tubular heart consisting of the paired primordia of the sinus venosus and a single atrium, ventricle and truncus (1). In the 16 somite embryo, the paired primordia fuse and a thickened portion of the endodermal lining of the foregut is then found to be in contact with the ventral and caudal walls of the midline sinus venosus (Fig 1). This thickened endodermal plate will shortly develop into the hepatic diverticulum.

DEVELOPMENT OF VENOUS STRUCTURES

Ventrally and on either side of the endodermal plate, the mesoderm of the septum transversum begins to "thicken" and as it does so, the hepatic diverticulum begins to project into it (2). Meanwhile blood islands have been developing within the mesoderm of the yolk sac and they link to form the vitelline venous plexus. As this grows larger and increases in extent, two large vitelline veins develop and join with the mesenteric veins to make the right and left omphalomesenteric veins. These veins join with the umbilical veins to produce paired omphaloumbilical trunks which pass through the septum transversum to join the sinus venosus (Fig 2). At the end of Horizon XI (20 somites, 25 days), the two sets of veins separate so that the medially positioned omphalo-mesenteric veins and the laterally positioned umbilical veins join the right and left horns of the sinus venosus individually.

The relationship between the developing liver parenchyma and the vessels draining the yolk sac and gut has been the subject of considerable controversy in man, not least because the possibility of inter-species variation was overlooked for many years.

17

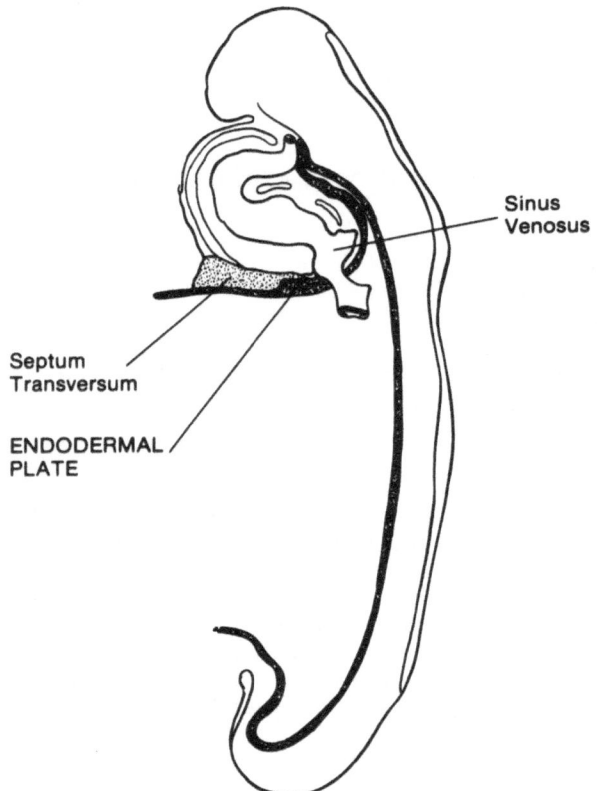

Fig. 1 *Longitudinal section of a human embryo at stage 11 of*
development (16 somites). The endodermal plate, which
will form the liver, projects into the septum transversum
and lies in contact with the ventral and caudal walls
of the sinus venosus.

The classical description of Minot (3) utilized the term
intercrescence to indicate the way in which the large omphalomesenteric vessels appeared to be invaded by cords or tubules of
liver parenchymal cells.   Each vein was divided up by the invading
cells and so transformed into a plexus of small vascular channels
which would ultimately become the hepatic sinusoids.

An alternative suggestion (Fig 3) was made in 1952 by Lipp
(4) and has since been supported by Elias (5) and Severn (2).
They observed the formation of many endothelially-lined blood
islands within the mesenchyme of the septum transversum and
especially in that part near to the wall of the hepatic diverticulum.

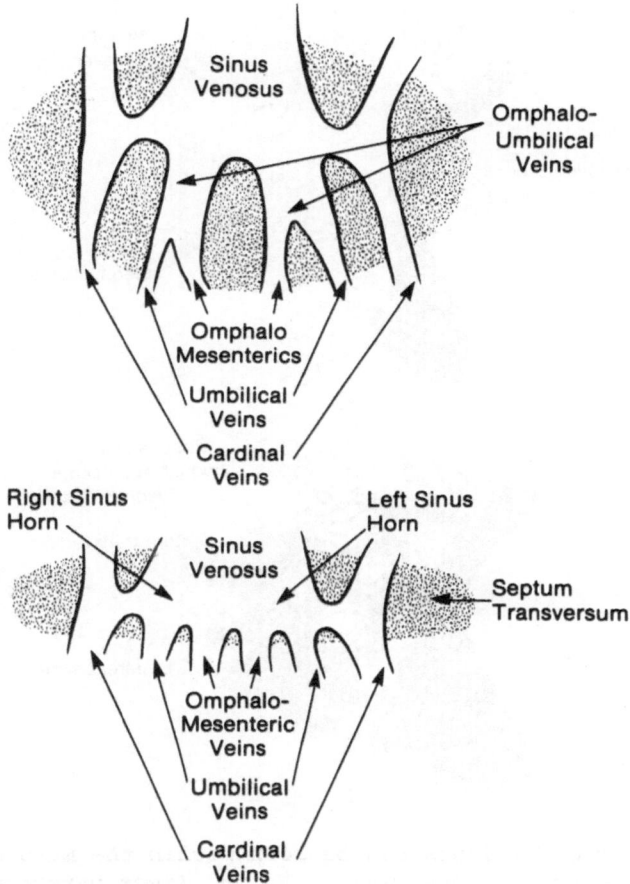

Fig. 2   *Schematic representation of the development of the
          venous channels draining into the sinus venosus.
          The stippled area indicates the presence of the septum
          transversum.   Note the changes in the omphalo-umbilical
          veins (above) which separate (below) to form separate
          omphalomesenteric and umbilical veins which then enter
          the sinus venosus individually.*

Here they seemed to be a little larger than those further away
from the diverticulum.   The parenchyma which develops from this
structure appears as an irregular mass of cords and tubules which
grows into the adjacent septum transversum and then spreads around
the pre-existing blood islands.   This process was termed inter-
polation by Lipp (4) and interstitial invasion by Elias (5).

    In man, therefore, in contrast to the classical interpretation

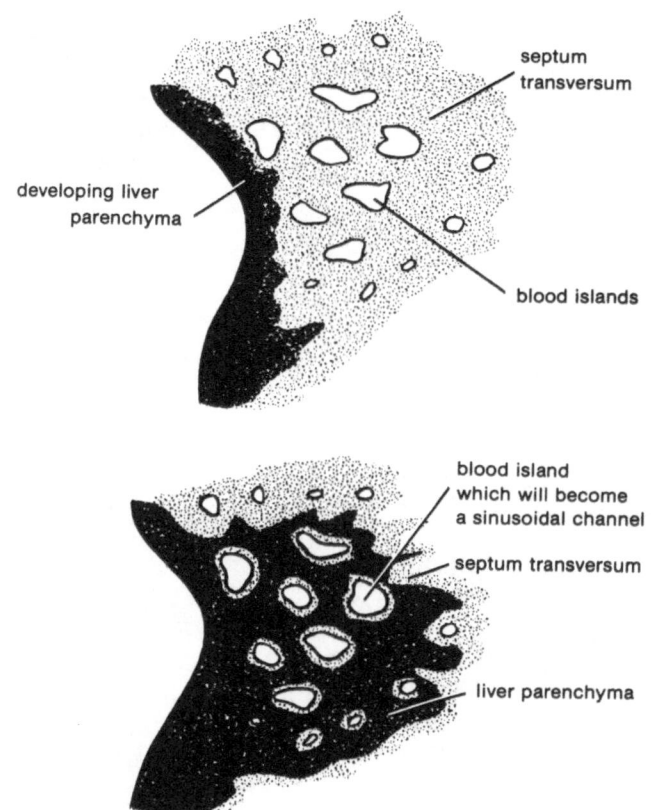

Fig. 3   *Above, blood islands can be seen within the mesenchyme*
         of the septum transversum.   Below, liver parenchyma,
         developing from the hepatic diverticulum on the left,
         grows into the septum transversum and then spreads around
         the blood islands.

it would seem that the mass of small vessels which will become the
sinusoids develops in situ, concurrent with the hepatic parenchyma,
and does not form as a result of the interruption of large preformed channels.

During days 26 and 27, while the endothelially-lined blood
islands have been forming, sprouts from the omphalomesenteric
veins grow out into the hepatic parenchyma and the mesenchyme of
the septum transversum (Fig 4).   These sprouts not only join the
developing sinusoids but also form anastomoses across the midline
and around the foregut.

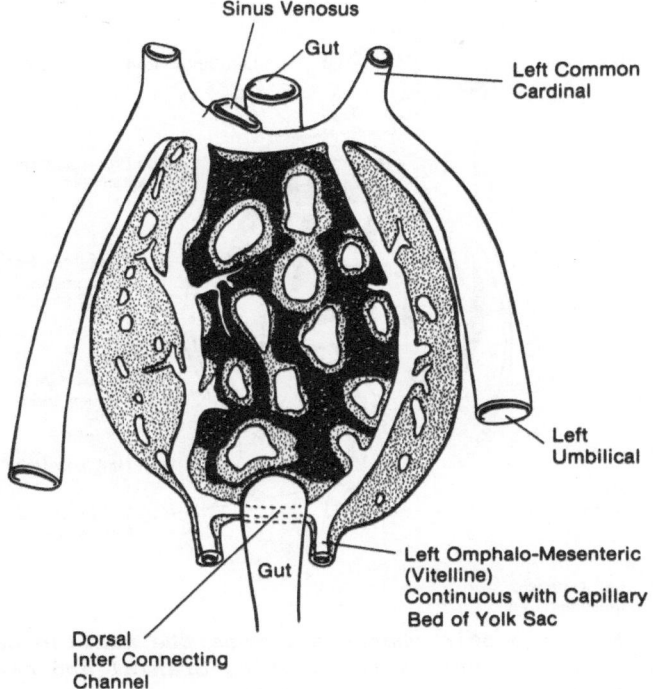

Fig. 4 *Sprouts from the omphalomesenteric veins grow into the*
hepatic primordium and the septum transversum.   These
sprouts link with the developing blood islands to form
sinusoids.   They also anastomose across the midline and
form channels such as the dorsal one seen caudally.

By days 30 and 31 (Horizon 13, 30 somites) the omphalomesenteric
veins are continuous with the sinusoidal channels and these are
completely surrounded by hepatic parenchyma (2) (Fig 5).   At this
time, there are four prominent anastomotic channels across the
midline (6).   One, the sub-diaphragmatic channel, is located under
the diaphragm between the proximal parts of the veins.   The other
three are found between more distal parts of the veins and develop
such that the most cephalic one is ventral to the gut, the next is
on the dorsal aspect while the third is also ventrally placed.
The most cephalic of these three channels is the first to develop
and will become the transverse portal sinus (sinus intermedius) of
the embryonic liver.

Hitherto, the paired umbilical veins have been carrying
placental blood to the sinus venosus as they travel through the
lateral body wall.   The right umbilical vein shortly drops out
and the left one remains as the single umbilical vein.   At this

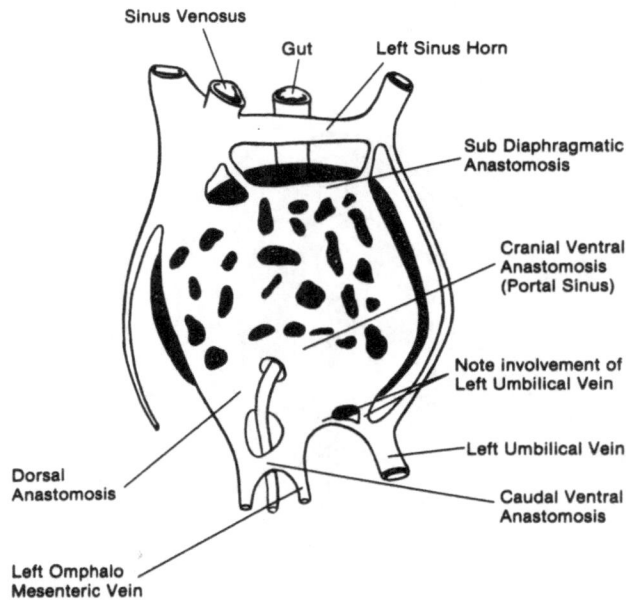

*Fig. 5   Four anastomotic channels across the midline can be
         identified: sub-diaphragmatic, cranial and caudal
         ventral, and dorsal.   Note the atrophy of the right
         umbilical vein with the cranial ventral anastomosis
         between the omphalomesenteric veins.*

stage, one noticeable feature of the developing embryo is the rapid
growth of the liver and one consequence of this is its fusion with
the body wall.   This permits the development of anastomoses between
the left umbilical vein and the portal sinus within the liver.   By
the time these are beginning to form, a progressively elongating
extension of the portal sinus is <u>already</u> seen within the liver in
the midline and this soon reaches and joins with the sub-diaphragmatic anastomosis.   This midline channel is the ductus venosus
(Figs 6, 7).   By the end of the fifth week of embryonic life, the
umbilical vein is discharging into the left side of the portal
sinus and Dickson (6) suggests that the left half of the sinus then
becomes an integral part of the umbilical vein.   From the portal
sinus, blood passes for the most part to the sinus venosus by the
ductus although some percolates through the sinusoids.

During this same week, the sinus venosus has shifted from its
original midline position towards the right side (Figs 5,8).   This
movement is associated with the gradual obliteration of the left
omphalomesenteric vein between the liver and the sinus venosus.
On the right side, that portion of the omphalomesenteric vein

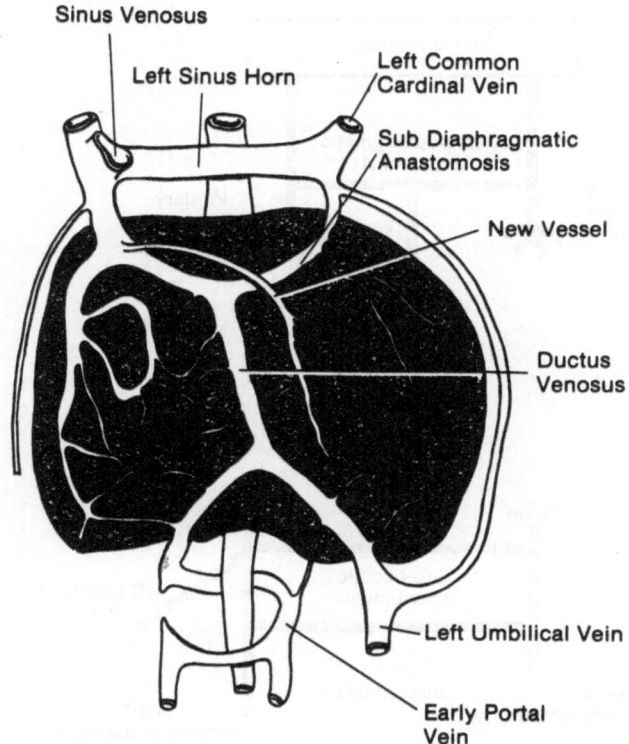

Fig. 6 *By the end of the fifth week, the left umbilical vein*
        drains into the left side of the portal sinus and from
        thence blood passes via the midline ductus venosus to
        the subdiaphragmatic anastomosis.   The new vessel
        joining the right half of this anastomosis is one of
        several which will become the middle and left hepatic
        veins.   Caudally, the development of the portal vein
        is seen resulting from selective atrophy.

between the liver and sinus venosus enlarges and it will become
the most cephalic part of the inferior vena cava (Fig 8).

    The left omphalomesenteric vein further atrophies as far
caudally as the anastomosis on the dorsal aspect of the duodenum.
The left half of the sub-diaphragmatic anastomosis however, remains
as a small vein (venula hepatica cranialis aut superior sinistra)
draining the dorsal cranial part of the left lobe.   The right half
of the sub-diaphragmatic anastomosis joins several newly developed
veins (the secondary left and middle hepatic veins) and so forms
connections with what will become the middle and left hepatic veins
of the adult (6) (Fig 9).

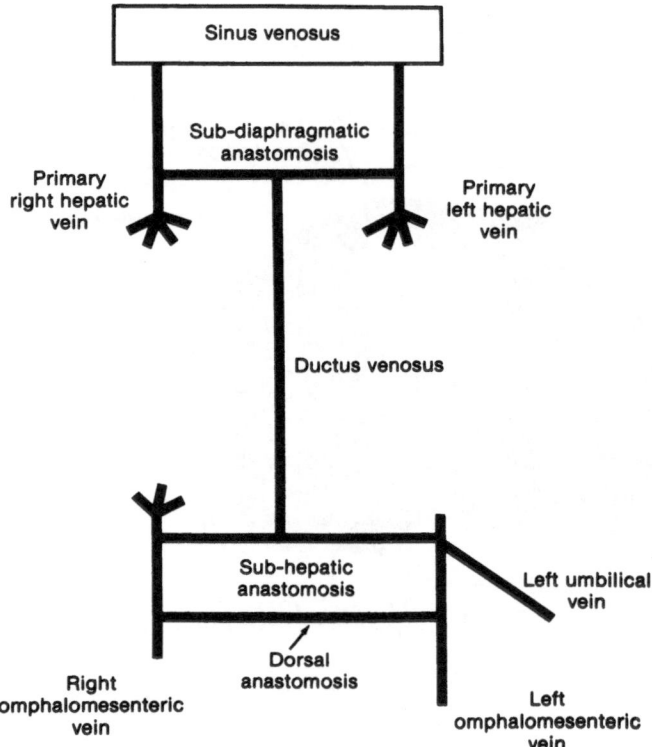

Fig. 7 The arrangement of the veins in the 5 mm human embryo
         (after Dickson).

        That part of the right omphalomesenteric vein within the liver
will form the right hepatic vein and the common hepatic vein (Fig 8).
The right half of the sub-diaphragmatic anastomosis is absorbed
into the common hepatic vein which thus receives all the hepatic
veins.   It is, generally, regarded as the forerunner of the
hepatic part of the inferior vena cava (6,7,8).

        A further consequence of the increasing size of the liver is
that its dextrodorsal surface comes into close proximity to the
posterior body wall.   Here the right suprarenal gland is developing
and it, therefore, lies in contact with the liver.   About this
time the inferior vena cava is forming, and as part of that process
the right and left subcardinal veins participate in anastomoses
across the midline and so venous blood from both sides of the body
below the adrenals can and does eventually flow into the right
subcardinal vein (Fig 10).   This vessel links with others in the
adjacent liver and so forms the remaining portion of the inferior
vena cava.   Barry (9) has suggested that the subcardinal vein

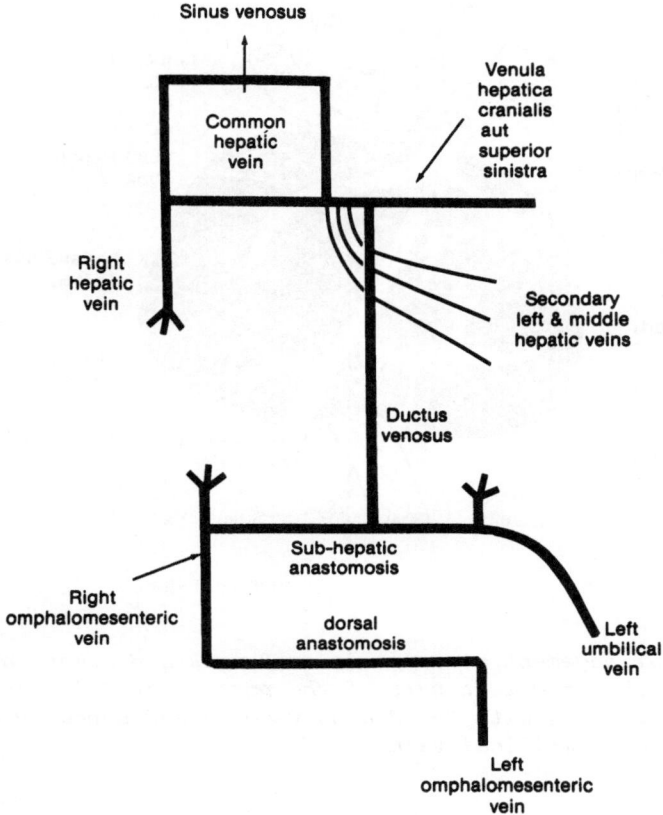

Fig. 8 The arrangement of the veins in the 7.75 mm human embryo (after Dickson).

connects especially with the right postero-caudate hepatic vein which lies between the right posterior and caudate segments during the 4th week.   As a result of increased flow, this vein increases in size and ultimately becomes at least a part of the hepatic portion of the inferior vena cava.   In the light of this suggested origin, it is not surprising that much of the caudate lobe drains directly into the inferior vena cava.   Barry also believes that this concept explains the variability of the level at which the right hepatic vein enters the inferior vena cava in the adult.   The level of confluence is the point at which these two hepatic veins joined in embryonic life and this, as he says, would be expected to be variable.

The portal vein develops from distal portions of the right and left omphalomesenteric veins and their dorsal anastomosis

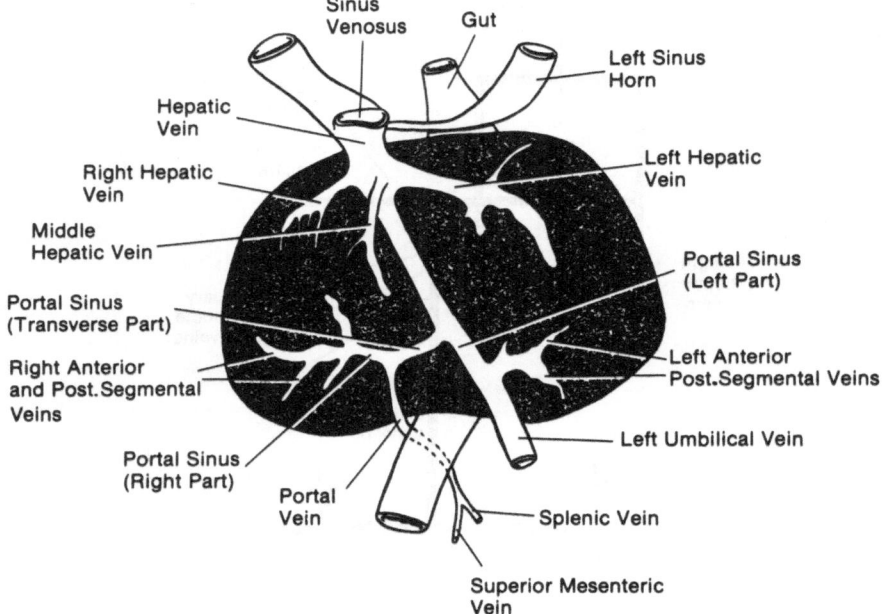

Fig. 9   The arrangement of veins in an 8 week old human fetus.
Note that the left part of the portal sinus is continuous
cephalically with the ductus venosus and caudally with
the left umbilical vein.

across the midline (Figs 5,6,9).   The distal part of the right
omphalomesenteric vein atrophies caudal to the dorsal anastomosis
while atrophy of the left omphalomesenteric vein occurs both
cranial and caudal to this anastomosis.   The remaining portions
of the omphalomesenteric veins together with their dorsal link
form an S-shaped vein which is the portal vein (6).

The superior mesenteric and splenic veins develop in situ
as separate and independent formations and join the left omphalomesenteric vein which thus become the starting point of the portal
vein.

By the eighth week of intrauterine life (30 mm crown rump
length) the venous vascular pattern is already complete in many
aspects (10) although even at birth the portal and hepatic venous
trees are still short and stunted as compared with those of the
adult (7).   Nevertheless, vascular development, both arterial and
venous, precedes that of the biliary tree (11).

The calibre and length of the sinusoids at term are comparable

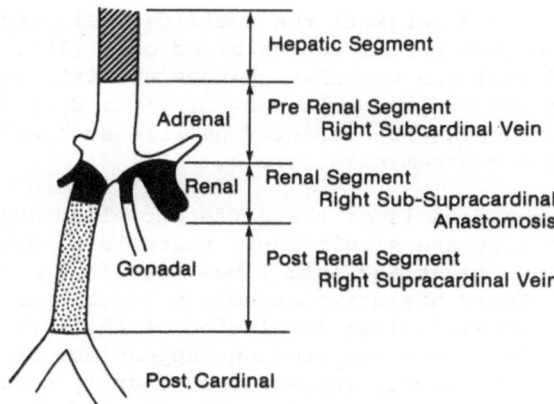

*Fig. 10   The development of the inferior vena cava is complex
          because it is derived from several sources.   The common
          iliac veins are remnants of the posterior cardinals and
          they join with the post-renal and pre-renal segments
          to form the caudal portion of the inferior vena cava.
          Each segment develops from a different embryonic vein.
          The hepatic segment links the pre-renal portion with
          the most cephalic part of the right omphalomesenteric
          vein to complete the formation of the cava.*

to those of the adult.   However, the sinusoids are clearly
arranged radially around the portal triad rather than around the
collecting veins.   This finding was an impetus for those who
maintained that the structural and functional unit of hepatic
tissue was the acinus arranged around the portal triad (10,12).

THE UMBILICAL VEIN AND DUCTUS VENOSUS

     Throughout fetal life, the umbilical vein gives off numerous
branches upon entering the liver.   Most of these supply the left
and quadrate lobes and much of the caudate lobe.   These parts of
the liver thus receive well oxygenated blood exclusively.   The
right lobe and caudate process receive some blood from the umbilical
vein but most of their supply comes from the portal vein (13).
The consequences of the differing sources of supply to the two
halves of the liver is a controversial subject.   The disparity
between the partial pressures of oxygen has been suggested as a
possible cause for anoxic damage being greater on the right side
than on the left (14).   However, under some circumstances, the
effects are more pronounced on the left side.   One reason suggested
for this is that because the left lobe is better supplied with
oxygen than the right, it is relatively more developed.   It may,
therefore, be particularly vulnerable to anoxic damage after

clamping of the cord cuts off the umbilical vein and causes the
left lobe to receive portal venous blood only (15).   It has also
been suggested that the vascular changes at birth may be responsible
to some degree for various evidences of liver dysfunction in the
first and second weeks of extrauterine life such as mild elevations
in bilirubin and transaminase levels.

Whatever the details of the different blood supplies are and
whether or not they are significant, there is no doubt that the
morphology of the right and left lobes are often markedly different
in neonates.   Emery has drawn attention to changes which amount
to a degree of physiological involution of the left liver.
Witzleben (16) has noted the frequent appearance of a line just
to the right of the ductus venosus that sharply demarcates the
right and left lobes of the liver.   To the left of the line, the
liver is darker, the hepatic trabeculae are narrower and the sinusoids wider than in the right lobe.   He also notes that haemo-
poiesis is more prominent on the right side than the left and
suggests that the two lobes should be studied almost as if they
are separate organs.

Ever since Vesalius discovered the ductus venosus in 1543,
it has been accepted that the ductus acts as a path for shunting
umbilical venous blood directly to the inferior vena cava.

Various authors such as Barron (17) and Chacko and Reynolds
(18) have reported the existence of a muscular sphincter at the
origin of the ductus from the portal sinus and it was suggested
that this sphincter might have some regulatory function in the
hepatic circulation.   In several more recent studies no evidence
has been found for a muscular sphincter in the ductus of man
although intimal lipping and subendothelial thickening have been
observed (9,19).

Lind (20) has shown that the ductus is functionally closed at
the time of birth and that there is little or no flow during the
first few days of life.   However, it should be noted that the
ductus may remain open in the presence of neonatal distress and
this may contribute to reduced sinusoidal perfusion.   The ductus
may also remain open when there is portal venous obstruction in
early extrauterine life.

After the function of the umbilical vein has ceased, it is
gradually transformed into a narrow, funnel-shaped duct with its
apex towards the umbilicus.   The peripheral end gradually obliter-
ates and becomes the ligamentum teres.   However, even in adults,
the lumen of the umbilical vein is preserved over a distance of
14-16 cm on the side of the left branch of the portal vein.   The
mean diameter of the umbilical vein at the hepatic end was found
by Obel (21) to be 2.3 mm.

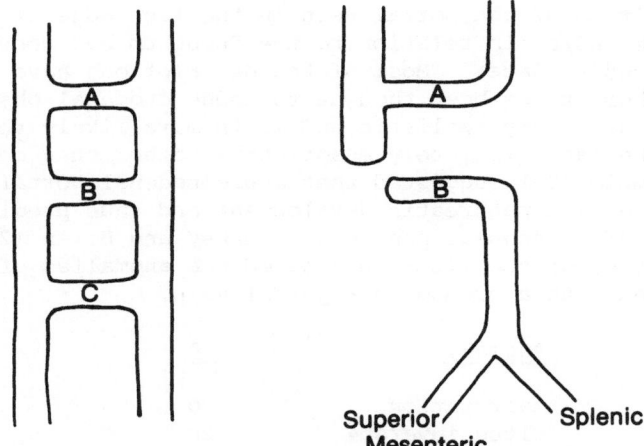

Fig. 11   *Schematic representation of the case described by*
          Johnson et al.   A, B and C are the midline anastomoses
          between the omphalomesenteric veins.   A and C are both
          ventral, A being cephalic to C while B is dorsal.   It
          is suggested that the anomaly seen in this case may
          represent failure of channel B to anastomose with the
          persisting portion of the right omphalomesenteric vein.

ANOMALIES OF VENOUS DEVELOPMENT

     Anomalies of the portal vein are rare.   Congenital absence
is most infrequent.   The most recent report (22) involved a 4½
year old girl who presented with a hepatoblastoma.   At operation
it was found that the superior mesenteric and splenic veins
drained into the left renal vein and thus bypassed the liver.
This patient also had short fifth fingers and toes and a clinically
insignificant ventricular septal defect.

     Duplication, atresia and stenosis have also been reported
(23,24).   However it is likely that only a minority of these are
truly congenital, the vast majority are almost certainly acquired.
However, Johnson et al (25) have recently reported on a 10 week
old girl who presented with features of extrahepatic portal hypertension.   Autopsy revealed a liver whose inferior surface was
grossly lobulated.   There was a dilated but normally formed portal
vein which ended blindly where a lobule of liver appeared to be
compressing it (Fig 11).   Whether the vascular anomaly was secondary
to pressure from the abnormal lobule or due to failure of formation
of anastomotic channels across the midline by the omphalomesenteric
veins or because of some other reason is unclear but this appears
to be a congenital anomaly rather than one secondary to infection.

Anteroposition of the portal vein in the free edge of the
lesser omentum and/or in relation to the duodenum has been described
in some 43 cases to date.   Most of the descriptions have been in
neonates in whom it has been thought to cause duodenal obstruction.
This does not seem very realistic and it is more likely that its
presence in the cases is merely associative rather than causative.
Beggs for example (26) suggested that a preduodenal portal vein
might interfere with pancreatic development and thus predispose to
the formation of an annular pancreas.   Makey and Bowen (27) in
their 1978 survey of the literature noted the anomalies of development associated with a preduodenal portal vein.

Anomaly	%
Malrotation	70
Situs inversus	28
Annular pancreas	23
Ladd's Bands	19
Duodenal diaphragm	16
Polysplenia	14
Biliary atresia	9
Duodenal stenosis	9

Preduodenal portal vein presumably represents persistence
of a ventral anastomotic channel rather than the more usual dorsal
one but clearly the developmental anomaly in many of the reported
cases is much more than simply the persistence of one anastomosis
rather than another.

The etiology of the cavernomatous type of portal venous
drainage has been the subject of some controversy also.   Simonds
(28) for example regards it as an acquired anamoly due to thrombosis
followed by recanalization.   Others (29,30) consider it an atypical
development of the plexus of veins between the omphalomesenteric
and hepatic veins during the second month of embryonic development.

Most recently, Leger et al (31) have stressed the importance
of the postnatal obliterative process in the umbilical vein and
the ductus and suggested that this might spread to the portal vein
and its tributaries.   More likely causes of this extensive obliteration are of the acquired type rather than the congenital and include
umbilical sepsis, dehydration and trans-umbilical transfusions (32,
33).

Hepatopedal flow from splenic and mesenteric veins is
maintained by the development of collateral veins in the lesser
omentum - constituting so-called cavernomatous transformation of
the portal vein.   These vessels are inadequate to prevent portal
hypertension and bleeding oesophageal varices is the most common
presentation in the circumstances (33).   In a recent case report

by Meredith et al (34) a 22 year old man presented with portal
hypertension following neonatal omphalitis and portal vein thrombosis.   This man was unusual because he also had obstructive
jaundice due to compression of the common bile duct by the varicose
collateral veins in the lesser omentum.

In fetal monsters the portal vein has been seen draining into
the umbilical vein and the superior vena cava and into the right
atrium.   Instances where it enters the inferior vena cava or the
azygos vein are not uncommon.   More complex anomalies of venous
drainage are also found, for example, Hellweg (35) reported absence
of the intrahepatic portal venous system and of the hepatic segment
of the inferior vena cava in a girl who died at 6 months.   The
splenic and superior mesenteric veins drained into a large vein
that passed posterior to the liver and joined the hepatic veins
to form the superior part of the inferior vena cava.   The lower
part of the inferior vena cava was normally formed, passed through
the diaphragm and joined the azygos vein.   The caudate and quadrate
lobes of the liver were absent - the former perhaps being associated
with absence of the right posterocaudate hepatic vein.

HEPATOPETAL COLLATERALS

When there is obstruction to flow in the extrahepatic portal
vein, blood may be rerouted by a variety of channels.   These
include: a) Epiploic veins in the lesser omentum hepatocolic and
hepatorenal ligaments, b) veins around the bile duct, c) veins
in the diaphragm, d) deep cystic veins, e) veins in the falciform
ligament, and f) the paraumbilical veins.

HEPATOFUGAL COLLATERALS

When the obstruction to portal flow is within the liver a
number of collaterals can move the blood from abdominal viscera
around the hepatic obstacle.

McIndoe (36) has classified these on an embryological basis
and they can be summarized here.

A) Veins located in the gastrointestinal tract at the junction
of absorbing epithelium, e.g. gastroesophageal junction, junction
of upper with lower anus.

B) Veins occurring at the site of the obliterated fetal
circulation.   These are the paraumbilical veins in the falciform
and round ligaments.   They anastomose with epigastric, internal
thoracic and azygos veins.   The vestige of the ductus venosus
may also canalize under these circumstances.

C) Veins which are found at the sites where the gut and the

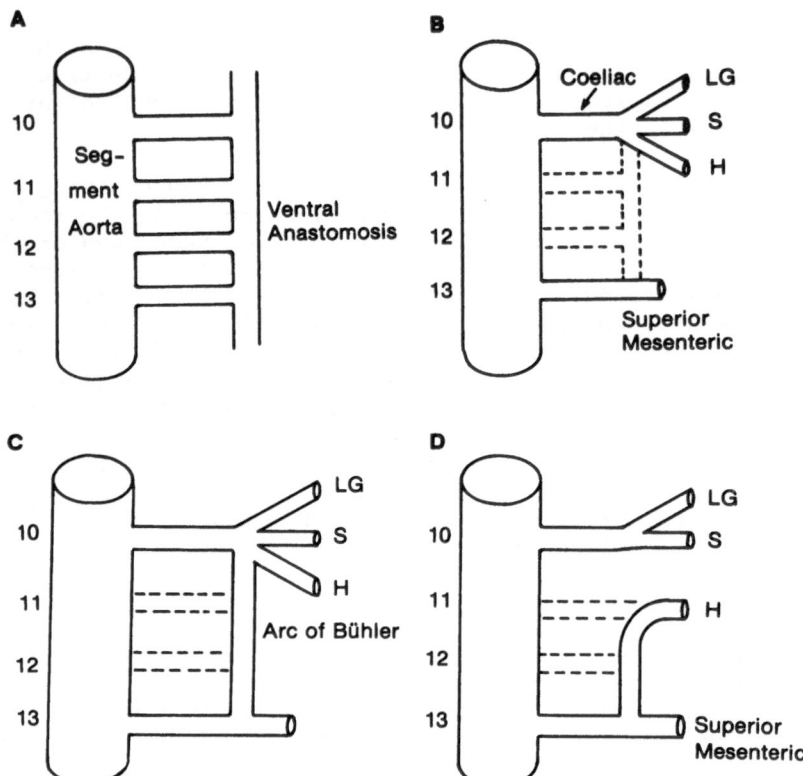

Fig. 12   *Diagrams to indicate the formation of the superior*
          mesenteric artery and the coeliac trunk and its branches.
          A – The four ventral segmental arteries derived from the
          *   aorta and their ventral anastomosis.*
          B – The usual pattern of atrophy in this early pattern
          *   to form the main arterial trunks.*
          C – Occasionally the ventral anastomosis persists and
          *   forms the Arc of Buhler.*
          D – When there is partial interruption of the ventral
          *   anastomosis, the hepatic artery arises from the*
          *   superior mesenteric artery rather than from the*
          *   coeliac trunk.*

glands derived from it which formed in mesenteries have become
retroperitoneal during development or as a result of some pathology.

These can arise from duodenum, small bowel, colon, pancreas,
spleen and omentum.   An example would be the portorenal plexus
which consists of anastomoses between the left renal vein and

the portal capillaries in the pancreas, spleen and splenic flexure
of the colon.

THE ARTERIAL SUPPLY OF THE LIVER

In early human embryos (4-17 mm, approximately 28-48 days)
the omphalomesenteric artery arises by four roots from the dorsal
aorta (Fig 12A).   The four roots are ventral segmental arteries
10, 11, 12 and 13 and all four are united by a longitudinal
ventral anastomosis which runs parallel to the aorta.   Normally
the greater part of the ventral anastomosis disappears as do
segmental arteries 11 and 12, thus leaving the first root to
become the stem of the coeliac artery and the last to become the
stem of the superior mesenteric artery (37) (Fig 12B).

Normally the three main branches of the coeliac axis arise
successively from the cranial end of the longitudinal anastomosis,
thus accounting for the fact that the left gastric artery arises
proximal to the origin of the hepatic and splenic arteries (Fig 12C).
If the ventral anastomosis is interrupted between the origins of
the left gastric and splenic arteries, then the left gastric will
arise from the aorta and the splenic and hepatic trunks will arise
from the superior mesenteric artery.   In a similar way, if the
anastomosis between the splenic and hepatic arteries is interrupted,
the left gastric and splenic arteries will arise from the aorta
while the hepatic artery will arise from the superior mesenteric
artery (Fig 12D).

Typically the hepatic artery, after giving off the gastro-
duodenal, divides into right, middle and left branches, the middle
artery usually being a branch of either the right or the left.
It is not known at which stage of embryonic life their branches
join the sinusoids. However, blood flow through the hepatic artery
is insignificant by comparison with that of the umbilical and
portal veins.

Michels (38) defined an aberrant hepatic artery as one arising
from any artery other than the coeliac. It may have a replaced
origin, in which it is the sole hepatic artery, or it may be an
accessory hepatic artery when it is present in addition to the
normal blood supply.

After a study of 200 human livers he described 10 basic types
of supply from the coeliac artery:

1) Right, middle and left - 55%

2) Right and middle only.   Left replaced from left
   gastric - 10%

3) Left and middle only.   Right replaced from superior
   mesenteric - 11%

4) Middle only - Right replaced from coeliac or
                 superior mesenteric
                                                                         1%
              - Left replaced from left gastric

5) Right, middle and left hepatus and accessor left
   from left gastric - 8%

6) Right, middle and left hepatus and accessory right
   from superior mesenteric - 7%

7) Right, middle and left hepatus and accessory left
   from left gastric and accessory right from superior
   mesenteric - 1%

8) Combination patterns of a) a replaced right hepatic
   and an accessory left; or b) an accessory right
   and a replaced left - 2%

9) Absence of celiacal hepatica.   Entire hepatic trunk
   derived from superior mesenteric - 4.5%

10) Absence of celiacal hepatica.   Entire hepatic trunk
    derived from left gastric - 0.5%

These variations in hepatic blood supply are common and they
are important surgically and radiologically.   Both replaced and
accessory hepatic arteries supply areas of liver that receive no
supply from any of the other hepatic arteries (38,39).   Surgical
ligation of aberrant vessels may thus cause hepatic damage.   It
should also be kept in mind that these aberrant vessels may also
give rise to the cystic arteries so that there is also the possibility of compromising the supply to the gallbladder.

Hepatic arteriography is of great value in the investigation
of hepatic trauma (40,41).   However, failure to opacify the entire
hepatic arterial supply on a selective hepatic or coeliac arteriogram may be due to atypical vascular anatomy rather than a haematoma.
Michel's findings (38) would suggest that if the non-opacified zone
lies in the region supplied by the right hepatic then a superior
mesenteric arteriogram should be performed.   On the other hand if
the "abnormality" is in the territory supplied by the left hepatic,
a main coeliac or a selective left gastric examination is indicated
instead.

THE HEPATIC ARTERIAL COLLATERAL SUPPLY

The liver which is slowly deprived of the hepatic artery develops a rich collateral arterial supply. The collaterals are formed from persistent modified vascular arcades which developed in relation to the embryonic gut in the dorsal and ventral mesenteries (42). Thus the gastro-epiploic, the pancreatic duodenal and the colic arteries represent parts of a dorsal anastomosis between the splanchnic branches of the aorta found in the dorsal mesentery. Similarly, the left and right gastric artery and the hepatic artery form a ventral anastomosis of the splanchnic arteries in the ventral mesentery of the foregut. As indicated earlier aberrant vessels are common and they too anastomose with the vascular arcades. The usual branches of the hepatic artery also anastomose extensively in the porta hepatis before sending their terminal branches into the liver (42).

SUMMARY

The development of the hepatic vasculature is complex. It involves the interaction of several groups of blood vessels with the hepatic parenchyma as this differentiates from the hepatic diverticulum.

The origin of the sinusoids in man is still not clearly understood. However, it is suggested that they are derived not by invasion of the omphalomesenteric veins, but rather that they form in situ and are then surrounded by the irregular mass of developing hepatic parenchyma. These early sinusoids are then linked to the omphalomesenteric veins which also form anastomoses across the midline.

Subsequent changes in the umbilical veins and the omphalomesenteric veins and their anastomotic connections are described to indicate the further development of the venous returns from the placenta and the gut. The origin and vascular links of the hepatic portion of the inferior vena cava are also examined. The early structure of the omphalomesenteric artery and the formation of the coeliac, superior mesenteric and hepatic arteries are briefly discussed.

Various types of anomalous development of the inferior vena cava, the portal vein and the hepatic arteries are mentioned and their clinical significance outlined.

REFERENCES

1. STREETER GL: Developmental horizons in human embryos. Description of Age Group XI, 13 to 20 somites, and Age Group XII, 21-29 Somites. Cont Embryo Carnegie Inst (Wash) 30: 211,1942.

2. SEVERN CB: A morphological study of the development of the
        human liver. II. Establishment of liver parenchyma,
        extrahepatic ducts and associated venous channels.
        Am J Anat 133: 85-93, 1972.

3. MINOT CS: On a hitherto unrecognized form of blood circula-
        tion without capillaries in the organs of vertebrata.
        Proc Boston Soc Nat Hist 29: 185-215, 1900.

4. LIPP W: Die fruhe Strukturentwicklung des Leberparechyms
        beim Menschen. Z mikr anat Forsch 59: 161-186, 1952.

5. ELIAS H: Origin and early development of the liver in various
        vertebrates. Acta Hepatol 3: 1-56, 1955.

6. DICKSON AD: Development of the ductus venosus in man and the
        goat. J Anat 91: 358-368, 1957.

7. WENDELIN H: Microangiography of the liver. An experimental
        study of sheep from the prenatal to the full grown period.
        Acta Paediatr Scand Suppl 233: 3-58, 1972.

8. HUNTINGTON GS, McCLURE CFW: The development of the veins in
        the domestic cat (Felis domestica). Anat Rec 20: 1-30,
        1920.

9. BARRY A: The development of hepatic vascular structures.
        Ann NY Acad Sci 111: 105-108, 1963.

10. MALL FP: A study of the structural unit of the liver.
        Am J Anat 5: 227-308, 1906.

11. HADCHOUEL M, HUGON RN, GAUTIER M: Reduced ratio of portal
        tracts to paucity of intrahepatic bile ducts. Arch
        Pathol Lab Med 102: 402, 1978.

12. RAPPAPORT AM, BOROWY ZJ, LOUGHEED WM, LOTTO WN: Subdivision
        of hexagonal liver lobules into a structural and functional
        unit; role in hepatic physiology and pathology. Anat
        Rec 119: 11-33, 1954.

13. VSEVOLODOV GF: Characteristics of the blood supply to the
        liver in the human fetus. Arkh Anat Gistol Embriol 55:
        34-40, 1968.

14. GRUENWALD P: Degenerative changes in the right half of the
        liver resulting from intra-uterine anoxia. Am J Clin
        Path 19: 801-813, 1949.

15. EMERY JL: Degenerative changes in the left lobe of the liver

in the newborn. Arch Dis Child 27: 558-561, 1952.

16. WITZLEBEN C: Liver. In Pathology of infancy and childhood. JM Kissane (ed). The CV Mosby Company, St. Louis, 1975. pp 267-308.

17. BARRON D: The "sphincter" of the ductus venosus. Anat Rec 82: 398, 1942.

18. CHACKO AW, REYNOLDS SRM: Embryonic development in the human of the sphincter of the ductus venosus. Anat Rec 115: 151-174, 1953.

19. MONTAGNANI CA: Intrahepatic vascular pattern in the newborn infant. Ann NY Acad Sci 111: 121-135, 1963.

20. LIND J: Changes in the liver circulation at birth. Ann NY Acad Sci 111: 110-120, 1963.

21. OBEL W: The umbilical vein in different periods of life in man. Folia Morphol (Warsz) 35: 173-179, 1976.

22. MAROIS D, VAN HEERDEN JA, CARPENTER HA, SHEEDY PF: Congenital absence of the portal vein. Mayo Clin Proc 54: 55-59, 1979.

23. MARKS C: Developmental basis of the portal venous system. Am J Surg 117: 671-681, 1969.

24. SNAVELY JG, BRECKELL ES: Fatal haemorrhage from esophageal varices; due to malformations and congenital stenoses in portal venous system. Am J Med 16: 459-464, 1954.

25. JOHNSON AO, OBISESAN AO, WILLIAMS AO: Extrahepatic portal hypertension due to congenital obstruction of the portal vein and associated gross hepatic lobulation. Clin Ped 18: 619-621, 1979.

26. BEGGS AS: Anomalous persistence in embryos of parts of peri-intestinal rings formed by vitelline veins. Am J Anat 13: 103-110, 1912.

27. MAKEY DA, BOWEN JC: Preduodenal portal vein: its surgical significance. Surgery 84: 689-690, 1978.

28. SIMONDS JP: Chronic occlusion of the portal vein. Arch Surg 33: 397-424, 1936.

29. BEITZKE H: Über einen Fall von kavernöser Umwadlung der Pfortader. Charité-Ann 34: 466-477, 1910.

30. FLEISCHHAUER H: Über den chronischen Pfortaderverschluss.
     Virchows Arch path Anat 286: 747-765, 1932.

31. LEGER L, COLIN A, SORS C, LEMAIGRE G: Les cavernomes de la
     veine porte: étude anatomique, physio-patho-génique.
     J Chir 84: 145-172, 1962.

32. WILSON KW, ROBINSON DC, HACKING PM: Portal hypertension in
     childhood. Brit J Surg 56: 13-22, 1969.

33. ROSCH J, DOTTER CT: Extrahepatic portal obstruction in child-
     hood and its angiographic diagnosis. Am J Roentgenol 112:
     143-149, 1971.

34. MEREDITH HC, VUJIC I, SCHABEL SI, O'BRIEN PH: Obstructive
     jaundice caused by cavernous transformation of the portal
     vein. Br J Radio 51: 1011-1012, 1978.

35. HELLWEG G: Congenital absence of intrahepatic portal venous
     system simulating Eck fistula; report of a case with
     necropsy findings. Arch Path 57: 425-430, 1954.

36. McINDOE AH: Vascular lesions of portal cirrhosis. Arch
     Path Lab Med 5: 23-42, 1928.

37. TANDLER J: Ueber die Varietäten der Arteria Coeliaca und
     deren Entwickelung. Anat Hefte Wiesb 25: 473-500, 1904.

38. MICHELS NA: Blood supply and anatomy of the upper abdominal
     organs. Lippincott and Company, Philadelphia, 1955.

39. GUPTA SC, GUPTA CS, GUPTA SB: Intrahepatic supply patterns
     in cases of double hepatic arteries - a study by corrosion
     casts. Anat Anz 146: 166-170, 1979.

40. NAHUM H, LEVESQUE M: Arteriography in hepatic trauma.
     Radiology 109: 557-563, 1973.

41. KONSTAM MA, NOVELLINE RA, ATHANASOULIS CA: Aberrant hepatic
     artery: A potential cause for error in the angiographic
     diagnosis of traumatic liver hematoma. Gastrointest
     Radiol 4: 43-45, 1979.

42. MICHELS NA: Collateral arterial pathways to the liver after
     ligation of the hepatic artery and removal of the celiac
     axis. Cancer 6: 708-724, 1953.

43. MICHELS NA: The hepatic, cystic and retroduodenal arteries and
     their relations to the biliary ducts with samples of the
     entire celiacal blood supply. Ann Surg 133: 503-524, 1951.

DISCUSSION

CHAIRMAN: E. CUTZ

LAUTT: The comment was made that the hepatic arterial flow is
very low in the fetus. Is it known at what stage the hepatic
arterial flow takes on normal proportions in relationship
with the total flow?

TAYLOR: No.

PETERS: I think it must be a gradual increase because at least
the size of the arterioles remains quite small. Even a month
or so after birth the arterioles are really quite small relative to their size in adults.

LAUTT: Is it known at what point the sympathetic nervous system
can be demonstrated in the liver?

PETERS: There is certainly not much known about what role
innervation of the liver plays and I don't know at what time
that innervation becomes evident.

TAYLOR: I can't really tell you about humans because I haven't
looked at human fetal livers late enough during gestation.
But in the rat you don't find any sympathetic ganglion cells
in the liver until 4 or 5 days after birth. You find a
similar sort of pattern in the heart.

MANLEY: What is the relationship between the ductus choledochus
which presumably forms the major intrahepatic bile ducts and
the more peripheral and smaller bile ducts which you said were
induced by mesenchymal tissue within the portal areas?

PETERS: Apparently the ductus choledochus doesn't extend as far
    out as we usually think.   I don't know the level at which it
    extends because it is hard to get fetuses of various ages for
    study.   The major ducts come off the ductus choledochus
    because one can see a couple of bifurcations.   But at the
    intralobular level the ducts seem to be developing from the
    parenchymal cords.   Even after birth there is a relative
    deficiency in duct structures compared with what one sees in
    adults.

TAYLOR: I agree.   I think one of the key things that comes out
    is that most of the human embryology books are hopelessly out
    of date in terms of the development of the liver, both in
    terms of the breakup of the omphalomesenteric veins and also
    with respect to the biliary tree.   It is about time that the
    embryologists got their act together and that hepatologists
    start to write the truth in their review articles.

MANLEY: Induction from the collecting ducts promotes the formation
    of more peripheral tubules within the kidney and the absence
    of appropriate induction may lead to cyst formation.   Can one
    make the **same** analogy with the liver and suggest that the
    ductus choledochus might be an inducer of intrahepatic bile
    ducts and that certain diseases like Caroli's might be due to
    problems in induction, or at least in the joining up of two
    different duct systems?

PETERS: It is an interesting thought and cystic conditions do
    seem to go hand in hand in both organs.   However in the
    kidney the first portion of the tubule is of mesenchymal
    origin and that isn't the case with the epithelial structures
    of the liver.   All of the duct structures and the parenchymal
    cells seem to come off at the endoderm whereas the kidney
    develops from the urogenital ridge which then is invaded by
    the ureteral bud.   So I don't think it is quite the same.
    In developing livers it doesn't look as though the duct itself
    is inducing the development of smaller intralobular ducts.

RAPPAPORT: Dr. Peters has suggested that, during development, the
    mesenchyme comes first, then the bile ductules and then the
    arterioles.   I wonder whether it isn't the reverse, first
    the arterioles, then the ductules, and then mesenchyma?
    I cannot imagine that these structures develop without a
    blood supply.   He also stated that in cirrhotic livers
    proliferating ductules are seen everywhere there is a scar.
    Because the scars cut off the ductules from sinusoidal flow
    it must be arterioles or arteriolar capillaries that supply
    the ductules.   The periductular arteriolar plexus is almost
    part and parcel of the wall of the ductules.   I have a feeling
    that in the development of the ductules the arterioles are leading.

PETERS: Whether or not the arteriole spirals around the bile ducts
    in the human liver as it does in the liver of certain other
    animals is unfortunately not known.   But in the developing
    human liver one finds portal areas in which there are small
    arterioles and no ducts and portal areas in which ducts are
    seen without good arterioles.   In general it seems that
    arterioles are there before ducts, I didn't mean to imply the
    other way.   But they are both developing over a long period
    of time and both are still somewhat immature by time of birth.

    Looking at the diseased livers of adults, I have been struck
    by the relative lack of arterial supply in some of the scarred
    areas.   You will recall that we see two kinds of apparent
    duct changes, one which is truly ductular with bile duct epi-
    thelium and one which is really hepatocellular.   These trans-
    formed hepatocyte cords I call pseudocholangioles.   They
    look very ductular but they still are hepatocytes and they seem
    not to have the same blood supply as the proliferating ducts.

SHARP: How does bile get from the canaliculus into the bile
    ducts which we see?

PETERS: The liver cords which migrate off in the very early stages
    have a canaliculus.   That canaliculus remains there and seems
    to be converted into an interlobular duct.   So I don't have
    any difficulty in seeing that connection.   What I have
    difficulty in understanding is how the interlobular ducts
    connect up with the major ducts.

TAYLOR: I haven't seen this at all in animals.   The difficulty
    in answering these questions points out the need for some
    experimental hepatology in the embryo.

SHANDLING: Do the speakers have any information comparing
    development in utero with development during regeneration?

PETERS: There is induction of some fetal enzymes during regenera-
    tion, for example of alpha-fetoprotein, but the picture is
    not clear.   For example, we know that the regeneration which
    follows certain types of toxic liver injury doesn't produce
    the same level of alpha-fetoprotein as the regeneration
    associated with viral hepatitis B.   Perhaps some of the latter
    induction is viral.   Many investigators, the Japanese in
    particular, talk about a reversion to more primitive type cells
    in very severe hepatic necrosis.   One can see cord-like
    structures of oval hepatocytes looking very much like ducts.
    In most regeneration that I see, say after ordinary viral
    hepatitis, the hepatocytes get very large and very hydropic
    and don't morphologically look like those in the fetus.

GREENE: I wonder if I misinterpreted something you said, namely
    that the mesenchyme has some sort of stimulatory effect on
    the development of the bone marrow, and that this effect can
    be interrupted during development.   If this is the case I
    wonder if a disease such as type IB glycogenosis, in which
    there is an association between liver, pancreatic and bone
    marrow involvement, could represent a developmental
    abnormality.

PETERS: The only thing I mentioned was that erythropoiesis
    within the liver seems to require the liver endodermal tissue,
    the hepatoblast, because the primitive mesenchyme will develop
    sinusoids on transplant but it won't develop the hematopoietic
    tissue.   Also the liver seems to be producing rather primitive
    erythroid tissue, the more adult erythroid and myeloid tissue
    coming a little later from the marrow.

COHEN: Dr. Taylor alluded to some disparity between the right
    and left lobes of the liver in developmental hematopoiesis.
    I was wondering whether or not we see that same disparity in
    extramedullary erythropoiesis associated with disease.

TAYLOR: I am afraid that I can't answer that.

PETERS: I haven't specifically looked for it, but it certainly
    isn't terribly obvious.

DEVELOPMENTAL ASPECTS OF BILE ACID METABOLISM AND HEPATIC FUNCTION

John B. Watkins

Department of Pediatrics, University of Pennsylvania
School of Medicine, and Division of Gastroenterology
and Nutrition, The Children's Hospital of Philadelphia
Philadelphia, Pennsylvania

INTRODUCTION

Bile acids represent the major solid constituents in bile.
They are essential for bile formation due principally to their
unique chemical and structural characteristics which permit the
solubilization and secretion of nonpolar lipids and potentially
toxic compounds into bile. In the fetus and developing infant,
major changes in the structural and functional characteristics of
the hepatocytes and in the organization of the liver occur. In
turn, biliary lipid secretion, the distribution and size of the bile
acid pool and the functional capacity of the infant to excrete
organic anions and absorb essential lipophilic nutrients are
markedly altered.

The focus of this discussion will be to review and emphasize
the physiological limitations and changes in bile acid metabolism
which occur normally in the developing fetus and infant. These
changes will be examined in view of the new advances in cell biology
and liver metabolism and will emphasize those factors which may
influence bile acid metabolism or the structure and function of
the hepatocyte.

FETAL BILE ACID METABOLISM

In the fetus and at birth, the hepatic uptake, intracellular
processing and secretion of lipophilic organic anions appear to be
poorly developed. From studies performed in utero, there is
increasing evidence that the placenta compensates for the fetal
hepatic immaturity by assuming a major detoxification and excretory

43

role until birth at which time the functional immaturity of the
liver assumes clinical significance.   Numerous approaches have
been devised to characterize the development of hepatic function
in the human fetus.   Since bile acids represent the major organic
anions synthesized only by the liver, many studies have focussed
upon the ontogeny of this process.   To date, it has been established
that bile acids in the human may be isolated from the gallbladder as
early as 14 to 16 weeks gestation (1).   In vitro, organ culture
studies of fetal hepatic function demonstrate that bile acid uptake,
conjugation and possibly secretion may occur as early as 12 weeks
gestation (2), although bile acid synthesis has not yet been demonstrated.   Studies designed to characterize the species of bile
acids available to or synthesized by the fetus have demonstrated
that fetal gallbladder bile at 22-26 weeks gestation contains principally the taurine conjugated dihydroxy bile acids.   Later in
gestation, at 28-30 weeks, small amounts of glycocholate have been
recovered.   Taurocholate and taurochenodeoxycholate are the pre-
dominant bile acids from 30 weeks gestation to birth (3).   The
importance of taurine conjugation in the fetus as well as the
possible influence of bile acid conjugate status on postnatal bile
acid metabolism are discussed subsequently.

The relative predominance of dihydroxy bile acids early in
gestation may indicate a possible deficiency of the 12-alpha
hydroxylase enzyme system (4).   Alternatively, it could reflect
the presence of alternate metabolic pathways for bile acid synthesis,
for example via the 26-hydroxy-cholesterol pathway, or differential
rates of placental bile acid transport (5).   In this regard, there
has recently been an increasing interest in bile acid synthesis
during fetal life, in the hope of defining the origin of some of
the unusual bile acids detected in adults and children with cholestatic syndromes.   Sophisticated gas chromatography-mass spectroscopy analyses have been performed to identify the bile acids found
in meconium or amniotic fluid of full term infants (6).   These
studies suggest that the fetal colon serves as a repository which
reflects the biosynthetic events during gestation, particularly as
the bile acids secreted into bile or excreted in urine before birth
could be reabsorbed in the fetal intestine and participate in an
intrauterine enterohepatic circulation.   The studies performed to
date have indicated that a large percent of the bile acids recovered
from meconium exists as bile acid sulfoconjugates.   This metabolic
alteration could serve a truly excretory function for the fetus,
since the sulfated bile acid conjugates might be poorly reabsorbed
from the fetal intestine.   The sulfation of neutral steroids such
as progesterone has been demonstrated to be a primary excretory
pathway in the human fetus.   Furthermore, the sulfated steroid
then serves as a substrate for a unique fetal metabolic pathway
which leads to further hydroxylation and inactivation of these
biologically active compounds.   A similar hydroxylation step or
other modification has not been demonstrated for bile acids,

although considerable bile acid sulfatase enzyme activity has been
isolated from the placenta, liver and small intestine of the fetus
(7).   Further evidence for unique fetal bile acid synthetic pathways lies in the detection, by analytical gas liquid chromatography-
mass spectroscopy, of unusual unsaturated C-24 monohydroxy bile
acids, of bile acids with various alterations in the steroid side
chain, and of considerable quantities of the better known secondary
bile acids: deoxycholic acid, ursodeoxycholic acid, and lithocholic
acid (6,7).   The high concentration of the secondary bile acids
may represent placental transfer of bile acids from the mother to
the fetus rather than fetal metabolism (8).   Attempts to delineate
the extent to which maternally derived bile acids contribute to
the total fetal bile acid pool are incomplete and difficult to extra-
polate to the human due to species differences in placental transport.   Nevertheless, in the fetal sheep, rat and dog, using tracer
quantities of ^{14}C cholesterol as substrate, only the synthesis of
the primary bile acids, cholic acid and chenodeoxycholate, could
be demonstrated (9).   Synthesis of the secondary bile acids,
deoxycholic and lithocholic acids, did not occur.   The recovery of
labeled secondary bile acids in fetal bile could be demonstrated
only if the maternal bile acid pool was labeled, suggesting that
their presence in the fetal bile is due solely to maternal to fetal
transfer (10).   By contrast, a bi-directional placental transfer
can be demonstrated for cholic acid and particularly for chenodeoxycholic acid.   Some degree of autonomous regulation of bile
acid synthesis can be demonstrated by the increased conversion of
cholesterol to bile acids in response to external biliary drainage.
Despite this synthetic response to bile acid depletion, the bile
acid pool size in the fetus, corrected for body weight or body
surface area, appears to be less than that of the adult, which
suggests that an immaturity in the regulation of bile acid synthesis
may exist in utero.

Direct investigation of the metabolism of bile acids has been
performed in utero utilizing an elegant surgical model devised by
Jackson and collaborators (11).   These studies demonstrated that
infused doses of ^{14}C cholic acid are efficiently taken up, conjugated
and secreted in the near term fetal dog and monkey.   The maximum
rate of bile acid secretion was somewhat less than in the adult,
equalling 83 vs 96 percent of the infusion rate, a difference mainly
accounted for by placental transfer.   There is considerable species
variation and the excretory role served by the placenta appears to
correlate with the maturity of the hepatic excretory function.
For example, in the fetal dog, less than 5 percent of the infused
cholic acid was excreted by the placental route, hepatic function
being relatively mature, with nearly 80 percent of the cholic acid
being conjugated and secreted into bile.   In the Rhesus monkey,
fetal placental excretion was much greater, equalling 30 percent
(range 18-40%) of the total excretion, with hepatic conjugation and
secretion accounting for less than 40 percent of the total excretion.

No free or unconjugated bile acids were secreted into bile and thus conjugation with taurine, the major bile acid conjugate formed by the fetus, does not per se appear to limit the rate of excretion.

In order to characterize further the relative hepatic maturity of the fetal dog, taurocholate, in amounts equal to 20 times the endogenous pool size, was infused.   During this infusion to determine the capacity of the fetus to excrete a load of bile acid, bile flow increased together with bile acid excretion rates which augmented by a factor of 30 over resting values.   Bile acid concentrations in bile increased four to five times, which demonstrated a relatively efficient handling by the fetus of an exogenously administered bile acid load, and a rather mature hepatic function (12).   These studies should be compared to those of Little and co-workers who demonstrated in the fetal rat that the bulk of the bile acid pool is contained within the liver and serum, and that effective redistribution of bile acids into the intestine occurs only following birth (13). Interestingly, this process may be accelerated by the administration of corticosteroids to and possibly by cholestasis in the mother. Further work will be necessary in order to determine which aspect of hepatic function is responsible for these maturation effects. Of particular interest in this regard are the studies of DeWolf-Peeters et al (14) who have related the degree of functional cholestasis which exists normally in the neonatal rat to a diminished surface area of the biliary canaliculi.   These developmental studies report an increase in relative surface area of the canaliculus with postnatal development, a change which corresponds to the normal course of maturation of the biliary secretory process.   The results suggest that morphometric analysis reflects indirectly the capacity of the liver near term to mature and develop the structural and enzymatic components necessary for bile acid synthesis and biliary lipid secretion.

Evidence for the secretion of bile into the intestine during fetal life presents the possibility that an enterohepatic circulation of bile acids exists in utero.   In order to study this process further, perfusion studies of the fetal jejunum and ileum have been performed in utero.   These studies demonstrated that a significant degree of passive reabsorption of conjugated bile acids may occur proximally in the jejunum even at the low concentrations observed normally in the intestinal contents of the neonate.   Furthermore, in several laboratories, it has now been established that there is reduced capacity for the active reabsorption of taurocholate in the fetal ileum.   These observations support the concept that a generalized and nonselective permeability for many substances exist in the fetal intestine, and that selective reabsorptive processes may well be poorly developed (15).   Persistence of this phenomenon post-natally would promote an inadequate intraluminal environment for the lipolysis and absorption of nonpolar nutritionally significant lipids.   Furthermore, a short-circuit or early return of secreted

bile acids to the liver might significantly alter the hepatic regulation of bile acid synthesis and influence bile acid kinetics in
postnatal life.

In summary, hepatic function in the fetus clearly differs from
the infant at term and the adult in several important parameters.
The bile acid pool is contracted and confined principally to the
liver.   Bile acid synthesis and bile acid secretion appear limited,
and the morphological function of the hepatocyte secretory apparatus
is reduced.   There is some evidence that fetal detoxification and
excretion of potentially toxic lipophilic bile acids (e.g. lithocholic acid) exist.   It is clear that the fetus experiences a major
change in the maturation of hepatic function near term, and that
much new information is needed in order to delineate each aspect
of this development.

NEONATAL BILE ACID METABOLISM

The functional significance of hepatic immaturity is measured
by organic anion conjugation and excretion.   It becomes immediately
apparent at birth when one considers the remarkable integration of
homeostatic and excretory functions necessary for the infant,
including a requirement for suitable nutrient intake and absorption.
This capacity is often severely limited in the premature infant of
30-36 weeks gestation.   For example, malabsorption of 10-20 percent
of fat intake is commonplace for a formula fed infant.   As intake
is often maximal and cannot be readily increased to compensate for
such losses, fat malabsorption may severely limit the calories
available to the infant for growth (16).   Recent investigations to
delineate the mechanisms for this fat malabsorption have established
that the intraluminal phase of fat digestion is incomplete in the
neonate.   Signer et al (17) and others have demonstrated that
dietary lipid composition and intraluminal bile acid concentrations
primarily influence the efficiency of fat absorption.   Numerous
studies have now demonstrated that in the pre-term infant, intraluminal bile acid concentrations are low, 1-2 mM/litre during meals.
These concentrations exhibit very little variation throughout the
day, and are in the range associated with poor fat absorption in
both infants and in adults.   Furthermore, as they are at or below
the critical micellar concentration, they are insufficient to
adquately solubilize the products of lipolysis or nonpolar dietary
lipids.   In order to determine the factors responsible for such
low intraluminal bile acid concentrations, it is necessary to
examine both the hepatic and intestinal aspects of neonatal bile
acid metabolism.

In the adult, there exists an efficient enterohepatic circulation for bile acids so that nearly 95-98% of the bile acid pool is
reabsorbed during each cycle and the amount lost is replaced by
new bile acid synthesis.   During meals bile acid reabsorption in

the jejunum represents a relatively minor proportion of the whole
so that bile acid concentrations are maintained at levels above the
critical micellar concentration (CMC). While bile acid reabsorption may occur passively in the jejunum, it is clear that there is
an active transport process localized to the distal ileum which
serves to maintain an efficient enterohepatic circulation. The
overall efficiency of this process is such that the bile acid pool
is well maintained, the liver clearly capable of compensating for
such fecal loss that does occur with new bile acid synthesis (18).
In the neonate, the activity of several sites which normally contribute to the maintenance of the bile acid pool in the adult appear
to be diminished. The ability of the gallbladder to concentrate
bile acids is lower than in the adult, and the proximal small
intestine appears to be unusually permeable with a diminished
capacity to transport actively glucose and a variety of compounds.
Following birth, the membrane structure of the small intestine and
its permeability to exogenous proteins may be significantly different
than in the adult (15). Intestinal permeability to lipids, bile
acids, and other lipophilic compounds has been largely unstudied
in the infant. The maturation of distal ileal function, specifically for bile acid transport, has now been determined in the rat,
guinea pig, rabbit, and man (17,18,19,20). In each instance, an
active transport system for bile acids is either absent or relatively
inefficient at birth. In an animal model, kinetic analysis of
the active transport process in vitro suggests that the increase in
ileal surface area postnatally is important for the functional
maturation of this process. Preliminary studies in rats and in
the human indicate that increased transport capacity may be induced
by steroid administration either before weaning or prenatally (21).
Recent studies using isolated ileal enterocytes demonstrate that
this may be due to stabilization of the sodium-potassium ATPase
system at the basolateral membrane (18). However, to date there
are no studies which examine the role of hormonal influences or
diet on this aspect of intestinal maturation.

     In order to examine directly the composite of hepatic and
intestinal functions which influence intraluminal bile acid
concentrations, numerous investigators have determined the bile
acid pool size using the isotope dilution technique described by
Lindstedt (22). In the neonate, the bile acid pool size has been
determined without radiation hazard using stable isotopes and
deuterium or ^{13}C bile acids. These investigations demonstrate
that the bile acid pool in the neonate is reduced. For example,
at three days of age, the cholic acid pool in the full term
infant averages 41 mg or, expressed in terms of body surface,
290 ± 36 mg/m^2, compared to a cholic acid pool size in the adult
of 605 ± 122 mg/m^2. Cholic acid synthesis in these infants was
found to be 23 mg/day (i.e. 110 ± 20 mg/m^2/day compared to $194 \pm$
28 mg/m^2/day in the adult) or, expressed as a fractional turnover
rate, 43% of the pool/day. In the infant, pool size appears to

correlate directly with intraluminal bile acid concentrations during
meals.   Thus, it appears that the recycling or secretion rates are
maximum and do not increase as in the adult in order to compensate
for variations in bile acid pool size;   accordingly, the reduced
pool size in infants appears to limit intraluminal bile acid concentrations.   This reduction may be due to a disordered regulation of
bile acid synthesis or an excessive loss of bile acids in the enterohepatic circulation either via the urine or the intestinal tract.
Urinary bile acid losses are reported to be low in newborn infants
(0.1 - 2.3 mM/24 hr) and are considerably less than the values
reported for infants with cholestatic liver disease (23).   These
data should now be examined in view of the recent findings which
demonstrate that in the first several days following birth, there
is a marked increase in serum bile acid levels to values two to
three times those normally found in adults following meals (24,25).
Interestingly, these elevated values are maintained until six to
seven months of age, and may indicate that a relatively large
proportion of the bile acid pool escapes uptake by the liver, that
the infant is relatively cholestatic for the first several months
of life.

    The fecal excretion of bile acids has been shown to vary with
diet and with the degree of steatorrhea.   For the premature and
full term infant, these values have been quoted in the range of
3-4 mg/kg/day (26), amounts which are less than the synthetic rate
calculated by an isotope dilution technique.   This would imply
that the enterohepatic circulation may not yet be in a steady state
and that some infants following birth undergo a rapid expansion of
their bile acid pool.   Therefore, although the fetus at term is
capable of bile acid conjugation and bile acid synthesis, the
transition to an extrauterine existence is accompanied by an increase
in bile acid synthesis in order to establish an effective bile acid
pool.   Evidence for this hypothesis lies in the observation of
infants whose mothers are treated with dexamethasone before birth
(to induce pulmonary maturity and thus prevent hyaline membrane
disease) and who exhibit a marked increase in intraluminal bile
acid concentrations during meals.   Furthermore, a four-fold increase
in bile acid pool size to values equal to those for larger more
mature full term infants was demonstrated.   Bile acid synthesis
and fractional turnover rates were reduced to values found in adults
and older more mature infants, implying the existence of new steady
state conditions.   To date, only preliminary data are available
which characterize in the same infant the rate of maturation of the
enterohepatic circulation and enlargement of bile acid pool following birth.   In a recent study, Watkins and collaborators reported
that in premature infants the intraluminal bile acid concentrations
and bile acid pool size are low initially, but increase during the
first six weeks following birth to levels found in full term infants.
Bile acid synthesis rates remain relatively constant at both time
points as the pool size enlarges, which suggests that either

synthesis is maximal or that with increasing postnatal age, the
regulation of the bile acid pool and its conservation within the
enterohepatic circulation become more efficient (27).

BILE ACID CONJUGATION: INFLUENCE OF DIET

    Conjugation of bile acids in the liver with glycine and/or
taurine significantly alters their physical-chemical properties,
and hence the concentrations of bile acids required to form a
micellar phase and possibly the site of bile acid reabsorption in
the intestine (28).   Taurine conjugates, as previously noted,
predominate in the fetus and at birth, whereas in the adult, glycine
conjugated bile acids predominate.   This pattern does not appear
to emerge in the infant until two to seven months of age.   Although
many of the factors which influence bile acid conjugation have not
yet been defined, glycine conjugation, characteristic of herbivorous
mammals, appears in evolutionary terms to be the most advanced form
of bile acid conjugation.   By contrast, taurine conjugation, which
is extremely sensitive to taurine availability, appears relatively
early in the evolutionary scheme.   Taurine levels are reported in
the fetal liver and blood to be higher than maternal levels but
fall quickly after birth.   Cysteine sulfanilic acid decarboxylase
activity, which is required for taurine synthesis, is reported to
be low in the fetal and neonatal liver.   In view of the immaturity
of the transulfuration pathway, it has been suggested that exogenous
taurine, which is present in breast milk, may be an essential amino
acid for the human neonate as it is for the cat (29).   Most dietary
formulations are relatively low in taurine, and several studies
have demonstrated that the type of bile acid conjugate formed is
directly dependent on the dietary availability of taurine.   Accordingly, where duodenal fluid bile acid conjugates have been analyzed,
infants fed breast milk or taurine supplemented formula formed
predominantly taurine conjugates, whereas in the non-enriched
formulas, glycine conjugates predominated after two to three weeks
of age, which correlated with the observed decrease in serum and
urinary taurine levels.

    Hepner and co-workers, using double labeled bile acid conjugates
to study independently the metabolism of the bile acid nucleus and
amino acid moiety, demonstrated that the glycine component of
cholylglycine turns over about three times more rapidly than the
steroid nucleus in all of the glycine conjugated bile acids (30).
Furthermore, taurocholate deconjugation appears to be relatively
slower than glycocholate deconjugation in the adult.   In the neonate, the time course for the appearance of bacteria capable of
bile acid deconjugation has not been established; thus, the emerg-
ence of glycine conjugates may represent an imbalance between the
availability of substrate for conjugation and the loss of bile
acids from the enterohepatic circulation rather than being an
indication of the bacterial flora capable of bile acid deconjugation.

Furthermore, in the future a recently developed in vitro culture model may serve to elucidate better the inter-relationships and mechanisms required for the conservation of bile acids.

SUMMARY

The discussion has focussed upon bile acids as the major organic anions synthesized, conjugated and secreted by the liver. Their physiological importance has been emphasized. Central to this analysis has been consideration of the maturational factors which affect both the liver and intestine, which contribute to maintaining the enterohepatic circulation of bile acids, and which influence the metabolism of other compounds of nutritional and physiological importance, such as vitamin D, thyroid hormones and riboflavin.

More information is needed to evaluate those factors which limit or interfere with bile acid conservation, synthesis or excretion. Such studies may enable us to predict disease or further our understanding of the developmental processes influencing the liver in infancy and childhood.

ACKNOWLEDGEMENT

This work was supported by the National Institutes of Health through grants # HD 13932 and HD 13913.

REFERENCES

1. BONGIOVANNI AM: Bile acid content of gallbladder of infants, children and adults. J Endocrin & Metab 25: 678-685, 1965.

2. DeBELLE RC, BLACKLOW NR, BAYLAN M, LITTLE JM, LESTER R: Bile acid conjugation in fetal hepatic organ culture. Gastroenterology 69: 815, 1975.

3. POLEY JR, DOWER JC, OWEN CA, STICKLER GB: Bile acids in infants and children. J Lab Clin Med 63: 838-845, 1964.

4. SHARP HL, PELLER J, CAREY JB, KRIVET W: Primary and secondary bile acids in meconium. Pediatr Res 5: 274-279, 1971.

5. JAVITT NB: Cholestasis in infancy status report and conceptual approach. Gastroenterology 70: 1172-1181, 1976.

6. BACK P, WALTER K: Developmental pattern of bile acid metabolism as revealed by bile acid analysis of meconium. Gastroenterology 78: 671-676, 1980.

7. WATKINS JB, GOLDSTEIN E, CORYER R, BROWN ER, ERAKLIS A:

Sulfation of bile acids in the fetus. In The Liver: Quantitative Aspects of Structure and Function, R Preisig, J Berne (eds), 3rd International Gstaad Symposium, Gstaad. Dr. Madaus & Co., Berne, Switzerland, 1979.

8. LESTER R: Physiologic cholestasis. Gastroenterology 78: 864-865, 1980.

9. SMALLWOOD RA, JABLONSKI P, WATTS J McK: Bile salt synthesis in the developing sheep liver. Clin Sci & Molec Med 45: 403-406, 1972.

10. LESTER R, LITTLE JM, GRECO R, PIASECKI GT, JACKSON BT: Fetal bile salt formation. Pediatr Res 6: 375a, 1972.

11. JACKSON BR, SMALLWOOD RA, PIASECKI GH, BROWN AS, RAUSCHECKER HF, LESTER R: Fetal bile salt metabolism. I. The metabolism of sodium cholate-^{14}C in the fetal dog. J Clin Invest 50: 1286-1294, 1971.

12. SMALLWOOD RA, LESTER R, PIASECKI GH, KLEIN PD, GRECO R, JACKSON BT: Fetal bile salt metabolism. II. Hepatic excretion of endogenous bile salt and of a taurocholate load. J Clin Invest 51: 1388-1397, 1972.

13. LITTLE JM, RICHEY JE, VAN THIEL DH, et al: Taurocholate pool size and distribution in the fetal rat. J Clin Invest 63: 1042-1049, 1979.

14. DE WOOLF-PEETERS C, DE VOS R, DESMET V: Electron microscopy and histochemistry of canalicular differentiation in fetal and neonatal rat liver. Tissue Cell 4: 379-388, 1972.

15. GRAND RJ, WATKINS JB, TORTI FM: Development of the human gastrointestinal tract. A review. Gastroenterology 70: 790-810, 1976.

16. WATKINS JB: Bile acid metabolism and fat absorption in newborn infants. Pediatr Clin N America 21: 501-512, 1974.

17. LESTER R, SMALLWOOD RA, LITTLE JM, BROWN AS, PIASECKI GJ, JACKSON BT: Fetal bile salt metabolism. J Clin Invest 59: 1009-1016, 1977.

18. DeBELLE RC, VAUPSHAS V, VITULLO BB, HABER LR, SHAFFER E, MACKIE GG, OWEN H, LITTLE JM, LESTER R: Intestinal absorption of bile salts: immature development in the neonate. J Pediatr 94: 472-476, 1979.

19. HEUBI JE, WOLCOTT RH: Perinatal maturation of intestinal bile

acid transport in guinea pigs. Gastroenterology 78: 1182a, 1980.

20. KELTS D, BOEHM C, WATKINS JB: Bile acid (BA) transport and maturation of distal ileal function. Gastroenterology 78: 1193a, 1980.

21. WATKINS JB, SZCZEPANIK P, GOULD JB, KLEIN PD, LESTER R: Bile salt metabolism in the human premature infant. Preliminary observations of pool size and synthesis rate following prenatal administration of dexamethasone and phenobarbital. Gastroenterology 69: 706-713, 1975.

22. LINDSTEDT S: The turnover of cholic acid in man: Bile acids and steroids 51. Acta Physiol Scand 40: 1-9, 1957.

23. WATKINS JB, PERMAN JA: Bile acid metabolism in infants and children. Clin Gastroenterol 6: 201-218, 1977.

24. SUCHY FJ, BALISTRERI WF, HEUBI JE, SEARCY JE, LEVIN RS: Physiologic cholestasis: Evaluation of the primary serum bile acid concentrations in normal infants. Gastroenterology 80: 1037-1041, 1981.

25. BARNES S, BERKOWITZ G, HIRSCHOWITZ BI, WIRTSCHAFTER D, CASSADY G: Postnatal physiologic hypercholemia in both premature and full term infants. J Clin Invest: (In press)

26. ROY CC, STE-MARIE M, CHARTRAND L, WEBER A, BARD H, DORAY B: Correction of the malabsorption of the preterm infant with a medium-chain triglyceride formula. J Pediatr 86: 446-450, 1975.

27. WATKINS JB, JARVENPAA AL, RAIHA N, SZCZEPANIK P, VAN-LEEUWEN P, KLEIN PD, RASSIN DK, GAULL G: Regulation of bile acid pool size: Role of taurine conjugates. Pediatr Res 13: 410a, 1979.

28. SCHIFF ER, SMALL NC, DIETSCHY JM: Characterization of the kinetics of the passive and active transport mechanisms for bile acid absorption in the small intestine and colon of the rat. J Clin Invest 51: 1351-1362, 1972.

29. HAYES KC, CAREY RE, SCHMIDT SY: Retinal degeneration associated with taurine deficiency in the cat. Science 188: 949-951, 1975.

30. HEPNER GW, HOFMANN AF, THOMAS J: Metabolism of steroid and amino acid moieties of conjugated bile acids in man. I. Cholylglycine. J Clin Invest 51: 1889-1905, 1972.

HEPATIC DRUG-METABOLIZING ENZYMES DURING EMBRYONIC AND

FETAL DEVELOPMENT

Allan B. Okey and Daniel Nebert

Division of Clinical Pharmacology, Dept. Paediatrics
The Hospital for Sick Children, Toronto, Ontario, and
Developmental Pharmacology Branch, National Institute
of Child Health and Human Development, National
Institutes of Health, Bethesda, Maryland

INTRODUCTION

Twenty or thirty years ago, it was believed that all drugs
(and other environmental pollutants) were "toxic", or pharmacologically active, in their parent (non-metabolized) form. The function
of all drug-metabolizing enzymes was therefore regarded as detoxication, i.e. to "inactivate" the active parent drug. More recently
it has become increasingly evident that although some drugs are,
indeed, active in their nonmetabolized parent form, many drugs are
inactive until being metabolized (1,2). A delicate balance exists,
therefore, between detoxication and toxification.

During embryonic and fetal development, most drug-metabolizing
enzymes are totally absent, or at least exist at undetectable levels.
If the drug is toxic without being metabolized (for example, chloramphenicol or theophylline), the neonate - and especially the
premature - will be at increased risk due to its developmental
deficiency in drug metabolism. On the other hand, if the drug is
toxic only after metabolism (for example, polycyclic hydrocarbons
present in cigarette smoke), the individual with the highest enzyme
level will be at greatest risk. It therefore becomes moot whether
"higher levels of enzyme" are advantageous or disadvantageous to
the individual; one must first understand all detoxication and
toxification pathways of the drug being studied. The same reason-
ing also would apply during early embryonic and fetal development,
except in this case "drug toxicity" would be reflected as abortions,
stillbirths, and various anatomical and developmental birth
defects.

Drug-metabolizing enzymes therefore can be pictured as "double-edged swords), detoxifying one drug while potentiating another drug via metabolism to a reactive intermediate.   This problem may be important in understanding drug-related pediatric liver disease, as we shall illustrate in this Chapter.   How many different drug-metabolizing enzymes exist?   How do these enzymes contribute to liver disease and teratology?   How early during embryonic development do these enzymes exist?   In an attempt to provide answers to these questions, we describe an experimental model system in the mouse.   This system, the Ah locus, principally represents a genetic difference in receptor concentration.   Because of this defect, we have demonstrated large differences in the biotransformation and pharmacokinetics of certain drugs, resulting in important variations in risk toward birth defects, drug toxicity, mutation, and certain types of malignancy.   By means of our greater understanding of the Ah locus, we might also provide some insight into the relationship between the developmental expression of other drug-metabolizing enzymes and pediatric disease, including birth defects.

HOW MANY DIFFERENT DRUG-METABOLIZING ENZYMES EXIST?

Most drugs and other environmental pollutants are so fat-soluble that they would remain in the body indefinitely were it not for the metabolism resulting in more water-soluble derivatives. These enzyme systems, located principally in the liver (but also probably present to some degree in virtually all tissues of the body), are usually divided into two groups: Phase I and Phase II. During Phase I metabolism, one or more water-soluble groups (such as hydroxyl) are introduced into the fat-soluble parent molecule, thus allowing a "handle", or a position, for the Phase II conjugating enzymes to attack.   Many Phase I products, but especially the conjugated Phase II products, are sufficiently water-soluble so that these chemicals are excreted readily from the body (1).

In Table I we have listed a large number of potentially relevant metabolic reactions that may be important in detoxication or toxification, leading to drug-induced disease.   Basically, any time a chemical bond is cleaved and/or electrons are passed one at a time, the possibility exists for unwanted reactions of such inter-mediates with nucleic acids or proteins.   The reactions can be complicated, including the degree of stability of short-lived chemical intermediates, the redox state, movement of unpaired electrons from one molecule to another (free radicals), and lipid peroxidation.   Generally, reactions involving DNA are believed to be most important for carcinogenesis, as is true for metagenesis, but absolute experimental proof of this hypothesis is still lacking. Reactions involving proteins and cell membrane surfaces may be more important than those involving nucleic acids for toxicity and teratogenesis, but experimental proof of this hypothesis is also lacking.

A. Phase I Metabolism

1. What is "cytochrome P-450"?

The majority of all Phase I oxidations (1) is performed by
cytochrome P-450. "Cytochrome", derived from Greek, literally
means "colored substance in the cell". The color is derived from
the properties of the outer electrons of transition elements such
as iron, and indeed cytochromes appear reddish in color when
sufficient concentrations exist in a test tube.

"P-450" denotes a reddish pigment with the unusual property of
having its major optical absorption peak (Soret maximum) at about
450 nm, when the material has been reduced and combined with carbon
monoxide (3). Although the name P-450 was intended to be temporary
until more knowledge about this substance was known, the terminology
has persisted for 16 years because of the increasing complexity of
this enzyme system with each passing year and because of the lack
of agreement on any better nomenclature.

Cytochrome P-450 clearly represents a family of hemoproteins
(heme-containing proteins similar in some ways to hemoglobin)
possessing catalytic activity toward thousands of substrates. This
collection of enzymes is known to metabolize: almost all drugs and
laboratory reagents; small chemicals such as benzene, thiocyanate,
or ethanol; polycyclic aromatic hydrocarbons such as benzo(a)pyrene
(ubiquitous in city smog, cigarette smoke and charcoal-cooked foods)
and biphenyl; halogenated hydrocarbons such as polychlorinated and
polybrominated biphenyls, defoliants, insecticides, and ingredients
in soaps and deodorants; certain fungal toxins and antibiotics;
many of the chemotherapeutic agents used to treat human cancer;
strong mutagens such as N-methyl-N'-nitro-N-nitrosoguanidine and
nitrosamines; aminoazo dyes and diazo compounds; various chemicals
found in cosmetics and perfumes; numerous aromatic amines, such as
those found in hair dyes, nitro aromatics, and heterocyclics; N-
acetylaryl-amines and nitrofurans; wood terpenes; epoxides; carba-
mates; alkyl halides; safrole derivatives; anti-oxidants, other
food additives, and many ingredients of foodstuffs and spices; both
endogenous and synthetic steroids; prostaglandins; and other endogenous compounds such as biogenic amines, indoles, thyroxine, and
fatty acids.

Until recently the general consensus among most laboratories
(4) has been that two, or four, or certainly less than one dozen,
forms of P-450 exist and that overlapping substrate specificity
accounts for all diversity seen when thousands of different chemicals
are metabolized. At the other extreme, it has been postulated (5)
that organisms have the genetic capacity to produce as many distinct
forms as there are inducers of P-450. Possessing the genetic
capacity to synthesize hundreds or thousands of different forms of

TABLE I

POTENTIALLY IMPORTANT METABOLIC REACTIONS THAT MAY PLAY A ROLE IN LIVER DISEASE

A. Oxidations (Phase I metabolism)

   1. Aromatic or aliphatic C-oxygenations (epoxidations, hydroxylations)

   2. N-, O-, or S-dealkylations

   3. N-oxidations or N-hydroxylations

   4. S-oxidations

   5. Deaminations

   6. Dehalogenations

   7. Metallo-alkane dealkylations

   8. Desulfurations

   9. Alcohol or aldehyde dehydrogenations

  10. Xanthine (and other purines) oxidations

  11. Tyrosine hydroxylation

  12. Monoamine (including catecholamine) oxidations

B. Reductions (Phase I metabolism)

   1. Azo reductions

   2. Nitro reductions

   3. Arene oxide reductions

   4. N-hydroxyl reductions

   5. Quinone reductions

   6. Carbonyl sulfide reduction by carbonic anhydrase

C. Hydrolyses (Phase I metabolism)

1. Hydrolyses of esters
2. Hydrolyses of amides
3. Hydrolyses of peptides

D. Conjugations (Phase II metabolism)

1. Glucuronidations
2. Sulfate conjugations
3. Glutathione conjugations
4. Acetylations
5. Glycine conjugations
6. Serine conjugations
7. N-, O-, or S-methylations
8. Ribonucleoside or ribonucleotide formations
9. Glycoside conjugations
10. "Water conjugations"

E. Beyond Phase II metabolism

1. C-oxygenations
2. Glucuronidations
3. Glycosidations
4. Deacetylations

F. Direct chemical reactions (oxidation/reduction)

P-450 does not imply that all of them would exist at any one time. In this respect, the P-450 system would be to the hundreds of thousands of environmental chemicals as the immune system is to the approximately one million antigens on this planet; in other words, as a new chemical or antigen enters the body, a new drug-metabolizing enzyme or antibody is mobilized in response to this stimulus. Further work is needed to confirm or disprove this interesting hypothesis (5) about multiple forms of P-450.

2. What is "monooxygenase activity"?

Monooxygenases are enzymes that insert one atom of atmospheric oxygen into their substrates (6,7). The various forms of P-450 represent a large subset of all monooxygenases. To perform this monooxygenation, the P-450 hemoprotein receives two electrons from the cofactors NADPH and/or NADH, and these electrons are received one at a time, usually via reductases (flavoproteins). In certain bacteria such as Pseudomonas, the entire electron chain (NADH, reductase, an iron-sulfur protein, and P-450· is in the cytosol (soluble cytoplasm). In most organisms, however, the electron chain is deeply embedded principally in the endoplasmic reticulum (and to some degree in the inner mitochondrial membrane and nuclear envelope). The endoplasmic reticulum centrifuged at 100,000 x $\underline{g}$ for an hour becomes the "microsomal pellet". The microsomal electron chain contains reductase and P-450, but the mitochondrial electron chain is more similar to bacteria, containing reductase, iron-sulfur protein (called "adrenodoxin"), and P-450.

In sum, P-450-mediated monooxygenase activities are ubiquitous in virtually all living things - some kinds of bacteria, and presumably all plants and animals. For example, certain bacteria are being developed to destroy oil spills in the ocean; this catalytic activity by definition represents Phase I metabolism and reflects P-450-mediated monooxygenase(s).

3. Oxidations, reductions, and hydrolyses

P-450-mediated monooxygenase activities (Table I) include: aromatic and aliphatic hydroxylations of carbon atoms; N-, O-, and S-dealkylations; N-oxidations and N-hydroxylations; S-oxidations; deaminations; dehalogenations; metallo-alkane dealkylations; desulfurations; certain purine and monoamine oxidations; certain azo and nitro reductions; and certain arene oxide (8) and N-hydroxyl (9) reductions. Removal of methyl or ethyl groups from substrates (dealkylations) can result in the methylation or ethylation (alkylation) of nucleic acid or protein, a potentially important mechanism for tumorigenesis or drug toxicity. Tetra-ethyl lead in gasoline, for example, is metabolized by P-450 in this manner to a reactive intermediate which is toxic to the central nervous system (1).

Human liver alcohol dehydrogenase catalyzes the oxidation of
the 3β-hydroxyl group of digitoxigenin and related derivatives;
after oxidation of the 3β-hydroxyl group, cardiac activity of these
digitalis-related genins is decreased by more than 90% (10).
Genetic differences, or ethanol-induced differences, in alcohol
dehydrogenase may therefore alter the required loading and maintenance doses of digitalis due to this potentially important detoxication pathway. Liver alcohol dehydrogenase may also toxify chemicals,
metabolizing allyl alcohol to the extremely neurotoxic acrolein (11)
and several xylyl alcohols to aldehydes that are much more toxic
to lung than liver tissue (12). Alcohol dehydrogenase is therefore
an excellent example of the dual nature of an enzyme designed to
metabolize endogenous substrates: the enzyme not only is capable
of detoxifying certain drugs or other foreign chemicals but is also
capable of toxifying certain other drugs.

Quinone reduction by DT diaphorase (13) has been postulated to
be an important step leading to glucuronide conjugation. Quinone-
derived free radicals might also be generated by this catalytic
activity or by some similar activity other than DT diaphorase.
Carbonyl sulfide has recently been shown (14) to be metabolized to
hydrogen sulfide by carbonic anhydrase; hydrogen sulfide is responsible for carbonyl sulfide toxicity. Carbonic anhydrase therefore
represents a reductase capable of toxification, i.e. potentiating
toxicity.

B. Phase II Metabolism

Drugs and other foreign chemicals are most commonly conjugated
with glucuronide (15), sulfate, or glutathione (Table I). "Direct"
bilirubin, for example, is the water-soluble conjugate. Glutathione
transferases (16) act on a seemingly endless number of chemicals -
including arene oxides, epoxides, chlorodinitrobenzene, bromosulfo-
phthalein (for testing liver function), and bilirubin; at least
six glutathione transferases have been isolated and characterized
so far. Epoxide hydrolase adds water to arene oxides or epoxides
to form dihydrodiols (17). This "water conjugation" occurs, for
example, during phenytoin metabolism.

C. Beyond Phase II Metabolism

Although dihydrodiols are, in general, readily excreted, it is
now clear (2) that diol-epoxides are formed and that these highly
reactive intermediates may be important in toxicity, tumorigenesis,
and birth defects (2,17,18). Diols can therefore undergo further
C-oxygenations (Table I).

Once a conjugate has been formed, the general belief has been
that the drug is excreted irreversibly. Glucuronides treated with
β-glucuronidase have been shown (19), however, to form reactive

intermediates capable of binding covalently with nucleic acids and proteins.   Of interest, β-glucuronidase activity is extremely high in kidney and bladder.   By a similar mechanism, one might postulate that glycosides may react with various glycosidases, resulting in reactive intermediates capable of binding covalently with nucleic acids and proteins.   Evidence in favor of this mechanism enhancing mutagenesis in vitro has just been reported (20).   Following conjugation with acetic acid, many drugs can be deacetylated (Table I) to form reactive intermediates (2).

D. Direct Chemical Reactions (Oxidation/Reduction)

Some chemicals by their inherent chemical properties possess a high redox potential.   o-Aminophenol, for example, is capable of oxidizing ferro- to ferri-hemoglobin.   Nitrates also cause methemoglobinemia, and methylene blue (because of its redox potential) reduces the ferri- back to ferro-hemoglobin.   Such one-electron chemical reactions may possibly play a role in liver disease and birth defects.

In sum, a few enzymes may exist in the body only to take care of foreign chemicals.   Many enzymes designed for normal-body substrates, however, apparently also handle many foreign drugs and chemicals.   The result is a combination and delicate balance of detoxication and toxification.

HOW DO THESE ENZYMES CONTRIBUTE TO LIVER DISEASE?

Table II includes a list of disorders reflecting increased sensitivity to drugs, increased resistance to drugs, disease exacerbated by enzyme-inducing drugs, and changes in the balance of detoxication/toxification.   The list is not intended to be complete and may raise more questions than it provides answers. Some of these disorders have been discussed recently in detail (52).

Hyperbilirubinemia may occur on the basis of a genetic defect such as the Crigler-Najjar syndrome or on the basis of immature development, as commonly occurs in the premature.   Induction of the glucuronidase which conjugates bilirubin in the newborn can be successful by phenobarbital treatment of the mother for several days prior to delivery (53);   the disadvantage of the sedative effect of the enzyme-inducing barbiturates is undoubtedly the reason why such therapy has not become routine for neonatal hyperbilirubinemia.

Among newborns and especially prematures with respiratory distress syndrome, the induction of lung surfactant by steroid administration to the mother (54) has become clinically applicable. In this case, the "maturing" developmental process is being speeded up by corticosteroids for reasons not known.   Although side effects from steroids might occur - including latent unknown changes in differentiation - so far the successful treatment of respiratory distress syndrome has outweighed the liabilities. Vaginal adenocarcinoma and other genito-urinary tract anomalies among offspring whose mothers had received diethylstilbestrol therapy during pregnancy (55,56) remains the most serious known example of a latent effect occurring as the result of treatment during pregnancy.

The toxicity in the premature infant by bilirubin and drugs such as chloramphenicol and theophylline (Table II) is a combination of deficiency in the liver of drug-metabolizing enzymes and decreased renal clearance due to immaturity of the kidney. The clinical implications of developmental differences in drug metabolism have also been discussed in several excellent reviews (26, 57-66).

A liver N-acetyltransferase requiring acetyl-CoA (21) is an excellent example of the double-edged sword nature of drug-metabolizing enzymes (Table II). About 50% of the United States population are slow acetylators (an autosomal recessive trait), and the other 50% are rapid acetylators. Because of decreased detoxication in slow acetylators, hydralazine or phenelzine may cause liver disease known as the lupus syndrome and isoniazid may cause toxic peripheral neuropathy (67). On the other hand, because of increased toxification among rapid acetylators, isoniazid can cause hepatic necrosis that is sometimes fatal. If one examines the phenotype of patients with idiopathic systemic lupus erythematosis (68), the preponderance of slow acetylators is statistically significant. Such a study suggests that unknown agents in the environment (possibly azo dyes in foods and cosmetics that require acetylation for detoxication), in combination with a predisposition in the patient for developing the autoimmune disorder, result in this life-shortening disease. A quart of cherry soda having 0.01% azo dye, for example, represents about 100 mg of azo dye.

There are dozens of important drug-drug interactions, competing at a receptor site, at the enzyme active-site, or in an unknown manner. The effect of erythromycin is to elevate theophylline levels, for example, thus prolonging theophylline action and/or toxicity (69). This combination of drugs is one of many that can lead to serious clinical consequences.

Many drugs induce their own metabolism (70,71). With chronic dosage, one might therefore observe an enhancement of detoxication - undoubtedly a form of drug dependence or addiction explainable by enzyme induction. On the other hand, one might observe increased toxicity, if the induced enzyme metabolizes an increased amount of drug to important reactive intermediates. Drug-induced sensitivities such as light-sensitive dermatitis, chemical hepatitis, and perhaps even auto-immune disease may fall into this latter category.

TABLE II

POSSIBLE ROLE OF DRUG METABOLISM IN PEDIATRIC LIVER DISEASE

	References
A. Disorders with increased sensitivity to drugs	
1. Enzyme deficiencies resulting in decreased detoxication	
a. "Lupus syndrome" in slow acetylators of hydralagine	21
b. Crigler-Najjar syndrome	22
c. Dicumarol sensitivity	23
d. Sulfite oxidase deficiency	24
2. Enzyme deficiencies resulting in decreased detoxication due to insufficient "development" at time of drug exposure	
a. Grey syndrome (chloramphenicol)	25
b. Neonatal hyperbilirubinemia	26
c. Theophylline toxicity magnified in premature	27
d. Other possible drug idiosyncracies	
3. Disorders of unknown etiology	
a. Malignant hyperthermia	28
b. Norethisterone-induced jaundice	29
c. Reye's syndrome	30
d. Other possible drug idiosyncracies	
B. Disorders resulting from increased resistance to drugs	
1. Possibility of defective receptor	
a. Coumarin resistance	31
b. Familial hypercholesterolemia	32
2. Defective absorption	
a. Juvenile pernicious anemia	33

It is common knowledge that many chemicals administered chronically influence the effects of a second chemical.   For example, cigarette smokers require several times more coffee to feel the same caffeine effect.   The bones of children on chronic anti-seizure medication may become osteoporotic (decreased calcium content due to changes in vitamin D metabolism caused by the drug).   The egg shells of birds exposed chronically to various insecticides may become brittle, presumably due to the interference by these environ-mental chemicals in normal sex steroid metabolism.   Conney's extensive review 14 years ago (70) listed more than 200 drugs, carcinogens, other environmental chemicals - and even normal body steroids - that induce their own metabolism and/or that of other substrates via P-450 induction.   Much research is still needed to understand the relationship between the induction of drug-metaboliz-ing enzymes and clinical disease.

HOW EARLY DURING EMBRYONIC DEVELOPMENT DO THESE ENZYMES EXIST?

There is a common misconception that P-450 and other drug-metabolizing enzymes do not exist developmentally in the liver of laboratory animals until just prior to birth.   AHH[1] activity, a P-450-mediated monooxygenase activity, however, is detectable in 5-week-old embryos of women who smoke cigarettes during pregnancy (72).   Just because an enzyme level is undetectable, by the experimental methods employed, does not necessarily indicate that the enzyme level is "zero".   The Avogadro number is 6.023×10^{23} molecules in one mole.   If the limits of an enzyme assay are 6×10^{-12} moles (6 picomoles), for example, there still might exist 10^{11} molecules of a reactive intermediate or a product that would escape detection by the usual experimental techniques.   The exist-ence of undetectable - but important - amounts of drug-metabolizing enzymes among critical tissues of the developing embryo is an important consideration in the cause of certain birth defects; this subject will be expanded upon in the latter portion of the next Section.

Figure 1 illustrates the developmental expression of three different P-450-mediated activities which hydroxylate testosterone in three different positions.   Totally empirical, the data demons-trate that each enzyme may have its own developmental curve of increasing, decreasing, or remaining the same, as a function of age in any tissue of the embryo, fetus, or neonate.   The possible role of detoxication and/or toxification in each tissue therefore depends upon developmental expression of appropriate drug-metabolizing enzymes and may be important in pediatric disease or teratogenesis.

The birth process itself initiates maturation of certain enzymes - such as tyrosine aminotransferase and P-450-mediated mono-oxygenase activites (74) - by means of a totally unknown mechanism. Such data therefore suggest that a 1-month-old premature will have

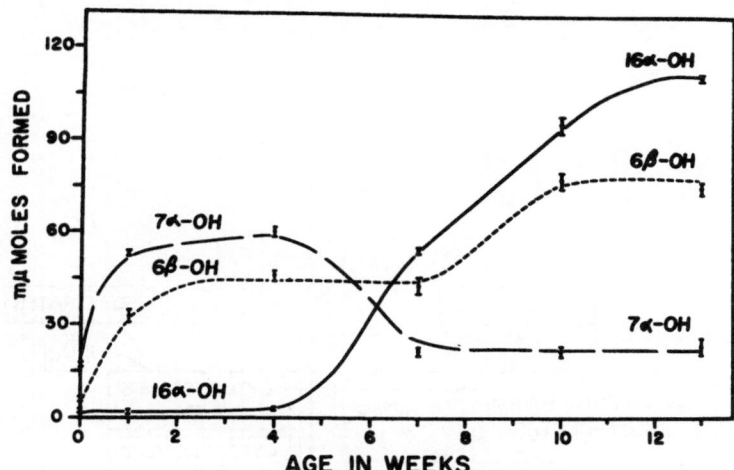

Fig. 1 *Ontogenic expression of three distinct testosterone*
hydroxylase activities in the liver of untreated male
rats (73). (Reproduced with permission from Academic
Press).

much higher levels of various liver enzymes, compared with a term
newborn, when both babies were conceived on the same day.

AN EXPERIMENTAL MODEL SYSTEM IN THE MOUSE: THE Ah COMPLEX

In summary of the previous Sections (Figure 2), P-450-mediated
monooxygenases represent a major class of Phase I drug metabolism.
Drugs may be pharmacologically active or toxic in their nonmetabolized forms, and metabolism will render them less active or innocuous
(detoxication).   Alternatively, drugs that are inert may be metabolized to pharmacologically active or toxic intermediates (toxification). Exploitation of a particular genetic difference in mice,
termed the Ah complex, represents an excellent example of the fine
balance between detoxication and toxification, and the possible role
of drug metabolism and developmental enzymology in pediatric disease
and teratogenesis.   The Ah complex is viewed as a combination of
regulatory, structural, and probably temporal genes which may or
may not be linked.

A. Initial Studies

The Ah complex (Figure 3) regulates the induction of numerous
drug-metabolizing enzymes in virtually all mammalian tissues.
"Responsiveness" to aromatic hydrocarbons was first characterized
in the C57BL/6 inbred mouse strain (B6, responsive, Ah[b]), and

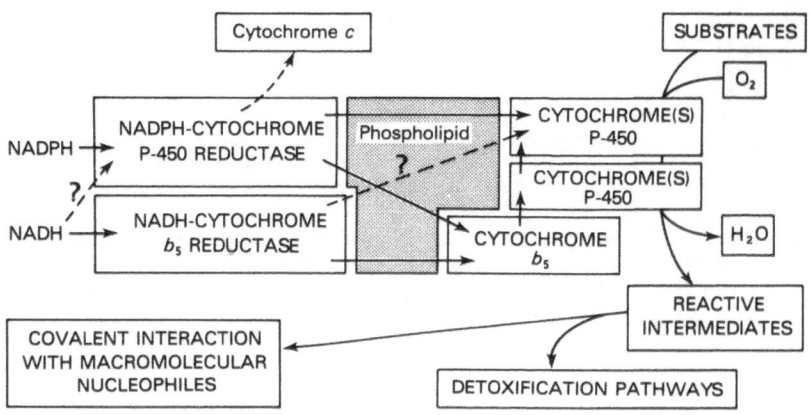

Fig. 2   *Scheme for the P-450-mediated membrane-bound multicomponent*
monooxygenases and the various possibly important pathways
for fat-soluble substrates (75).   For any given substrate,
the relative balance between detoxication and toxification
likely would differ among various tissues, strains and
species.   Age, genetic expression, nutrition, hormone
concentration, diurnal rhythm, pH, saturating versus non-
saturating conditions of the substrate, K_m and V_{max} for
each enzyme, subcellular compartmentalization of each
enzyme, efficiency of DNA repair, and the immunological
competence of the animal - may all be important factors
affecting this balance.   (Reproduced with permission from
National Institue of Environmental Health Sciences.)

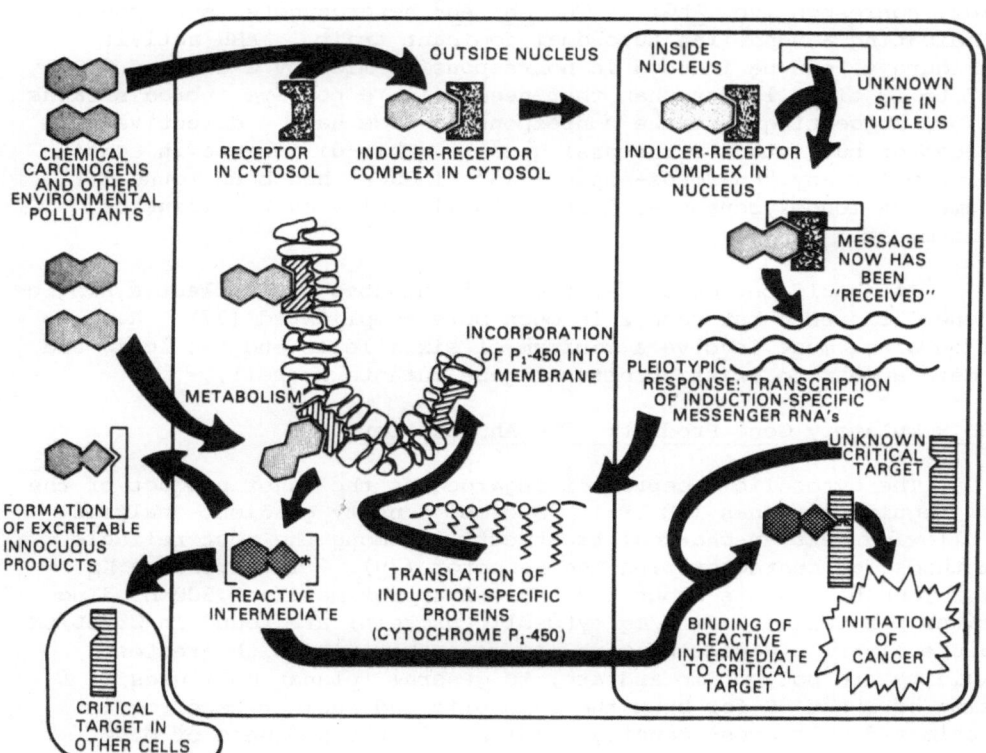

Fig. 3 Diagram of a cell and the hypothetical scheme by which a
        cytosolic receptor, a product of the regulatory Ah gene,
        binds to inducer (5).   The resultant "pleiotypic response"
        includes greater amounts of cytochrome P_1-450 (and numerous
        other forms of P-450 still being characterized), leading to
        enhanced steady-state levels of reactive intermediates,
        which are associated with genetic increases in birth defects,
        drug toxicity, or chemical carcinogenesis. Depending upon
        the half-life of the reactive intermediate, important
        covalent binding may occur in the same cell in which meta-
        bolism took place, or in some distant cell. Although the
        "unknown critical target" is illustrated here in the nucleus,
        there is presently no experimental evidence demonstrating
        unequivocally the subcellular location of a "critical
        target(s)" required for the initiation of drug toxicity or
        cancer or, for that matter, whether the "target" is nucleic
        acid or protein.
        (Reproduced with permission from Dr. W. Junk b.v.
        Publishers.)

DBA/2 was the first nonresponsive mutant inbred strain characterized
(D2, nonresponsive, Ah^d).   The Ah^b/Ah^d heterozygote is responsive,
indicating a Mendelian autosomal dominant trait.   AHH activity
(Figure 4) can be induced in nonresponsive mice by a dose of TCDD
12 to 18 times larger than that needed in responsive inbred strains
(76), suggesting that the nonresponsive mice have a defective Ah
receptor but intact structural genes.   This difference in sensitivity for any "Ah-locus-associated" inducer has been found for
numerous monooxygenase activities in virtually every tissue of
the mouse.

It should be noted that the Ah locus does not reflect a single-
gene difference but rather is much more complicated (77).   Regulation alone must involve a minimum of six alleles and two loci, and
there appear to exist structural gene mutants as well.

B. Regulatory Gene Product: The Ah Receptor

The cytosolic receptor is regarded as the major product of the
Ah regulatory genes (78,79).   Sucrose density gradient analysis,
following dextran-charcoal treatment, is among the most reliable
methods for characterizing the receptor (79).   The apparent K_d
for TCDD binding is about 0.7 nM, and approximately 5,500 binding
sites per cell (60 fmol/mg cytosolic protein) are found in C57BL/6N
mouse liver.   Representative inducers that bind with greatest
avidity are polycyclic and are, in general, planar molecules.   A
size of about 6S for both the cytosolic and nuclear receptor is
estimated on sucrose density gradients in the presence of 0.4M
KCl (79,80).   All nonresponsive strains so far examined have no
detectable Ah receptor.   It remains possible that these nonresponsive mice have as many as 100 "normal" receptor molecules per cell,
because this number is not detectable in our assay.   Alternatively,
these strains may have larger numbers of receptor molecules per
cell but with poorer affinity toward TCDD.

There is a good structure-activity relationship between
biologic response and the chemical's capacity to displace (^3H)TCDD
from the Ah receptor (Table III).   Dozens of endogenous compounds,
including glucocorticoids and sex steroids, do not displace the
radioligand from its receptor - even at 1,000-fold excess concentrations.   Presence of the Ah^b allele correlates well with the apparent
nuclear translocation of the inducer-receptor complex (Figure 5).
With the use of cells in culture, we have recently demonstrated the
apparent temperature dependence (Figure 6) of this nuclear translocation of the inducer-receptor complex.

C. Multiple Structural Gene Products: Induced Forms of P-450

The induction of at least two dozen monooxygenase activities
appears to be under the control of the same Ah receptor.   These

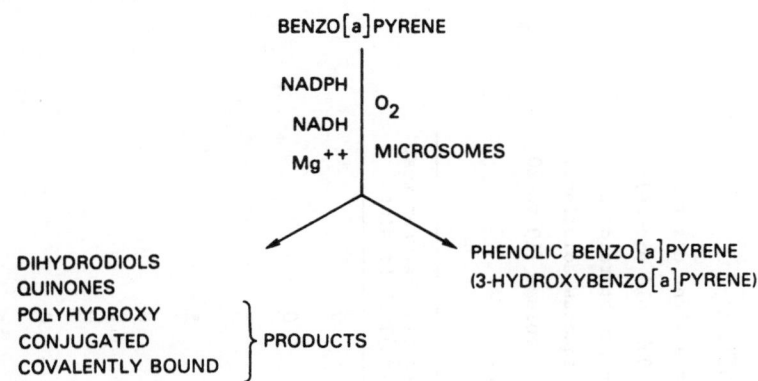

Fig. 4 Current concept of the "AHH" activity". The substrate
benzo(a)pyrene is oxygenated to arene oxides which
rearrange nonenzymically to phenols or are oxygenated
by direct oxygen insertion to phenolic derivatives.
The 3- and 9- phenols have the strongest fluorescence
in alkali. Other oxygenated derivatives of benzo(a)
pyrene, including dihydrodiols and quinones, are not
measured by this assay.

activities include: C-hydroxylations of benzo(a)pyrene and several
other polycyclic hydrocarbon carcinogens, biphenyl, zoxazolamine,
acetanilide, naphthalene, aflatoxin B_1, and theophylline; O-de-
ethylations of 7-ethoxycoumarin, phenacetin, and ethoxyresorufin;
O-demethylation of p-nitroanisole; N-demethylations of 3-methyl-
4-methylaminoazobenzene and theophylline; and as yet undetermined
oxygenations of β-naphthoflavone, α-naphthoflavone, ellipticine,
lindane, niridazole, caffeine, and theobromine (77). These substrates are highly variable in size and shape, and the question was
therefore raised long ago (82) whether these induced activities
represent the relatively nonspecific metabolism by a single form
of polycyclic aromatic-induced P-450 or the more specific metabolism
by a whole family of individual enzymes.

Most laboratories have been hesitant to accept the possibility
that there might exist more than a single form of "induced cytochrome P-448" in a MC-treated animal - in spite of clear evidence
to the contrary for more than 5 years (71). With the use of two
detergents and two column chromatographic steps, P-450 from MC-
treated B6 mouse liver microsomes was recently separated into 16
fractions, and many reconstituted monooxygenase activities were
studied (83). Practically every MC-induced activity was dissociable

TABLE III

SPECIFIC (^{3}H)TCDD BINDING TO B6 CYTOSOL RECEPTOR IN THE PRESENCE OF COMPOUNDS THAT HAVE
VARIED POTENCIES FOR HEPATIC CYTOCHROME P_1-450 INDUCTION

Specific binding was determined by sucrose density gradient analysis after dextran-
charcoal treatment using 10 mm [^{3}H]TCDD [79]. Each compound tested (1,000-fold excess)
was added to cytosol 15 min before [^{3}H]TCDD, using ethanol as a vehicle for steroids or
polycyclic aromatic hydrocarbons. Bilirubin and hematin were added as aqueous solutions,
and p-dioxane was used as a solvent for all dibenzo-p-dioxins. An equal volume (10 to 20
μl/ml) of the appropriate solvent was added to cytosol in control tubes.

Compound tested	Potency as an inducer of P_1-450[a]	Per cent competition between test compound and [^{3}H]TCDD binding
Bilirubin	0	0
Hematin	0	0
Cholesterol	0	5
Cholic acid methyl ester	0	5
Phenobarbital	0	0
Pregnenolone-16α-carbonitrile	0	0
Dexamethasone	0	0
β-Methasone	0	10
Progesterone	0	0

Estradiol-17β	0	5
Dihydrotestosterone	0	0
p,p'-DDT	+	65
α-Naphthoflavone	++	30
β-Naphthoflavone	+++	75
Benzo[a]pyrene	+++	100
3-Methylcholanthrene	+++	100
Benz[a]anthracene	+++	100
TCDD	++++	100
2,3-Dichlorodibenzo-p-dioxin	+	55
1,2,4-Trichlorodibenzo-p-dioxin	++	55
1,2,3,4,7,8-Hexachlorodibenzo-p-dioxin	+++	85
Octachlorodibenzo-p-dioxin	0	0

[a]Data taken from our laboratories [A.B. Okey, G.F. Kahl, T.M. Guenthner, N.M. Jensen, and D.W. Nebert, unpublished data] and from Refs. 78 and 81.

[Reproduced with permission from American Society of Biological Chemists].

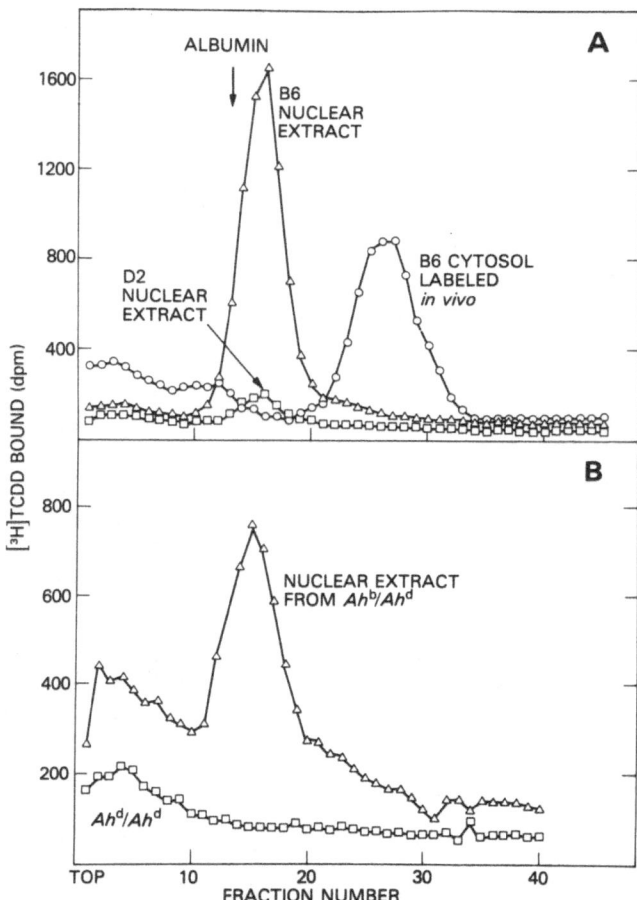

Fig. 5 Genetic differences in the nuclear binding of (^{3}H)TCDD
        in vivo (79). _A_, nuclear extracts from responsive B6 and
        nonresponsive D2 liver were treated with dextran-charcoal
        and then centrifuged on sucrose density gradients. B6
        cytosol (labeled in vivo) was treated with dextran-charcoal
        and centrifuged as usual on a gradient. _B_, hepatic nuclear
        extracts from a responsive _Ah^b/Ah^d_ and a nonresponsive
        _Ah^d/Ah^d_ individual from the B6D2F$_1$ x D2 backcross. The
        extracts following dextran-charcoal treatment were centri-
        fuged on gradients.   The B6 and D2 mouse had each received
        2 ug of (^{3}H)TCDD (approximately 0.3 umol/kg body weight)
        and were killed 2 h later.   The backcross animals had each
        received 5 ug of (^{3}H)TCDD (about 9.75 umol/kg body weight)
        and were killed 3 h later.
        (Reproduced with permission from American Society of
        Biological Chemists.)

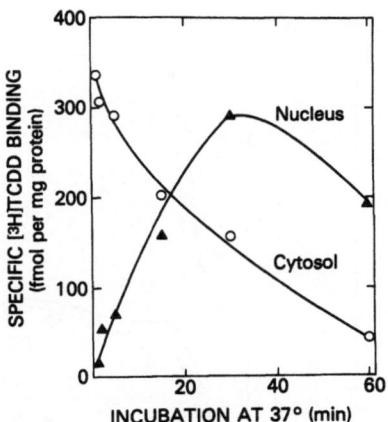

Fig. 6   Temperature-dependent cytosol-to-nucleus translocation of
         specific (³H)TCDD binding sites in intact Hepa-1 cells (80).
         Cells were incubated with 1 nM (³H)TCDD for 1 hour in
         culture at 4°C; the tissue culture dishes then were trans-
         ferred to the surface of a 37° water bath for the indicated
         intervals of time, after which the dishes were placed on
         ice before harvesting the cells. (Reproduced with permission
         from American Society of Biological Chemists.)

from every other MC-induced activity.   Hence, "biphenyl 2-hydroxy-
lase activity" is not synonymous with "P-448", nor is "AHH activity"
or "ethoxyresorufin O-deethylase activity" synonymous with "P-448".
By two-factor analysis of variance, it was concluded that the data
can be explained statistically by a lower limit of about 20 different
groups of P-450.   In fact, this estimate is probably very much on
the low side.

    P-450-mediated monooxygenase activities known not to be
associated with the Ah locus include the induced and control
metabolism of: aminopyrine, d-benzphetamine, phenytoin, hexobarbital
aniline, benzenesulfonanilide, chlorcyclizine, ethylmorphine, pento-
barbital, estrogen, and testosterone.   Also not associated with
the Ah locus is the induction of NADPH cytochrome c reductase and
NADPH-P-450 reductase, epoxide hydrolase, and glutathione transferase.

    Other inducible enzymes that are not monooxygenases but which
appear to be metabolically coordinated and associated with the Ah^b
allele include microsomal UDP glucuronosyltransferase and cytosolic
reduced NAD(P):menadione oxidoreductase (77).   Cytosolic ornithine
decarboxylase becomes markedly enhanced early during the induction
process and is also associated with the presence of the Ah receptor
(84).

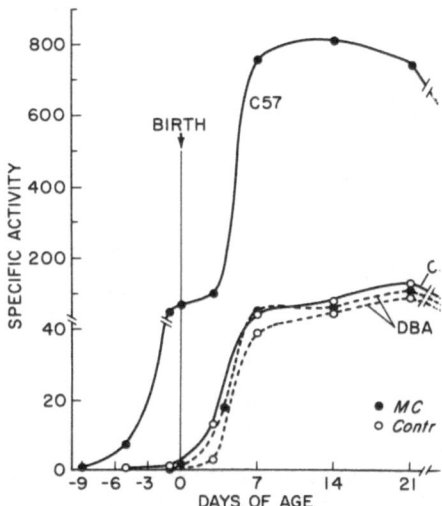

Fig. 7   *Hepatic levels of the basal AHH activity and of the enzyme
activity in response to MC treatment of C57BL/6N (C57) and
DBA/2 (DBA) mice, as a function of age (85). Each <u>closed</u>
<u>circle</u> represents the mean AHH specific activity from
individual livers of 6 to 15 mice 24 hours after the intra-
peritoneal administration of 80 mg of MC per kilogram of
body weight. Each <u>open</u> <u>circle</u> represents the mean enzyme
activity from individual livers of 5-12 mice 24 hours after
treatment with corn oil alone. The <u>closed</u> <u>circles</u> depicting
AHH activity before birth represent the average specific
activity found in 5 or more individual livers from a litter
of fetuses whose mother had received MC intraperitoneally
24 hours before. The <u>closed</u> <u>circles</u> on day zero indicate
the mean AHH activity from individual mice born within
24 hours after their mother had received the MC. Specific
activity on the ordinate represents units per milligram of
total liver homogenate protein. A unit of AHH activity is
defined as that amount of enzyme catalyzing in 1 min at 37°C
the formation of products the fluorescence of which is
equivalent to 1 pmole of 3-hydroxybenzo(a)pyrene recrystal-
lized standard. (Reproduced with permission from Macmillan
Journals Ltd.)*

D. Suggestive Evidence for Temporal Genes: Developmental Differences
   in P-450 Induction

     It was known years ago (85) that MC-induced AHH activity
develops in the embryonic mouse at least as early as there is
detectable liver tissue to assay (Figure 7). Developmental data

in rabbit (86), rat (87), and mouse (87,88) liver have demonstrated differences in the induction of different forms of P_1-450 by poly-cyclic aromatic compounds - in the apparent presence of sufficient Ah receptor.   The rabbit is most interesting, because the Ah receptor is detectable early in gestation and throughout adulthood (89) - yet one form of P-450 but not another is inducible in the newborn, and the reverse is true in the adult liver.   Some type of temporal control therefore must be operational, in order to explain these developmental findings.   In view of the apparent presence of adequate Ah receptor, most likely temporal control affects the expression of structural gene products (i.e. transcription of mRNA for these enzyme proteins) rather than regulatory gene products.   Further studies, however, are necessary in order to understand this interest-ing developmental system.

E.   Use of the Ah Complex in Teratology

Numerous drugs have been implicated in causing birth defects in man, although experimental proof is of course difficult.   Most notably, "drug-induced syndromes" have been described for phenytoin, warfarin, trimethadione, and alcoholism.   The clinical features of one syndrome often overlap with those of another; some investigators maintain, however, that clear-cut distinctions exist for each of these syndromes (90).   Of interest, only one child may be afflicted with such a syndrome when the mother has received the same medication for two or more pregnancies.   There have also been cases of one fraternal (dizygotic) twin being affected but not the other and cases of identical (monozygotic) twins both being affected with a drug-induced syndrome.   The situation clearly sounds like a complex combination of genetic and environmental factors.

In studies involving the association of the Ah locus with birth defects (18), the routine use of offspring from appropriate crosses between B6 and D2 parent strains is ideal, because expression of high AHH inducibility by MC most closely approximates a single-gene diff-erence, similar to the dominant red color trait in the garden pea. Children from the F_1 x D2 backcross and from the F_1 x F_1 intercross therefore exhibit 50% and 75%, respectively, the dominant phenotype. In other words, the Ah^b/Ah^b and Ah^b/Ah^d individuals have sufficient Ah receptor and therefore are highly inducible for AHH activity and associated P_1-450; the Ah^d/Ah^d individuals have no detectable Ah receptor and are poorly inducible for AHH.   One therefore can determine whether this single allelic difference is advantageous or disadvantageous with respect to risk for birth defects when all embryos receive the same dose of the same drug.   Hence, we can evaluate the possible importance of steady-state levels of reactive intermediates in the mechanism of chemically induced birth defects among individuals sharing the same uterus.   This genetic probe is a particularly powerful experimental model system in the research area of teratology, because the test compounds studied often cause

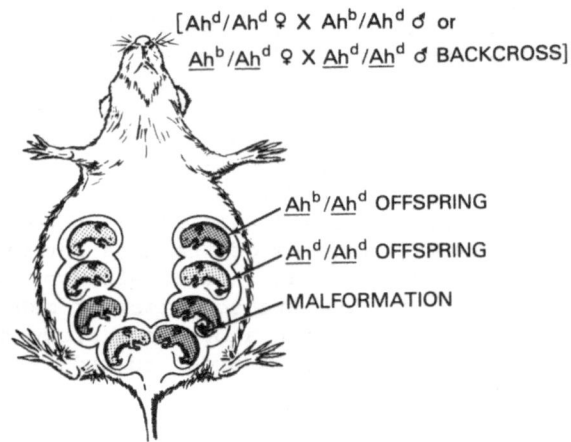

*Fig. 8 Diagrammatic illustration in which embryos of two distinct
genotypes reside in the uterus of a mother of either one
or the other genotype (91).   With either backcross, the
expected distribution of responsive-to-nonresponsive embryos
is one-to-one.   (Reproduced with permission from Springer-
Verlag.)*

undesirable side effects (e.g. sedation, diarrhea, malnutrition,
hormonal imbalance, etc) that are hard to distinguish from specific
teratogenic effects of the compounds.

   About 7 years ago, we wondered if we could demonstrate the
importance of a genetic component with the use of the Ah locus and
inbred strains of mice.   For example, could the genetic predisposition of a particular embryo be more important than maternal influences
in causing or preventing a birth defect?

   Benzopyrene (BP) was chosen because it is known to be a good
inducer of AHH activity and associated P_1-450, and it is known to
be metabolized by P_1-450 to toxic intermediates.   By determining
the genotype of offspring from the F_1 x recessive parent backcross
(Figure 8), we can prove whether the Ah^b allele is correlated
specifically with dysmorphogenesis.   There are two ways to generate
progeny from the backcross: one is with a nonresponsive Ah^d/Ah^d
mother;   the other is with a responsive Ah^b/Ah^d mother.   When BP
is given to the nonresponsive mother, Ah^b/Ah^d embryos exhibit more
birth defects, stillborns, and resorptions and decreased weight
gain than Ah^d/Ah^d embryos in the same uterus.   When BP is given to
the responsive Ah^b/Ah^d mother, on the other hand, genetic differences among embryos in the uterus are cancelled, presumably because
of the overwhelming contribution of BP metabolites from maternal

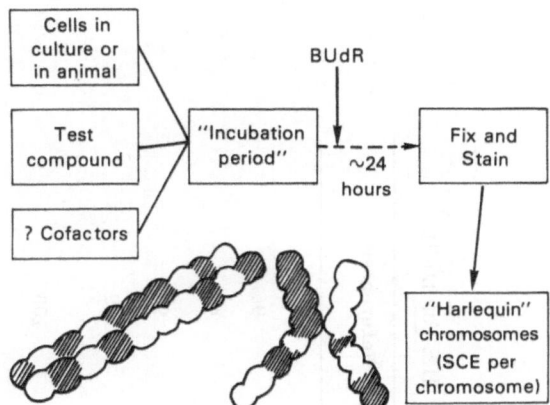

*Fig. 9   Schematic diagram of the principles of sister chromatid
         exchange (92).   BUdR, 5-bromodeoxyuridine.   Cells in
         culture can be exposed to a test compound, with or without
         cofactors.   Following exposure of the animal to a test
         compound, cells (e.g. lymphocytes) can also be removed from
         the animal and cultured.   (Reproduced with permission from
         Raven Press.)*

tissues.   Of particular interest in this study (18) is the fact
that the mother and father both must be of a particular genotype
before differences in teratogenesis among embryos (due to their
genotype) will be expressed.   These data are offered as an example
in attempting to explain clinically why only one child may be
afflicted with an apparent "drug-induced syndrome" although the
mother has taken the same dose of a particular drug during more
than one pregnancy.

F.   Evidence for Drug-Metabolizing Capability in Embryo Even
     Before Implantation

Most recently mouse embryos have been cultured at day $3\frac{1}{2}$, $5\frac{1}{2}$,
$7\frac{1}{2}$, and $8\frac{1}{2}$ in medium containing BP and supplemented with 5-bromo-
deoxyuridine to allow detection of sister chromatid exchanges
(Figure 9).   This technique (93,94) was chosen because of its
exquisite sensitivity in detecting toxicity, in this case presumably
caused by BP metabolites formed by the induced AHH activity.   A
strong correlation was seen between increased sister chromatid
exchanges and the Ah^b allele among five inbred strains, one outbred
strain, and two recombinant inbred strains (95).   These data suggest
that Ah-responsive mouse embryos (late pre-implantation and early
post-implantation stages) possess the subcellular processes necessary
for induction of enzymes that metabolize BP to its chemically
teratogenic/toxic form(s).   Both the Ah regulatory gene product

TABLE IV

HUMAN DISORDERS THAT APPEAR TO BE ASSOCIATED WITH THE Ah LOCUS[a]

Disorder	Association with high or low AHH inducibility	References
Malignancy		
Bronchogenic carcinoma	High[b]	96
Bronchogenic carcinoma	No association found	97
Laryngeal carcinoma	High[c]	98
Cancer of oral cavity	High[c]	99
Cancer of renal pelvis or ureter	No association found	100
Cancer of urinary bladder	No association found	101
Acute leukemia of childhood	Low[b]	102
Toxicity		
Zoxazolamine-induced fatal hepatic necrosis	Unknown[d]	103

Earlier onset of menopause among cigarette smokers	Unknown[d]	104
Infertility among cigarette smokers	Unknown[d]	105
Acetaminophen-induced diffuse bilateral cataracts	Unknown[d]	106

[a]Reviewed in detail in Ref. 75. [Reproduced with permission from National Institute of Environmental Health Sciences].

[b]Consistent with genetic data from inbred strains of mice [77].

[c]Studies of these disorders in mice have not been specifically carried out, but the human data are consistent with what is known [107] about environmental carcinogens and their effect on local and distant tissue sites in genetically Ah-responsive and Ah-nonresponsive mice.

[d]Genetically Ah-responsive mice are at increased risk for these disorders [77]. In retrospect (or in studies to be designed in the future), it would have been (or would be) of interest to know the Ah phenotype of afflicted clinical patients.

(in other words, the cytosolic receptor) and the structural gene product (inducible P_1-450) therefore appear to be functional from an early embryonic age.

We thus believe that the genetic predisposition for the metabolism of a drug or other chemical <u>in a given tissue of an individual embryo or fetus</u> rather than in tissues of the mother can be important in the etiology of certain birth defects.   Such an hypothesis could explain why a birth defect is found in one child, for example, when the mother had received the same dose of the same drug during each of two or more pregnancies.   Other chemicals and drugs - known or suspected to interact with cytochrome(s) P_1 450 - are being planned for study in this experimental model system.

EVIDENCE FOR THE <u>Ah</u> COMPLEX IN THE HUMAN

With the use of 20 to 40 cc of drawn blood, peripheral lymphocytes have been cultured in the presence of mitogens and an inducer of AHH activity such as MC, in order to assess the human <u>Ah</u> phenotype. In spite of the shortcomings with this assay method (reviewed in ref. 51), a growing list of clinical disorders (Table IV) appears to be associated with the human <u>Ah</u> locus.

There clearly exists sufficient evidence that heritable variation of AHH inducibility occurs in man.   Experimental difficulties, however, make it impossible at this time to be certain of whether AHH induction is controlled by a single genetic locus or by two or more loci (i.e. polygenic).   Until one can increase the range of fold inducibility of AHH activity and/or decrease the magnitude of day-to-day variability of "control" AHH activity, however, AHH inducibility in cultured mitogen-activated lymphocytes or any other similar test system cannot be used as a promising biochemical marker for predicting who is at risk for aplastic anemia, leukemia, bronchogenic carcinoma, or other various types of environmentally-caused toxicity or malignancy.   We believe that a high ratio of P_1-450 to other forms of P-450 exists in many, if not all, extrahepatic tissues <u>in vivo</u>, just as appears to be the case in cultured lymphocytes, monocytes, pulmonary macrophages, and even skin fibroblasts.   An alternative assay for assessing the human <u>Ah</u> locus phenotype (such as a receptor assay, a radioimmunoassay for induced P_1-450, or a (^{32}P)cDNA probe for the P_1-450 gene) might be more successful than the existing commonly performed AHH inducibility assay.

SUMMARY

Cytochrome P-450-mediated monooxygenases represent a disproportionate amount of Phase I drug metabolism.   These enzymes metabolize a vast variety of drugs, environmental chemicals, and endogenous compounds such as: barbiturates, acetaminophen, warfarin, benzo(a) pyrene, polychlorinated and polybrominated biphenyl, pesticides,

aromatic amines, naturally-occurring and synthetic steroids, fungal
toxins and antibiotics. During the course of metabolism, sometimes
these substrates are detoxified and other times these chemicals are
toxified, i.e. converted into "reactive intermediates" which may be
toxic, teratogenic, mutagenic, or carcinogenic before they can be
conjugated and excreted.

In experimental animals and in the human, levels of cytochrome
P-450 generally are low in the embryo but increase rapidly in the
neonatal period.   The human fetal liver has considerable drug-
metabolizing capability from the first trimester.   Mouse embryos
appear to have drug-metabolizing capability even before implantation.

Many forms of cytochrome P-450 probably exist.   One of these,
P_1-450 (aryl hydrocarbon hydroxylase, "AHH") is highly induced by
exposure of "genetically responsive" mice to polycyclic aromatic
compounds (such as 3-methylcholanthrene, benzo(a)pyrene, polychlorinated biphenyls, and 2,3,7,8-tetrachlorodibenzo-p-dioxin).
P_1-450 has very high metabolic activity towards benzo(a)pyrene and
is strongly implicated in toxic responses to drugs and environmental
chemicals.   Induction of P_1-450 is under the control of the Ah
locus, a complicated group of genes regulating at least two dozen
related monooxygenase activities.

Recently we have characterized a receptor which binds inducing
chemicals in the cytoplasm and then translocates into the nucleus
where the inducer-receptor complex stimulates production of specific
RNA for P_1-450 synthesis.   Genetically "nonresponsive" mice appear
to have a defective receptor which fails to bind inducing chemicals
properly.

Evidence exists that the human population also exhibits heritable
variation in cytochrome P_1-450 inducibility.   This genetic polymorphism may have important implications for understanding individual
variations in susceptibility to toxicity from drugs and environmental
chemicals.

ACKNOWLEDGEMENT

The expert secretarial assistance of Ms. Ingrid E. Jordan is
greatly appreciated.

FOOTNOTE

Abbreviations used include: AHH, aryl hydrocarbon (benzo(a)
pyrene) hydroxylase; B6, the inbred C57BL/6N mouse strain; D2, the
inbred DBA/2N mouse strain; TCDD, 2,3,7,8-tetrachlorodibenzo-p-dioxin;
MC, 3-methylcholanthrene; BP, benzo(a)pyrene; and P_1-450, all forms
of P-450 induced by polycyclic aromatic compounds and under control by
the Ah^b allele. Recent evidence indicates that probably many more
than two such induced forms occur.

REFERENCES

1. GOLDSTEIN A, ARONOW L, KALMAN SM (eds): Principles of Drug
    Action, 2nd Edition. John Wiley & Sons, N.Y. 1974. 854 pages.

2. MILLER JA, MILLER EC: Perspectives on the metabolism of chemical
    carcinogens. In Environmental Carcinogenesis: Occurrence,
    Risk Evaluation and Mechanism. Netherlands Cancer Society,
    Amsterdam, Netherlands. 1979. pp. 25-50.

3. OMURA T, SATO R: The carbon monoxide-binding pigment of liver
    microsomes. I. Evidence for its hemoprotein nature.
    J Biol Chem 239: 2370-2378, 1964.

4. SATO R, OMURA T (eds): Cytochrome P-450. Academic Press, N.Y.
    1978. 233 pages.

5. NEBERT DW: Multiple forms of inducible drug-metabolizing
    enzymes. A reasonable mechanism by which any organism can
    cope with adversity. Mol Cell Biochem 27: 27-46, 1979.

6. MASON HS, FOWLKS WL, PETERSON E: Oxygen transfer and electron
    transport by the phenolase complex. J Amer Chem Soc 77:
    2914-2915, 1955.

7. HAYAISHI O, KATAGIRI M, ROTHBERG S: Mechanism of the pyro-
    catechase reaction. J Amer Chem Soc 77: 5450-5451, 1955.

8. SUGIURA M, YAMAZOE Y, KAMATAKI T, KATO R: Reduction of epoxy
    derivatives of benzo(a)pyrene by microsomal cytochrome
    P-450. Cancer Res 40: 2910-2914, 1980.

9. YAMAZOE Y, ISHII K, YAMAGUCHI N, KAMATAKI T, KATO R: Reduction
    of N-hydroxy-2-acetylaminofluorene by liver microsomes.
    Bochem Pharmacol 29: 2183-2188, 1980.

10. FREY WA, VALLEE BL: Digitalis metabolism and human liver
    alcohol dehydrogenase. Proc Nat Acad Sci USA 77: 924-
    927, 1980.

11. PATEL JM, WOOD JC, LEIBMAN KC: The biotransformation of allyl
    alcohol and acrolein in rat liver and lung preparations.
    Drug Metab Disp 8: 305-308, 1980.

12. PATEL J, HARPER C, DREW RT: The biotransformation of p-xylene
    to a toxic aldehyde. Drug Metab Disp 6: 368-374, 1978.

13. LIND C, VADI H, ERNSTER L: Metabolism of benzo(a)pyrene-3,6-
    quinone and 3-hydroxybenzo(a)pyrene in liver microsomes
    from 3-methylcholanthrene-treated rats. A possible role

of DT-diaphorase in the formation of glucuronyl conjugates. Arch Biochem Biophys 190: 97-108, 1978.

14. CHENGELIS CP, NEAL RA: Studies of carbonyl sulfide toxicity: Metabolism by carbonic anhydrase. Toxicol Appl Pharmacol 55: 198-202, 1980.

15. DUTTON GJ, WISHART G, CAMPBELL MT: Perinatal development of glucuronidation. In Advances in Pharmacology and Therapeutics: Drug-action Modification, Comparative Pharmacology, volume 8. E. Oliver (ed.) Pergamon Press, Ltd., Oxford, England. 1978. pp. 113-122.

16. JAKOBY WB: The glutathione S-transferases: a group of multifunctional detoxification proteins. In Advances in Enzymology and Related Areas of Molecular Biology. A. Meister (ed). John Wiley & Sons, Inc., N.Y. 1978. pp. 383-414.

17. OESCH F: Epoxide hydratase. In Progress in Drug Metabolism, volume 3. J.W. Bridges, L.F. Chasseaud (eds). John Wiley & Sons, N.Y. 1979. pp. 253-301.

18. SHUM S, JENSEN NM, NEBERT DW: The Ah locus: In utero toxicity and teratogenesis associated with genetic differences in benzo(a)pyrene metabolism. Teratology 20: 365-376, 1979.

19. KINOSHITA N, GELBOIN HV: β-Glucuronidase catalyzed hydrolysis of benzo(a)pyrene-3-glucuronide and binding to DNA. Science 199: 307-309, 1978.

20. TAMURA G, GOLD C, FERRO-LUZZI A, AMES BN: Fecalase: a model for activation of dietary glycosides to mutagens by intestinal flora. Proc Nat Acad Sci USA 77: 4961-4965, 1980.

21. EVANS DAP, WHITE TA: Human acetylation polymorphism. J Lab Clin Med 63: 394-403, 1964.

22. CRIGLER JF, NAJJAR VA: Congenital familial non-hemolytic jaundice with kernicterus. Pediatrics 10: 169-180, 1952.

23. SOLOMON HM: Variations in metabolism of coumarin anticoagulant drugs. Ann NY Acad Sci 151: 932-935, 1968.

24. SHIH VE, ABROMS IF, JOHNSON JL, CARNEY M, MANDELL R, ROBB RM, CLOHERTY JP, RAJAGOPALAN KV: Sulfite oxidase deficiency. Biochemical and clinical investigations of a hereditary metabolic disorder in sulfur metabolism. N Eng J Med 297: 1022-1028, 1977.

25. WEISS CF, GLAZKO AJ, WESTON JK: Chloramphenicol in the newborn
    infant. A physiologic explanation of its toxicity when
    given in excessive doses. N Eng J Med 262:   787-794, 1960.

26. KLINGER W: Development of drug metabolizing enzymes. In
    Drug Disposition During Development. P.L. Morselli (ed).
    Spectrum Publications, Inc., N.Y. 1977. pp. 71-88.

27. ARANDA JV, SITAR DS, PARSONS WD, LOUGHNAN PM, NEIMS AH:
    Pharmacokinetic aspects of theophylline in premature
    newborns. N Eng J Med 295: 413-416, 1976.

28. KALOW W, BRITT BA, RICHTER A: The caffeine test of isolated
    human muscle in relation to malignant hyperthermia.
    Can Anaesth Soc J 24: 678-694, 1977.

29. SOMAYAJI BN, PATON A, PRICE JH, HARRIS AW, FLEWETT TH: Nor-
    ethisterone jaundice in two sisters. Brit Med J 2:   281-283,
    1968.

30. MULLEN PW: Immunopharmacological considerations in Reye's
    syndrome: A possible xenobiotic initiated disorder?
    Biochem Pharmacol 27: 145-149, 1978.

31. O'REILLY RA: The second reported kindred with hereditary
    resistance to oral anticoagulant drugs. N Eng J Med 282:
    1448-1451, 1970.

32. BROWN MS, GOLDSTEIN JL: Receptor-mediated endocytosis:
    Insights from the lipoprotein receptor system. Proc Nat
    Acad Sci USA 76: 3330-3337, 1979.

33. McINTYRE OR, SULLIVAN LW, JEFFRIES GH, SILVER RH: Pernicious
    anemia in childhood. N Eng J Med 272: 981-986, 1965.

34. MARVER HS, SCHMID R: The porphyrias. In The Metabolic Basis
    of Inherited Disease: J.B. Stanbury, J.B. Wyngaarden,
    D.S. Frederickson (eds). McGraw-Hill. N.Y. 1972. pp. 1087-
    1140.

35. WANG YM, VAN EYS J: The enzymatic defect in essential pentos-
    uria. N Eng M Med 282: 892-896, 1970.

36. DE LUCA HF: Vitamin D metabolism and function. In Monographs
    on Endocrinology. F. Gross, A. Labhart, T. Mann, J. Zander
    (eds). Springer-Verlag, Berlin & N.Y. 1979. pp. 1-78.

37. BOSS GR, SEEGMILLER JE: Hyperuricemia and gout. Classification,
    complications and management. N Eng J Med 300: 1459-1468,
    1979.

38. LEE PA, PLOTNICK LP, KOWARSKI AA, MIGEON CJ: In Congenital
     Adrenal Hyperplasia. University Park Press, Baltimore, Md.
     1977.

39. BROWN BR, SIPES IG: Biotransformation and hepatotoxicity of
     halothane. Biochem Pharmacol 26: 2091-2094, 1977.

40. YUNIS AA: Chloramphenicol-induced bone marrow suppression.
     Sem Hematol 10: 225-234, 1973.

41. MITCHELL JR, JOLLOW DJ: Biochemical basis for drug-induced
     hepatotoxicity. Isr J Med Sci 10: 312-318, 1974.

42. BOIVIN P, GALAND C, BERNARD JF: Deficiencies in GSH biosynthesis.
     In Glutathione. L. Flohe, H.C. Benöhr, H. Sies, H.D. Waller,
     A. Wendel (eds). Academic Press, N.Y. 1974. pp. 146-157.

43. SPIELBERG SP, GARRICK MD, CORASH LM, BUTLER JD, TIETZE F,
     ROGERS LV, SCHULMAN JD: Biochemical heterogeneity in
     glutathione synthetase deficiency. J Clin Invest 61:
     1417-1420, 1978.

44. LÖHR GW, BLUME KG, RÜDIGER HW, ARNOLD H: Genetic variability
     in the enzymatic reduction of oxidized glutathione. In
     Glutathione. L. Flohe, H.C. Benöhr, H. Sies, H.D. Waller,
     A. Waller, A. Wendel (eds). Academic Press, N.Y. 1974.
     pp. 165-173.

45. NECHELES TF: The clinical spectrum of glutathione-peroxidase
     deficiency. In Glutathione. F. Flohe, H.C. Benöhr, H. Sies,
     H.D. Waller, A. Wendel (eds). Academic Press, N.Y. 1974.
     pp. 173-180.

46. BEUTLER, E: Disorders due to enzyme defects in the red blood
     cell. Adv Metab Disord 6: 131-160, 1972.

47. SCOTT EM: The relation of diaphorase of human erythrocytes to
     inheritance of methemoglobinemia. J Clin Invest 39:
     1176-1179, 1960.

48. HUEHNS ER, SHOOTER EM: Human haemoglobins. J Med Genet 2:
     48-90, 1965.

49. COMINGS DE: Hemoglobinopathies producing cyanosis. In
     Hematology. W.J. Williams, E. Beutler, A.J. Erslev, R.W.
     Rundles (eds). McGraw-Hill, N.Y. 1972. pp. 434-440.

50. SHAHIDI HT: Acetophenetidin-induced methemoglobinemia.
     Ann NY Acad Sci 151: 822-832, 1968.

51. NEBERT DW: The Ah locus. A gene with possible importance in
       cancer predictability. Arch Toxicol Suppl 3: 195-207, 1980.

52. NEBERT DW: Human genetic variation in the enzymes of detoxica-
       tion. In Enzymatic Basis of Detoxication, volume 1.
       W.B. Jakoby (ed). Academic Press, N.Y. 1980. pp. 25-68.

53. MAURER HM, WOLFF JA, FINSTER M, POPPERS PJ, PANTUCK E,
       KUNTZMAN R, CONNEY AH: Reduction in concentration of total
       serum bilirubin in offspring of women treated with pheno-
       barbitone during pregnancy. Lancet ii: 122-124, 1968.

54. LIGGINS GC: Premature delivery of foetal lambs infused with
       glucocorticosteroids. J Endocrinol 45: 515-522, 1969.

55. HERBST AL, ULFELDER H, POSKANZER DC: Adenocarcinoma of the
       vagina association of maternal stilbestrol therapy with
       tumor appearance in young women. N Eng J Med 284: 878-881,
       1971.

56. GREENWALD P, BARLOW JJ, NASCA PC, BURNETT WS: Vaginal cancer
       after maternal treatment with synthetic estrogens. N Eng
       J Med 285: 390-393, 1971.

57. DONE AK: Developmental pharmacology. Clin Pharmacol Ther 5:
       432-479, 1964.

58. SERENI F, MANDELLI M, PRINCIPI N, TOGNONI G, PARDI G, MORSELLI
       PL: Induction of drug metabolizing enzyme activities in
       the human fetus and in the newborn infant. Enzyme 15:
       318-329, 1973.

59. YAFFE SJ, JUCHAU MR: Perinatal pharmacology. Ann Rev Pharmacol
       14: 219-238, 1974.

60. GILLETTE JR, STRIPP B: Pre- and postnatal capacity for drug
       metabolite production. Fed Proc 34: 172-178, 1975.

61. MIRKIN BL (ed): Perinatal Pharmacology and Therapeutics.
       Academic Press, N.Y. 1976.

62. NEIMS AH, WARNER M, LOUGHNAN PM, ARANDA JV: Developmental
       aspects of the hepatic cytochrome P450 monooxygenase system.
       Ann Rev Pharmacol 16: 427-445, 1976.

63. PELKONEN O: Transplacental transfer of foreign compounds and
       their metabolism by the foetus. In Progress in Drug Metab-
       olism, volume 2. J.W. Bridges, L.F. Chasseaud (eds).
       John Wiley & Sons, London. 1977. pp 119-161.

64. HUNTER J, CHASSEAUD LF: Clinical aspects of microsomal enzyme
     induction. In Progress in Drug Metabolism, volume 1.
     J.W. Bridges, L.F. Chasseaud (eds). John Wiley & Sons,
     London. 1977. pp. 129-191.

65. NEUBERT D, BARRACH H-J: Special aspects of pre- and perinatal
     toxicology and pharmacology. In Advances in Pharmacology
     and Therapeutics: Drug-action Modification, Comparative
     Pharmacology, volume 8. E. Oliver (ed). Pergamon Press
     Ltd, Oxford, England. 1978. pp. 71-79.

66. PELKONEN O, KÄRKI NT, KORHONEN P, KOIVISTO M, TUIMALA R,
     KAUPPILA A: Inducibility of monooxygenase activities in
     the human fetus and placenta. In Advances in Pharmacology
     and Therapeutics: Drug-action Modification, Comparative
     Pharmacology, volume 8. E. Oliver (ed). Pergamon Press
     Ltd., Oxford, England. 1978. pp. 101-122

67. HUGHES HB, BIEHL JP, JONES AP, SCHMIDT LH: Metabolism of
     isoniazid in man as related to the occurrence of peripheral
     neuritis. Am Rev Tuberc 70: 266-273, 1954.

68. REIDENBERG MM, DRAYER DE, ROBBIN WC: Polymorphic drug acetyla-
     tion and systemic lupus erythematosus. In Advances in
     Pharmacology and Therapeutics: Clinical Pharmacology,
     volume 6. P. Duchene-Marullaz (ed). Pergamon Press,
     Oxford, England. 1979. pp. 51-56.

69. CUMMINS LH, KOZAK PP Jr, GILLMAN SA: Theophylline determina-
     tions. Ann Allergy 37: 450-451, 1976.

70. CONNEY AH: Pharmacological implications of microsomal enzyme
     induction. Pharmacol Rev 19: 317-366, 1967.

71. NEBERT DW, EISEN HJ, NEGISHI M, LANG MA, HJELMELAND LM, OKEY AB:
     Genetic mechanisms controlling the induction of polysubstrate
     monooxygenase (P-450) activities. Ann Rev Pharmacol
     Toxicol: in press, 1981.

72. PELKONEN O, JOUPPILA P, KÄRKI NT: Effect of maternal cigarette
     smoking on 3,4-benzpyrene and N-methylaniline metabolism
     in human fetal liver and placenta. Toxicol Appl Pharmacol
     23: 399-407, 1972.

73. CONNEY AH, LEVIN W, JACOBSON M, KUNTZMAN R: Specificity in
     the regulation of the 6β-, 7α- and 16α-hydroxylation of
     testosterone by rat liver microsomes. In Microsomes and
     Drug Oxidations. J.R. Gillette, A.H. Conney, G.J. Cosmides,
     R.W. Estabrook, J.R. Fouts, G.J. Mannering (eds). Academic
     Press, N.Y. 1969. pp. 279-302.

74. MANCHESTER DK, NEIMS AH: The effect of birth on the maturation
     of hepatic cytochrome(s) P-450 mono-oxygenase and tyrosine
     aminotransferase activities in the guinea pig. Biol Neonate
     31: 213-218, 1977.

75. NEBERT DW: Genetic differences in susceptibility to chemically
     induced myelotoxicity and leukemia. Env Health Perspect:
     in press, 1980.

76. POLAND AP, GLOVER E, ROBINSON JR, NEBERT DW: Genetic expression
     of aryl hydrocarbon hydroxylase activity. Induction of
     monooxygenase activities and cytochrome P_1-450 formation
     by 2,3,7,8-tetrachlorodibenzo-p-dioxin in mice genetically
     "nonresponsive" to other aromatic hydrocarbons. J Biol
     Chem 249: 5599-5606, 1974.

77. NEBERT DW, JENSEN NM: The Ah locus: Genetic regulation of the
     metabolism of carcinogens, drugs, and other environmental
     chemicals by cytochrome P-450-mediated monooxygenases.
     In CRC Critical Reviews in Biochemistry, volume 6.
     G.D. Fasman (ed). CRC Press, Inc., Cleveland, Ohio. 1979.
     pp. 401-437.

78. POLAND AP, GLOVER E, KENDE AS: Stereospecific, high affinity
     binding of 2,3,7,8-tetrachlorodibenzo-p-dioxin by hepatic
     cytosol. Evidence that the binding species is the receptor
     for the induction of aryl hydrocarbon hydroxylase.
     J Biol Chem 251: 4936-4946, 1976.

79. OKEY AB, BONDY GP, MASON ME, KAHL GF, EISEN HJ, GUENTHNER TM,
     NEBERT DW: Regulatory gene product of the Ah locus.
     Characterization of the cytosolic inducer-receptor complex
     and evidence for its nuclear translocation. J Biol Chem
     254: 11636-11648, 1979.

80. OKEY AB, BONDY GP, MASON ME, NEBERT DW, FORSTER-GIBSON CJ,
     MUNCAN J, DUFRESNE MJ: Temperature-dependent cytosol-to-
     nucleus translocation of the Ah receptor for 2,3,7,8-tetra-
     chlorodibenzo-p-dioxin in continuous cell culture lines.
     J Biol Chem: in press, 1980.

81. POLAND A, GLOVER E: Chlorinated dibenzo-p-dioxins: Potent
     inducers of δ-aminolevulinic acid synthetase and aryl
     hydrocarbon hydroxylase. II. A study of the structure-
     activity relationship. Mol Pharmacol 9: 736-747, 1973.

82. NEBERT DW, CONSIDINE N, OWENS IS: Genetic expression of aryl
     hydrocarbon hydroxylase induction. VI. Control of other
     aromatic hydrocarbon-inducible mono-oxygenase activities
     at or near the same genetic locus. Arch Biochem Biophys
     148-159, 1973.

83. LANG MA, NEBERT DW: Structural gene products of the Ah complex.
     Evidence for multiple forms of liver microsomal cytochrome
     P-450 from 3-methylcholanthrene-treated mice. J Biol Chem:
     in press, 1981.

84. NEBERT DW, JENSEN NM, PERRY JW, OKA T: Association between
     ornithine decarboxylase induction and the Ah locus in mice
     treated with polycyclic aromatic compounds. J Biol Chem
     255: 6836-6842, 1980.

85. NEBERT DW, GOUJON FM, GIELEN JE: Aryl hydrocarbon hydroxylase
     induction by polycyclic hydrocarbons: Simple autosomal
     dominant trait in the mouse. Nature New Biol (London) 236:
     107-110, 1972.

86. ATLAS SA, BOOBIS AR, FELTON JS, THORGEIRSSON SS, NEBERT DW:
     Ontogenetic expression of polycyclic aromatic compound-
     inducible monooxygenase activities and forms of cytochrome
     P-450 in the rabbit. Evidence for temporal control and
     organ specificity of two genetic regulatory sytems.
     J Biol Chem 252: 4712-4721, 1977.

87. GUENTHNER TM, NEBERT DW: Evidence in rat and mouse liver for
     temporal control of two forms of cytochrome P-450 inducible
     by 2,3,7,8-tetrachlorodibenzo-p-dioxin. Eur J Biochem 91:
     449-456, 1978.

88. NEGISHI M, NEBERT DW: Structural gene products of the Ah locus.
     Genetic and immunochemical evidence for two forms of mouse
     liver cytochrome P-450 induced by 3-methylcholanthrene.
     J Biol Chem 254: 11015-11023, 1979.

89. KAHL GF, FRIEDERICI D, BIGELOW SW, OKEY AB, NEBERT DW: Onto-
     genetic expression of regulatory and structural gene
     products associated with the Ah locus. Comparison of rat,
     mouse, rabbit, and Sigmoden hispedis. Devel Pharmacol
     Ther 1: 137-162, 1980.

90. SMITH DW (ed): Recognizable Patterns of Human Malformation.
     W.B. Saunders Company, Philadelphia, Pa. 1976. 504 pages.

91. NEBERT DW, LEVITT RC, JENSEN NM, LAMBERT GH, FELTON JS: Birth
     defects and aplastic anemia: Differences in polycyclic
     hydrocarbon toxicity associated with the Ah locus.
     Arch Toxicol 39: 109-132, 1977.

92. NEBERT DW: Etiology of birth defects. Potential importance
     of genetic differences in drug metabolism. In Determinants

of Drug Metabolism in the Immature Human. Raven Press,
N.Y. 1981. In press.

93. LATT SA, ALLEN JW, STETTEN G: In vitro and in vivo analyses
    of chromosome structure, replication, and repair using
    BrdU-33258 Hoechst techniques. In Proceedings of the
    First International Congress on Cell Biology. B.R. Brinkley,
    K.R. Porter (eds). Rockefeller University Press, N.Y. 1977.
    pp. 520-527.

94. WOLFF S: Sister chromatid exchange. Ann Rev Genet 11: 183-201,
    1977.

95. GALLOWAY SM, PERRY PE, MENESES J, NEBERT DW, PEDERSEN RA:
    Cultured mouse embryos metabolize benzo(a)pyrene during
    early gestation: Genetic differences detectable by sister
    chromatid exchange. Proc Nat Acad Sci USA 77: 3524-3528,
    1980.

96. KELLERMANN G, SHAW CR, LUYTEN-KELLERMANN M: Aryl hydrocarbon
    hydroxylase inducibility and bronchogenic carcinoma.
    N Eng J Med 289: 934-937, 1973.

97. PAIGEN B, WARD E, STEENLAND K, HOUTEN L, GURTOO HL, MINOWADA J:
    Aryl hydrocarbon hydroxylase in cultured lymphocytes of
    twins. Am J Hum Genet 30: 561-571, 1978.

98. TRELL E, KORSGAARD R, HOOD B, KITZING P, NORDEN G, SIMONSSON BG:
    Aryl hydrocarbon hydroxylase inducibility and laryngeal
    carcinomas. Lancet 2: 140, 1976.

99. TRELL E, KORSGAARD R: Smoking and oral carcinoma. Lancet 1:
    671, 1978.

100. TRELL E, OLDBRING J, KORSGAARD R, MATTIASSON I: Aryl hydro-
     carbon hydroxylase inducibility in carcinoma of renal
     pelvis and ureter. Lancet 2: 612, 1977.

101. TRELL E, OLDBRING J, KORSGAARD R, HELLSTEN S, MATTIASSON I,
     TELHAMMAR E: Aryl hydrocarbon hydroxylase inducibility
     and carcinoma of the urinary bladder. IRCS J Med Sci 6:
     138, 1978.

102. BLUMER JL, DUNN R, GROSS S: Lymphocyte aryl hydrocarbon
     hydroxylase (AHH) inducibility in acute leukemia of child-
     hood (AL). Proc Am Assoc Cancer Res 20: 310, 1979.

103. LUBELL DL: Fatal hepatic necrosis associated with zoxazolamine
     therapy. NY State J Med 62: 3807-3810, 1962.

104. JICK H, PORTER J, MORRISON AS: Relation between smoking and age of natural menopause. <u>Lancet 1</u>: 1354-1355, 1977.

105. VESSEY MP, WRIGHT NH, McPHERSON K, WIGGINS P: Fertility after stopping different methods of contraception. <u>Brit Med J 1</u>: 265-267, 1978.

106. COHEN SB, BURK RF: Acetaminophen overdoses at a county hospital: A year's experience. <u>So Med J 71</u>: 1359-1364, 1978.

107. NEBERT DW: The <u>Ah</u> locus: Genetic differences in toxic response to foreign compounds. In <u>Microsomes, Drug Oxidations, and Chemical Carcinogenesis, volume II</u>. M.J. Coon, A.H. Conney, R.W. Estabrook, H.V. Gelboin, J.R. Gillette, P.J. O'Brien (eds). Academic Press, N.Y. 1980. pp. 801-812.

DISCUSSION

CHAIRMAN: M.M. THALER

ROY: Dr. Okey, have you looked at binding to a steroid receptor?

OKEY: We have tested this very carefully.   We think that this receptor is functioning very much like steroid receptors but it is not a known steroid receptor.

ROY: Is the receptor induced?

OKEY: We haven't seen any evidence that the receptor itself is induced.

ROY: Have human placentas been studied for their capacity to hydroxylate things like benzopyrene and dioxane etc, and particularly in areas where the population has been exposed to high levels of these chemicals?

OKEY: Placenta has been studied a good deal and it has, in some cases, extraordinary capabilities to metabolize benzopyrene. However, various studies have been clouded by other drugs and unknown factors, possibly genetic variability.   My suspicion is that the human population is heterogeneous; there are responsive people and nonresponsive people.   In the mouse, the genetics of the two strains I talked about are straight-forward with a simple autosomal dominant strain.   When we do crosses with other strains, the genetics get messy.   I think that part of the variability in human response to toxic substances is because of genetic differences in the capability of their enzyme system.   We are now working with cultured human cells where we can put inducers in culture and study induction phenomena.

A CLINICAL APPROACH TO CRYPTOGENIC CHOLESTASIS OF THE NEWBORN

Ross C. deBelle

The Montreal Children's Hospital
Montreal, Quebec

One of the most difficult clinical problems faced by
pediatricians is neonatal cholestasis. The reasons for the
clinical dilemma arise primarily from the array of disorders which
may be associated with the syndrome, the lack of specific clinical
tests and technology for precisely identifying the underlying
disorder and the urgency for specific treatment in certain clinical
entities before irreversible damage has been done to a young and
potentially viable liver. In reviewing the clinical nature of
this problem for presentation, it occurred to me that at the heart
of the dilemma lies our present lack of knowledge regarding the
pathophysiology of the majority of disorders which lead to neonatal
cholestasis.

It is encouraging to all of us that the people whom the
Canadian Liver Foundation has drawn here for this conference are
all actively engaged in investigations which are directed at
clarifying this problem and which will ultimately lead to improved
diagnosis and management of neonatal cholestasis. I will attempt
to provide an overview of the clinical problems with which we are
faced and, in particular, outline certain of the so-called cryptogenic disorders which may be either forgotten or which are poorly
understood. The other speakers in this program will outline for
you some of the exciting recent advances which have been made in
improving our understanding of what were previously considered
"cryptogenic" areas related to prolonged cholestasis of the newborn.

Prolonged cholestasis is defined by the persistence of jaundice
of variable intensity, dark urine and acholic stools for more than
ten days. With all due respect to the neonatologists, the neonatal
period as it involves the liver is considered up to 3 months of age.

97

TABLE   I

CAUSES OF CONJUGATED HYPERBILIRUBINEMIA IN INFANCY

Structural defects

        Bile duct
        abnormalities

                Biliary atresia
                Spontaneous perforation
                  of bile duct
                Choledochal cyst
                Bile duct stenosis
                Biliary hypoplasia
                  syndromes
                Choledocholithiasis
                Cholangiolitis

        Polycystic disease
        Vascular lesions

                Veno-occlusive disease
                Poor perfusion syndromes
                Hemangioendothelioma
                Lymphatic defects

        Chromosomal
        abnormalities

Metabolic defects
Infections
Post-hemolytic
  disorders
Toxic or deficiency
  disorders

        Intravenous nutrition
        Drugs

Familial syndromes
Neonatal hepatic
  necrosis
Idiopathic

Adapted from A.L. Mowat: Liver disorders in childhood. Butterworth,
London, 1979,p. 43.
    Table I lists the various causes of conjugated hyperbilirubin-
emia under the headings Structural Defects, Metabolic Defects,
Infections, Post-hemolytic Syndromes, Toxic or Deficiency Disorders,
Familial Syndromes, Neonatal Hepatic Necrosis and Idiopathic.

    First, with regard to bile duct abnormalities, Drs. Alagille,
Witzleben and Lilly will discuss the very real problem of biliary
atresia, the necessity for rapid and accurate diagnosis, the tools
available for diagnosis, and the potential for corrective surgery.
I might add that although computerized tomography and ultrasound

have greatly improved our diagnostic skills in identifying lesions
of the extrahepatic biliary tree in infants, there is still a great
need for a procedure such as retrograde cholangiography which has
so greatly expanded the diagnostic capabilities for biliary tract
lesions in adults.

The second group of disorders, Metabolic Defects such as
galactosemia and congenital fructosemia, are again extremely
important in terms of rapid and accurate diagnosis because of the
potential for immediate treatment and often cure of these infants.
This topic will be discussed in detail in the session on Metabolic
Liver Disease.

I would now like to focus on the problem of Infections as
related to neonatal cholestasis. With the development of vastly
improved facilities for caring for sick newborns in Neonatal
Intensive Care Units, it has become possible to treat effectively
infants with sepsis who previously would have become part of the
neonatal mortality statistics. Fortunately, many infants with
necrotizing enterocolitis and neonatal sepsis can be effectively
treated with antimicrobials, intravenous nutrition and surgery
when appropriate. However along with these advances have come
problems relating to prolonged obstructive liver disease which, at
present, are poorly understood. The difficulty is that the presence
of jaundice during the course of a neonatal infectious process may
or may not reflect hepatic involvement. Furthermore, the bacterial
etiology of hepatitis is often difficult to prove. A classic
example is the cholestatic potential of urinary tract infections
in newborns which should be recognized as a frequent cause of
prolonged jaundice and failure to thrive and which does not,
primarily, affect the liver. On the other hand, pathogenic E. Coli,
Listeria monocytogenes and more rarely, group B streptococci, have
become recently identified in the pathogenesis of neonatal septic
hepatitis. In addition, infants with necrotizing enterocolitis
may develop prolonged jaundice associated with ascending cholangitis.
When the clinical condition including coagulation status permits,
liver biopsies should be done in these infants in an attempt to
identify causative organisms by culture, immuno-fluorescence studies
or electron-microscopy, because in many cases recovery from septic
hepatitis may be possible with the early introduction of massive
intravenous antibiotic therapy. Furthermore, increased availability
of liver tissue for histopathology will lead to a better understanding of the prognosis in many of these infants.

Let us look next at the problem of Neonatal Hepatitis. This
condition is considered distinct from neonatal septic hepatitis in
that we are here dealing with specific hepatotrophic viruses and
infective agents, that is with infectious disorders which are mani-
fested primarily in the liver. In the past neonatal hepatitis
was considered as a catch-all for almost any condition that did not

include bile duct abnormalities and was defined mainly by a
characteristic liver histology which included hepatocellular
necrosis, giant cell transformation of hepatocytes and a portal
infiltrate composed primarily of chronic inflammatory cells
including plasma cells and lymphocytes. For these reasons, the
condition was also considered under the heading of "giant-cell
hepatitis" or "lupoid hepatitis" because of the plasma cell infiltrate. It has become apparent, however, that many toxic, genetic
and metabolic disorders involving the liver, for example fructosemia
or α-1-antitrypsin deficiency, may have a similar liver histology
and, therefore, were previously included under the heading Neonatal
Hepatitis. This is why it is of utmost importance to consider the
cause of cholestasis in infants as I have outlined and use the
liver biopsy as an adjunct in diagnosis and management.

Table II lists the various infectious etiologies of the hepatitis
syndrome in infants as well as the appropriate investigations to
define the agent and the clinical manifestations of disease. In
all cases it is important to attempt to diagnose the agent by
culture and serologic investigations in the infant and mother.
Liver biopsy in the infant is also important to identify precisely
the causative organism in the hepatocytes by culture, immunofluorescence or electron microscopy. The clinical manifestations
of disease provide an important tool to make the often difficult
distinction between neonatal hepatitis and biliary tract disorders
such as biliary atresia. You will note that most infants with
hepatitis present clinically with failure to thrive, often have
splenomegaly and frequently are incompletely obstructed and pass
yellow-colored stools. On the other hand, infants with biliary
atresia usually thrive initially, rarely have splenomegaly or
other generalized signs of infection, and usually pass only clay-
colored stools. These simple clinical signs can be very helpful
during the initial investigation of these children when early
laparotomy for a correctable surgical lesion is so important.
Conversely in an infant with cholestasis and the clinical manifestations of hepatitis it may be wiser to proceed with investigations
aimed at determining an infectious etiology before considering
surgery. Dr. Alagille will discuss investigations that should be
performed in infants with cholestasis in order to determine the
possibility of bile duct abnormalities. However, I would mention
that a properly conducted Rose Bengal I^{131} dye excretion test has
proven to be probably the most reliable indication of complete
bile duct obstruction in biliary atresia.

I want to point out that the viruses which are associated with
hepatitis in older infants and children, the Hepatitis A and B
viruses, are rarely identified as a cause of neonatal hepatitis.
Some of the possible reasons for this may be discussed during the
session on Viral Hepatitis. To date the hepatitis A virus has
not been implicated in neonatal hepatitis and hepatitis B surface

TABLE II

INFECTIOUS CAUSES OF THE HEPATITIS SYNDROME OF INFANCY

Infecting agents	Screening investigations	Definitive investigations	Principal extrahepatic clinical manifestations
Cytomegalovirus	CF antibody in serum	Isolation from urine and liver with demonstration of virus in liver by IF	Small for dates; microcephaly; meningo-encephalitis; intracranial calcification; neonatal thrombocytopenic purpura; splenomegaly; retinitis, deafness
Rubella virus	CF and HAI antibodies in serum	Specific IgM antibody, virus isolation from nasopharynx and liver	Small for dates; cataracts, retinitis; congenital heart defects; microphthalmia, buphthalmos and corneal edema; myocarditis; neonatal thrombocytopenic purpura; spleno-megaly; osteopathy; lymphadenopathy
Hepatitis B virus	Antigen and antibody in mother	Hepatitis B antigen in infant Demonstration of hepatitis B antigen in liver by IF and EM	None described
Herpes simplex virus	Perinatal herpes in mother	Isolation and demonstration of virus from superficial lesions and liver	Splenomegaly; heart failure, pneumonitis; skin vesicles; meningoencephalitis
Coxsackie B virus	Isolation from res-piratory tract and feces	Isolation from liver	Myocarditis; meningoencephalitis; pneumonitis
Varicella zoster virus	Demonstration of virus from superficial lesions	Demonstration of virus in the liver	Disseminated infection as in herpes simplex; skin lesions more obvious
Bacterial infection		Blood culture, urine culture, CSF	Anemia; any other system may be involved
Listeria		Isolation of organisms from blood culture, CSF or liver	Septicemia; meningitis; pneumonitis; purpura
Treponema pallidum	VDRL or TPI, particularly in mother	Demonstration of Treponema by dark ground illumination	Rhinitis; skin rash; bone lesions; anemia; lymphadenopathy; meningoencephalitis
Toxoplasma gondii	CF antibody in serum	Rising antibody titre in infant; specific IgM antibody; isolation of organisms from liver and CSF; visualization of organism from liver and CSF	Microcephaly; macrocephaly; meningo-encephalitis; intracranial calcification; chororetinitis; thrombocytopenia; purpura

CF = Complement fixing; HAI = Hem. agglutination inhibition; IF = Immunofluorescence microscopy; EM = Electron microscopy; CSF = Cerebrospinal fluid

antigen is being identified in only a small number of infants with
hepatitis, very few develop clinical or ongoing liver disease.   The
infection is usually derived from a carrier mother or a mother who
has had clinical hepatitis in the first, or more commonly the last
trimester of pregnancy.   The exact mode of infection is not clear
and may be transplacental, intrapartum or post-partum.   Preliminary
studies suggest that the occurrence of the "e" antigen in the mother
is associated with a high incidence of antigenemia in the infant.
In most cases the disease is either anicteric or clinically mild
with an elevation in serum transaminases;   the infant may become
a chronic carrier.   However, early fulminant hepatitis has been
observed in infants born of an asymptomatic carrier.

When considering post-hemolytic cholestasis (Table I) it
should be mentioned that transient conjugated hyperbilirubinemia
may occur during the recovery phase in erythroblastosis.   In this
instance it has been postulated that bilirubin is taken up by the
liver and conjugated faster than it can be excreted.   In these
neonates, liver function tests are normal.   Certain cases have
been described in which there has been a marked hemolytic anemia
or in which the unconjugated hyperbilirubinemia has been protracted.
The clinical picture in these cases mimics the hepatitis syndrome
of infancy and liver biopsy may show the cholestasis, hepatocellular
degeneration and giant-cell transformation previously described.
From the published results of follow-up it appears that the prognosis is excellent in these infants.   It is possible that certain
of these infants represent what was formerly referred to as the
"Inspissated Bile Syndrome".

The problem of neonatal cholestasis as related to Toxic or
Deficiency Disorders and particularly as it relates to the use of
intravenous alimentation in premature infants and in sick newborns
will be considered by Dr. Thaler.

The increasing identification of prolonged obstructive jaundice
in infants with genetic or familial syndromes represents a fascina-
ting area where recent investigations have done much to uncover
what were previously considered cryptogenic causes of cholestasis.
Dr. Alagille will discuss a group of infants which he has investigated with persistent cholestasis during the first three months of
life, dysmorphic features, marked abnormalities of serum lipids,
and liver histology characterized primarily by hypoplasia of the
intrahepatic bile ductules.   Dr. Weber will present her studies
on a familial form of cholestasis in North American Indian children
and Dr. Cox will discuss α-1-antitrypsin deficiency, a metabolic
disorder which may present as a clinical syndrome mimicking neonatal
hepatitis.   Dr. Russ Hanson and his colleagues have recently
described a family in which there was an inherited disorder of
bile acid metabolism such that the cholesterol side chain of the
bile acid sterol nucleus was incompletely metabolized.   The

resultant abnormal bile acids have been implicated in the mechanism of cholestasis. Abnormal bile acids have also been considered to play a role in the cholestasis observed in "Byler's Disease". Dr. Sharp will discuss these alterations of bile metabolism and their potential role in the development of cholestasis in infants and children. Finally under this heading one should mention the very rare occurrence of cystic fibrosis presenting primarily as obstructive liver disease in newborn infants. For this reason a sweat test should be included early in the work-up.

Acute Neonatal Hepatic Necrosis is a rare condition during the first few weeks of life. It begins with spontaneous hemorrhage and is rapidly followed by overwhelming liver disease. Liver biopsy when obtainable shows features of massive hepatic necrosis. The cause is usually not determined but may rarely be associated with Viral Hepatitis B.

The last heading "Idiopathic" unfortunately represents the majority of infants with cholestasis and for these we have as yet no clear idea of the etiology or pathogenesis.

In summary, recent research has defined certain specific causes of hepatobiliary disease in infancy. Unfortunately, the etiology of many disorders associated with prolonged jaundice in infancy is poorly understood. This has created a clinical dilemma in the differential diagnosis of neonatal cholestasis. Certain of the disorders which may be associated with this syndrome have been considered and others will be discussed in detail during the remainder of this conference. The priority in diagnosis is the immediate detection of medically treatable infections, especially with bacteria, syphilis or toxoplasmosis, and of the metabolic disorders for which effective dietary treatment is available. Urgent consideration must be given to excluding surgically correctable disorders such as bile duct abnormalities including choledochal cyst. Precise identification of the other specific causes may influence management of the individual case and may give information with prognostic or genetic implications.

Finally, consideration must be given not only to the environmental and genetic factors which either independently or together may produce neonatal cholestasis but also to the interaction between the cell types within the liver. An injury to any one of the cell types may disturb the functions of the other. Research into the causes of liver disease in infants must be directed not only at agents which damage the hepatocytes, but also at factors affecting other cells within the liver, including the reticulo-endothelial system and bile ductules. It is this type of research which will elucidate what are still cryptogenic causes of neonatal cholestasis.

THE ROLE OF BILE ACIDS IN PEDIATRIC CHOLESTASIS

Harvey L. Sharp, Deborah K. Freese, Russell F. Hanson

University of Minnesota Health Sciences Center
Departments of Pediatrics and Medicine
Minneapolis, Minnesota 55455

Bile acid metabolism is clearly altered by liver disease. The converse, however, as to whether bile acids contribute to the pathogenesis of liver disease is cloudy. Hepatobiliary disease will result from the administration of bile acids, particularly lithocholic acid, to lower animal species. Does a human counterpart exist? This chapter reexamines the role of bile acids in cholestasis by considering four areas: 1) physiological cholestasis of the newborn; 2) bile acid related cholestasis; 3) inborn errors of bile acid metabolism; and 4) our results with medical therapy in pediatric cholestatic conditions.

PHYSIOLOGICAL CHOLESTASIS OF THE NEWBORN

Lester recently reviewed in an editorial our understanding of bile acid metabolism by the immature liver (1). The relevance to humans of developmental bile acid metabolic studies in animals was initially demonstrated by Watkins. The normal human newborn showed a decreased cholic acid synthesis rate and pool size. These values were even lower in the premature infants (2). The bile acid metabolic status of the fetus is a more complex situation, see Table I. There are even preliminary indications that the enterohepatic circulation of bile acids is altered during pregnancy on the maternal side of the maternal-fetal unit. In the pregnant human the fasting gallbladder volume is larger and the rate of emptying of the gallbladder is slower (3).

In fetal animals, the bile acid synthesis rate appears decreased. In addition, there is reduced intestinal uptake and hepatic transport of bile acids into the biliary system (4,5,6). The concentration and distribution of bile acids have been examined in tissue available

TABLE I

BILE ACID COMPARTMENT CONSIDERATIONS

OF MATERNAL ⟵⟶ FETAL (NEWBORN UNIT)

LIVER	P	LIVER
BILIARY SYSTEM	L A	BILIARY SYSTEM
INTESTINE	C	INTESTINE
GUT BACTERIA	E	MECONIUM
BLOOD	N T	BLOOD
URINE	A	AMNIOTIC FLUID

to monitor human fetal bile acid metabolism including bacteria free
meconium, blood, and amniotic fluid.   For example, elevated
concentrations of bile acids in amniotic fluid have been proposed
as a method for detecting intestinal obstruction in utero (7).
However the complexities of bi-directional placental transfer
must be considered in interpreting fetal metabolic studies.

The following animal studies illustrate the variability of
placental transfer to the mother of sterols injected into the
fetal circulation.   Following an injection of labeled cholesterol
into the fetal circulation of sheep during the latter half of
gestation, labeled cholesterol or bile acids could not be detected
in the maternal bile.   However, labeled taurocholate and taurochenodeoxycholate were present in very low concentration in fetal
bile.   The presence of unlabeled deoxycholic acid and glycine
conjugated bile salts in fetal bile suggested maternal-fetal
transfer of bile acids.   Fetal bile acid synthesis and transport
into bile appears to be very immature in this study (8).   In a
different species, Little et al. demonstrated a 30% fetal to maternal
transfer of labeled cholate injected into near term fetal monkeys.
More variable was the low secretion range (14-58%) of the labeled
cholate into fetal gallbladder and intestine (5).

The liver, the intestine and its luminal contents, and less
crucially, the kidney, all exert an influence on normal bile salt
metabolism.   When considering the maternal-fetal unit, the placenta
also contributes to bile acid conjugation as well as transport (9).
The kidney assumes a larger role in bile acid excretion during
cholestasis.   Elegant GLC-Mass Spectrometry (GLC-MS) work by
Almé et al. compared the bile acids present in the urine of normal
and cholestatic patients (10).   The normal daily excretion of bile

acids into the urine is only 6.4 - 11 μmoles.   Twenty-six bile
acids positively identified in normal urine include 3-monohydroxyl-
ated, 14-dihydroxylated, and 9-trihydroxylated bile acids and
sterols.   The three monohydroxylated bile acids (lithocholate,
allolithocholate, and 3β-hydroxy-5-cholenoate) are presumably
secondary bile acids.   However, it is interesting that occasionally
significant quantities (0.08 - 0.75 μmoles/day) of 3β-hydroxy-5-
cholenoate can be detected.   The excretion of the mono- and di-
hydroxylated bile salts is normally facilitated by sulfation.
During cholestasis the total bile acid excretion is increased.
Tetrahydroxycholanic acids and sulfated trihydroxy bile acids are
unique to the cholestatic urine.

The three monohydroxy bile acids previously mentioned are
found in significant quantities in the urine of severely cholestatic
infants including patients with extrahepatic biliary atresia.
3β-hydroxy-5-cholenoic acid alone may account for 30% of the total
bile acids excreted via the kidney when significant derivation from
the gut bacteria is excluded indicating a primary synthesis pathway
for this monohydroxy bile acid within the liver.   Mitropoulos and
Myant have previously identified a mitochondrial pathway in the
rat liver in which cholesterol underwent oxidation of the side
chain at carbon 26 resulting in the formation of an isopropyl unit
before any modification of the ring system (12).   Subsequently
this pathway was demonstrated to be present in normal human liver(13).

We propose that the fetal liver has an alternate pathway
through the mitochondria as illustrated in Figure 1.   Our interest
in fetal bile acid metabolism began when we documented the presence
of lithocholic acid (by GLC-MS) and deoxycholic acid in normal
meconium.   At that time we suggested that these secondary bile
acids were maternal in origin and were transferred via the placenta
to the fetus (14,15).   However, now we must also consider the
possibility of a fetal liver origin for these bile acids via the
alternate mitochondrial pathway (Fig. 1).   Subsequent to our
observations, Watkins examined meconium utilizing better extraction
methodology which detected sulfated conjugates comprising 40-60%
of the total bile acid content (16).   Lithocholic acid comprised
60% of the sulfated conjugates and 15% of the non-sulfated conjugates.   Back and Ross also examined meconium from both prematures
and full-term newborns (17).   They also found significant quantities of deoxycholic and lithocholic acid.   Although there was no
significant difference between premature and full-term meconium
for these two bile acids, more 3β-hydroxy-5-cholenoic acid was
present in the premature meconium suggesting higher utilization
of this pathway during fetal development.   The sulfation fraction
of bile salts was smaller than that found by Watkins and contained
less lithocholic acid than 3β-hydroxy-5-cholenoic acid.

Similar findings were present in the amniotic fluid samples

CHOLESTEROL   5-CHOLESTENE-3β,26-DIOL

CHOLEST-5-ENE-3β,7α-DIOL   3β-HYDROXY-5 CHOLESTENOIC ACID

7α-HYDROXYCHOLEST-4-ENE-3-ONE   3β-HYDROXY-5 CHOLENOIC ACID

CHOLIC ACID   CHENODEOXYCHOLIC ACID   LITHOCHOLIC ACID

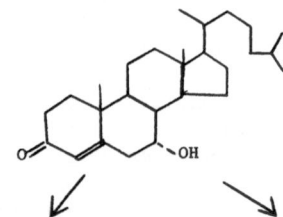

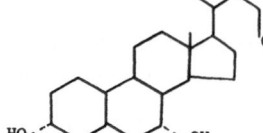

Fig. 1   Fetal Liver Bile Acid Pathways

obtained at 32-37 weeks of gestation compared to the 38-41 weeks
gestational period (18).   3β-hydroxy-5-cholenoic acid comprised
39% of the 1.31 μM of total bile acids in the earlier gestational
age samples as opposed to 20% of the 2.06 μM of total bile acids
in the later gestational age samples. The peak percentage appeared
to be around 36 weeks where the range was 68-74% of 1.7 μM of total

bile acids.   Total bile acids in amniotic fluid and cord blood
are increased during cholestasis of pregnancy (19).   Although
increased fetal risk is documented during this state, there is no
good evidence that liver disease in the fetus or newborn is associated with these elevated levels of bile acids.   We have wondered
whether amniocentesis might predict inherited forms of liver disease
by measurement of elevated total or abnormal composition of bile
acids.   Amniotic fluid was obtained at 38 weeks gestation from a
mother undergoing this procedure for low estradiols.   Her previous
son had arterio-hepatic dysplasia (20).   Both the total concentration of bile acids and their distribution documented by GLC-Mass
Spectrometry were normal (21).   Since the infant was subsequently
diagnosed for this disorder in the nursery, we were disappointed
that our first evaluation of amniotic fluid was unrewarding.
Perhaps fetal blood samples might be a more worthwhile screening
procedure.

        Normal maternal serum bile acid levels are lower than venous
cord bile acid levels (19).   Sulfated bile acids are only detected
in the cord blood.   Lithocholic acid, deoxycholic acid, and 3β-
hydroxy-5-cholenoic acid are only detected under normal circumstances
in cord blood.   During cholestasis of pregnancy both maternal and
cord bile acids are elevated in both the sulfated and non-sulfated
fractions, but under these circumstances the bile acid levels are
significantly higher in the maternal venous samples.   That
physiologic cholestasis exists is further suggested by the higher
concentrations of conjugates of cholic acid in the serum in premature
infants (22).   However, this study does not document the length
of time during infancy that physiologic cholestasis persists.
Suchy et al. suggest that normal serum levels of bile acids are
reached by eight months of age (23).

BILE ACID RELATED CHOLESTASIS

        The hepatobiliary toxicity of lithocholic acid (LCA) has been
known since 1941 (24), popularized in 1960 (25), and recently
summarized in 1979 (26,27).   The current hypothesis of LCA pathogenesis is related to membrane alterations and to precipitable
material in the bile canaliculus.   Bile acid induced hepatocellular
cholestasis has been primarily related to the monohydroxy bile acids
(LCA and 3β-hydroxy-5-cholanoic acid) (28).   The role of other
bile acids has only recently been examined.   A study by Drew and
Priestly evaluated bile flow in the rat under constant rate
infusions (54 μl/min) with increasing concentrations of taurine
conjugated bile salts (29).   Deoxycholate stimulated bile flow
at a concentration of 1 μmole/min/kg but the rats became cholestatic
at 5 μmoles/min/kg.   Chenodeoxycholate stimulated bile flow up
through concentrations of 5 μmoles/min/kg but caused cholestasis at
10 μmoles/min/kg.   Cholate stimulated bile flow up to 20 μmoles/min/
kg but after 100 minutes of infusion suddenly produced cholestasis.

Very little has been reported concerning the differences that amino acid conjugation might have on bile flow. Mechanistically for instance, taurine conjugated LCA (TLCA) is not incorporated into the bile canalicular membrane whereas LCA is (30). Glyco-deoxycholate is less choleretic than deoxycholate or taurodeoxy-cholate (31). Interaction of the bile acids appears very important in bile flow. The simultaneous administration of TLCA and taurochenodeoxycholate to the rat results in stimulation of bile flow and more TLCA secretion. TLCA causes cholestasis with less TLCA in bile and the cholestasis can be complete when the rat becomes bile salt depleted (28).

Yousef et al. reported sex differences in the composition of 5β-bile acids in rat bile (32). A smaller percentage of muri-cholate, deoxycholate, and hyodeoxycholate are present in the bile salt pool of the female than male rats. More striking and consis-tent is the observation that female rats excrete five to ten times more sulfated bile acids than male rats (33). Most sulfated bile acids have a 5α-configuration. Bile salt sulfatase is low in guinea pig and human fetal liver (34). The induction of liver injury by LCA during fetal development in animal models may in part be related to poor sulfation ability (35,36). The lack of liver toxicity during the administration of chenodeoxycholate to man for gallstones appears to be related to the ability to sulfate LCA. Monkeys which form bile acid sulfates poorly (37) are more susceptible to liver damage from chenodeoxycholic acid administra-tion. The sulfate ester of taurolithocholate reduces bile flow only half as much as other forms of LCA (38). Sulfation of bile salts enhances their fecal and urinary excretion and therefore may represent a protective mechanism in patients with cholestasis (39, 40).

Glucuronidation of bile salts, like sulfation, forms very polar metabolites with increased solubility in water and therefore may be similarly protective. The average 24-hour urinary bile salt excretion in 10 patients with extrahepatic biliary obstruction is 40 mg/day of which 50% are sulfates and 12.5% are glucuronides (41). The average 24-hour urinary excretion of bile salts in intrahepatic cholestasis is 34 mg, of which 50% is sulfated and 20% is glucuronidated. Since only trace amounts of bile salts are normally glucuronidated, this pathway appears to be important in man during cholestasis.

INBORN ERRORS OF BILE ACID METABOLISM

An inborn error of bile acid metabolism, presenting as a liver disease, would suggest that abnormal bile acids are the etiologic agents. The best defined entity is cerebrotendinous xanthomatosis, which has the following clinical manifestations: 1) progressive neurological dysfunction; 2) tuberous and tendon xanthomas; 3)

premature atherosclerosis;   4) pulmonary insufficiency;   5) cataracts;
and 6) endocrine hypofunction (42).   The following abnormalities
of cholesterol metabolism are found in this disorder: a) total
bile acid production is low (only 50% of normal), b) cholic acid
predominates in the bile (less than 10% is chenodeoxycholic acid),
c) unusually low concentrations of deoxycholic acid and lithocholic
acid exist and d) 25-hydroxylated bile alcohols are found in the
bile and feces.   Oftebro et al. have defined the metabolic defect
as the absence of mitochondrial 26-hydroxylase activity for 5β-
cholestane-3α,7α,12α-triol (43).   Liver function is normal in
these patients with the only abnormality being a pigment accumulating in the cytoplasm (44).

However, another inborn error of cholic acid synthesis,
characterized by the inadequate conversion of trihydroxy-coprostanic
acid (THCA) to cholic acid presents as cholestasis of infancy
(45,46).   This presumed autosomal recessive defect also presents
with failure to thrive, rickets, and decreased intrahepatic bile
ducts and it ends fatally with cirrhosis and liver failure.   No
pruritus ever develops.   Gallbladder drainage, cholestyramine
and phenobarbital do not alter the course of this disease.   THCA
is the main bile acid (55-100%) of the total bile acids in the
serum, bile, urine and feces.   The defect appears to be the
result of a decreased ability to convert THCA to varanic acid
(24-hydroxylated THCA).   Since dihydroxycoprostanic acid (DHCA)
does not accumulate and the mitochondria appear morphologically
normal, a single enzyme defect in acyl dehydrogenase appears quite
likely.   However, determination of the level of this enzyme in
homozygotes and heterozygotes has not yet been accomplished.
Nevertheless these patients are presently the closest example of
a bile acid induced liver disease.

The Cerebro-Hepato-Renal syndrome of Zellweger is an autosomal
recessive disorder which can be confused with the disorder just
discussed.   These patients present in the nursery with severe
hypotonia and feeding difficulties (47).   They continue to fail
to thrive with marked psychomotor retardation and seizures ending
in death within the first six months of life.   Our interest in
this disorder was prompted by the abnormal mitochondria consisting
of dense matrix and twisted cristae (48).   We therefore looked
at the urinary bile acid patterns over a period of time in three
patients.   As their disease progressed, we found THCA, DHCA, and
varanic acid present in the urine of these patients (49).   Thus
it appears that side chain beta oxidation occurs in the mitochondria.
Hepatomegaly is found in 75% of these patients with the interesting
observation that 23% manifest a paucity of the cholangioles.   Some
of these patients progress to a micronodular cirrhosis(50).   It is
easy to speculate but difficult to prove in these two disorders
that the abnormal trihydroxy bile acids alter the intrahepatic
bile ducts.

MEDICAL THERAPY IN PEDIATRIC CHOLESTATIC CONDITIONS

Another method to evaluate whether bile acids cause liver disease is to alter bile salt metabolism and reevaluate the hepatic disorder.   Our first clue that this might be feasible was in a patient with paucity of the intrahepatic bile ducts when both common bile duct drainage and later gallbladder drainage not only relieved pruritus but improved liver function and growth (51). Cholestyramine was tried in this patient as a medical alternative to this procedure and worked (51,52).   Phenobarbital had been shown to increase bile flow in rats (53).   In 1968 we tried phenobarbital for the first time in this same patient after we documented that he had developed essentially non-secretion of bile salts into the biliary tree (54).   Because of the gratifying response with this patient, 27 other children with various chole-static conditions received either or both medication (55).   All patients had at least one month of trial therapy, with a majority receiving the medication for over one year.   Changes in the follow-ing parameters were evaluated relative to therapy: 1) pruritus, 2) liver function, 3) hepatosplenomegaly (including liver biopsy in most), and 4) height and weight deviations.

The effect of cholestyramine on bile acid metabolism has been studied in a few normal humans.   It reduces the chenodeoxycholic pool size and increases the cholic acid pool size (56).   The same appears true in liver disease patients (57).   The results of phenobarbital studies are not as clear-cut, but in three normal humans increased cholesterol synthesis was found along with induced enzymes of cholesterol metabolism (58).   In primates phenobarbital increases both the bile salt-dependent and independent fraction of bile flow (59).   In patients with liver disease phenobarbital increases the synthesis and pool size of chenodeoxycholic acid (57, 60).   After the three regimens used in this series of patients were reviewed, only cholestyramine alone was consistently beneficial and significantly only for children with either a paucity of the intrahepatic bile ducts or the familial syndrome of cholestasis with lymphedema (61).

SUMMARY

Fetal bile salt metabolism is immature and probably involves pathways through the mitochondria which result in more monohydroxy bile acids.   The newborn bile acid pool size, synthesis rate, and duodenal concentrations are at levels below those of the adult. Therefore there are good indications that the newborn not only has physiologic jaundice but also physiologic cholestasis.   Develop-mental cholestasis may predispose to the increased incidence of cholestatic liver disease during infancy.   Immature enzymatic capabilities to sulfate or glucuronidate monohydroxy bile acids may also play a role.

Clinical proof that bile acids may cause rather than just reflect cholestasis is still unclear.   An inborn error of bile acid metabolism could provide a definitive answer.   Presumptive evidence for such a disorder emanates from investigations in cholestatic children with increased amounts of the cholic acid precursor trihydroxycoprostanic acid (THCA).   A specific metabolic block in the 24-hydroxylating enzyme necessary to convert THCA to varanic acid is postulated, but enzyme assays on these families for absolute proof have not been reported.   This disease should not be confused with Zellweger Syndrome where progressive diffuse mitochondrial defects contribute to excessive amounts of THCA, DHCA, and varanic acid.   Nevertheless, both diseases have been documented to have an alteration in bile duct structure.

Alteration of bile salt metabolism with cholestyramine in patients with the more benign forms of paucity of the intrahepatic bile ducts and cholestasis with lymphedema results in significant clinical improvement of the liver disease in addition to relief of pruritus.   These data constitute the best present evidence that bile acids may contribute to the pathogenesis of these human disorders.

REFERENCES

1. LESTER R: Physiologic cholestasis. Gastroenterology 78: 864-870, 1980.

2. WATKINS JB, INGALL D, SZCZEPANIK P, KLEIN PD, LESTER R: Bile-salt metabolism in the newborn. Measurement of pool size and synthesis by stable isotope technic. N Eng J Med 288: 431-434, 1973.

3. EVERSON G, McKINLEY C, SHOWATER R, JOHNSON M, DeMARK B, SZCZEPANIK P, VAN LEEUWEN P, KLEIN P, KERN F: Bile acid kinetics and gallbladder function in pregnancy: the apparent regulatory role of the gallbladder. Gastroenterology 78: 1162, 1980

4. LITTLE JM, RICHEY JE, VAN THIEL DH, LESTER R: Taurocholate pool size and distribution in the fetal rat. J Clin Invest 63: 1042-1049, 1979.

5. LITTLE JM, SMALLWOOD RA, LESTER R, PIASECKI GJ, JACKSON BT: Bile salt metabolism in the primate fetus. Gastoenterology 69: 1315-1320, 1975.

6. LESTER R, SMALLWOOD RA, LITTLE JM, BROWN AS, PIASECKI GJ, JACKSON BT: Fetal bile salt metabolism: the intestinal absorption of bile salt. J Clin Invest 59: 1009-1016, 1977.

7. DÉLÈZE G, SIDIROPOULOS D, PAUMGARTNER G: Determination of
    bile acid concentration in human amniotic fluid for pre-
    natal diagnosis of intestinal obstruction. Pediatrics
    59: 647-650, 1977

8. SMALLWOOD RA, JABLONSKI P, WATTS J McK: Bile acid synthesis
    in the developing sheep liver. Clinical Sciences and
    Molecular Medicine 45: 403-406, 1973.

9. WATKINS JB: Developmental aspects of bile acid metabolism and
    hepatic function. In Pediatric Liver Disease: 43-54. MM
    MM Fisher and CC Roy (eds). Plenum Press, NY, 1983.

10. ALMÉ B, BREMMELGAARD A, SJÖVALL J, THOMASSEN P: Analysis of
    metabolic profiles of bile acids in urine using a lipo-
    philic anion exchanger and computerized gas-liquid
    chromatography-mass spectrometry. J Lipid Res 18: 339-362,
    1977.

11. MAKINO I, SJÖVALL J: Excretion of 3β-hydroxy-5-cholenoic and
    3α-hydroxy-5α-cholanoic acids in urine of infants with
    biliary atresia. FEBS LETT 15: 161-164, 1971.

12. MITROPOULOS KA, MYANT NB: The formation of lithocholic acid,
    chenodeoxycholic acid and α- and β-muricholic acids from
    cholesterol incubated with rat liver mitochondria.
    Biochem J 103: 472-479, 1967.

13. ANDERSON KE, KOK E, JAVITT NB: Bile acid synthesis in man:
    Metabolism of 7α-hydroxycholesterol-^{14}C and 26-hydroxy-
    cholesterol-[3]H. J Clin Invest 51: 112-117, 1972.

14. SHARP HL, CAREY JB Jr, PELLER J, KRIVIT W: Lithocholic acid
    in meconium. Pediat Res 2: 293, 1968.

15. SHARP HL, PELLER J, CAREY JB Jr, KRIVIT W: Primary and
    secondary bile acids in meconium. Pediat Res 5: 274-279,
    1971.

16. WATKINS JB: Fetal and neonatal hepatic function. The role
    of bile acids in neonatal hepatitis and biliary atresia.
    In DHEW Publication No. (NIH) 79-1269, NB Javitt (ed)
    pp 269-276.

17. BACK P, ROSS K: Identification of 3β-hydroxy-5-cholenoic acid
    in human meconium. Hoppe-Seyler's Zeitschrift für Physio-
    logische Chemie 354: 83-89, 1973.

18. DÉLÈZE G, PAUMGARTNER G, KARLAGANIS G, GIGER W, REINHARD M,
    SIDIROPOULOS D: Bile acid pattern in human amniotic

fluid.   Eur J Clin Investigation 8: 41-45, 1978.

19. LAATIKAINEN TJ, LEHTONEN PJ, HESSO AE: Fetal sulfated and
     nonsulfated bile acids in intrahepatic cholestasis of
     pregnancy. J Lab Clin Med 92: 185-193, 1978.

20. ALAGILLE D, ODIÈVRE M, GAUTIER M, DOMMERGUES JP: Hepatic
     ductular hypoplasia associated with characteristic facies,
     vertebral malformations, retarded physical, mental, and
     sexual development, and cardiac murmur. J Pediatr 86:
     63-71, 1975.

21. Unpublished observations.

22. SONDHEIMER JM, BRYAN H, ANDREWS W, FORSTNER GG: Cholestatic
     tendencies in premature infants on and off parental
     nutrition. Pediatrics 62: 984-989, 1978.

23. SUCHY FJ, BALISTRERI WF, SEARCY JE, LEVIN RS: Physiologic
     elevation of the primary serum bile acids during infancy.
     Pediatr Res 14: 511, 1980.

24. IVY AC: The applied physiology of bile secretion and bile
     salt therapy.   JAMA 117: 1151-1154, 1941.

25. HOLSTI P: Cirrhosis of the liver in rabbits induced by gastric
     instillation of desiccated whole bile. Acta Pathol Micro-
     biol Scand (Supp) 113: 1-67, 1956.

26. FISHER MM: Biochemical basis for toxic liver injury; litho-
     cholate hepatotoxicity. In Toxic Injury of the Liver,
     Part A. E Farber, MM Fisher (eds).Marcel Dekker Inc. 1979,
     pp 155-192.

27. PHILLIPS MJ, ODA M, FUNATSU K: Reactions of the liver to injury:
     cholestasis, its ultrastructural aspects. In Toxic Injury
     of the Liver, Part A. E Farber, MM Fisher (eds). Marcel
     Dekker Inc. 1979, pp 333-383.

28. JAVITT NB, EMERMAN S: Effect of sodium and taurolithocholate
     on bile flow and bile acid excretion. J Clin Invest 47:
     1002-1014, 1968.

29. DREW R, PRIESTLY BG: Choleretic and cholestatic effects of
     infused bile salts in the rat. Experientia 35: 809-811,
     1979.

30. YOUSEF IM, KAKIS G, FISHER MM: Biochemical differences between
     lithocholate and taurolithocholate induced intrahepatic
     cholestasis. Gastroenterology 72: 1153, 1977.

31. KLAASSEN CD: Comparison of the choleretic properties of bile
     acids. Europ J Pharm 23: 270-275, 1973.

32. YOUSEF IM, KAKIS G, FISHER MM: Bile acid metabolism in mammals.
     III. Sex difference in the bile acid composition of rat
     bile. Can J Biochem 50: 402-408, 1972.

33. ERICKSON H, TAYLOR W, SJÖVALL J: Sex difference in sulfation
     and excretion of 5α-cholanoic acids in rats. In Bile Acid
     Metabolism in Health and Disease. G Paumgartner, A Stiehl
     (eds). MTP Press, England, 1977. pp 75-78.

34. CHEN L-J, THALER MM, BOLT RJ, GOLBUS MS: Enzymatic sulfation
     of taurolithocholate in human and guinea pig fetuses and
     adults. Life Sciences 22: 1817-1820, 1978.

35. SILVERBERG M, SOLOMON L, EHRLICH JC: The hepatotoxic effects
     of lithocholic acid in the newborn hamster. Gastroent-
     erology 60: 753, 1971.

36. BUJANOVER Y, THALER MM: Malformations of intrahepatic bile
     ducts induced by intrauterine exposure to lithocholate.
     Gastroenterology 73: 1214, 1977.

37. GADACZ TR, ALLAN RN, MACK E, HOFMANN AF: Impaired lithocholate
     sulfation in the rhesus monkey: A possible mechanism for
     chenodeoxycholate toxicity. Gastroenterology 70: 1125-
     1129, 1976.

38. FISHER MM, MAGNUSSON R, MIYAI K: Bile acid metabolism in
     mammals. I. Bile acid-induced intrahepatic cholestasis.
     Lab Invest 25: 88-91, 1971

39. PALMER RH: The formation of bile acid sulfates: a new path-
     way of bile acid metabolism in humans. Proc Nat Acad
     Sci 58: 1047-1050, 1967.

40. STIEHL A: Bile salt sulphates in cholestasis. Europ J Clin
     Invest 4: 59-63, 1974.

41. FRÖHLING W, STIEHL A: Bile salt glucuronides: identification
     and quantitative analysis in the urine of patients with
     cholestasis. Europ J Clin Invest 6: 67-74, 1976.

42. SALEN G, SHEFER S, ZAKI FG, MOSBACH EH: Inborn errors of
     bile acid synthesis. Clinics in Gastroenterology 6:
     91-100, 1977.

43. OFTEBRO H, BJÖRKHEIM I, SKREDE S, SCHREINER A, PEDERSEN J:
     Cerebrotendinous xanthomatosis. A defect in mitochondrial

26-hydroxylation required for normal biosynthesis of cholic acid. J Clin Invest 65: 1418-1430, 1980.

44. SALEN G, ZAKI FG, SABESIN S, BOEHME D, SHEFER S, MOSBACH EH: Intrahepatic pigment and crystal forms in patients with cerebrotendinous xanthomatosis. Gastroenterology 74: 82-89, 1978.

45. EYSSEN H, PARMENTIER G, COMPERNOLLE F, BOON J, EGGERMONT E: Trihydroxycoprostanic acid in the duodenal fluid of two children with intrahepatic bile duct anomalies. Biochem Biophys Acta 273: 212-221, 1972.

46. HANSON RF, ISENBERG JN, WILLIAMS GC, HACHEY D, SZCZEPANIK P, KLEIN PD, SHARP HL: The metabolism of $3\alpha,7\alpha,12\alpha$-trihydroxy-5β-cholestan-26-oic acid in two siblings with cholestasis due to intrahepatic bile duct anomalies, an apparent inborn error of cholic acid synthesis. J Clin Invest 56: 577-587, 1975.

47. BOWEN P, LESS CS, ZELLWEGER H, LINDENBURG R: A familial syndrome of multiple congenital defects. Bull Johns Hopkins Hosp. 114: 402-414, 1964.

48. GOLDFISHER S, MOORE CL, JOHNSON AB, SPIRO AJ, VALSAMIS MP, WISNIEWSKI HK, RITCH RH, NORTON WT, RAPIN I, GARTNER LM: Peroxisomal and mitochondrial defects in the cerebro-hepatorenal syndrome. Science 182: 62-64, 1973.

49. HANSON RF, SZCZEPANIK-VAN LEEUWEN P, WILLIAMS GL, GRABOWSKI G, SHARP HL: Defects of bile acid synthesis in Zellweger's syndrome. Science 203: 1107-1108, 1979.

50. GILCHRIST KW, GILBERT EF, GOLDFARB S, GOLL U, SPRANGER JW, OPITZ JM: Studies of malformation syndromes of man XIB: The cerebro-hepato-renal syndrome of Zellweger: Comparative pathology. Eur J Pediatr 121: 99-118, 1976.

51. LOTTSFELDT FI, KRIVIT W, AUST JB, CAREY JB: Cholestyramine therapy in intrahepatic biliary atresia. New Eng J Med 269: 186-189, 1963.

52. SHARP HL, CAREY JB, WHITE JG, KRIVIT W: Cholestyramine therapy in patients with a paucity of the intrahepatic bile ducts. J Pediatr 71: 723-736, 1967.

53. ROBERTS RJ, PLAA GL: Effect of phenobarbital on the excretion of an exogenous bilirubin load. Biochem Pharm 16: 827-835, 1967.

54. SHARP HL, MIRKIN BL: Effect of phenobarbital on hyperbiliru-
     binemia, bile acid metabolism and microsomal enzyme
     activity in chronic intrahepatic cholestasis of childhood.
     J Pediatr 81: 116-126, 1972.

55. SHARP HL, KANE W: Medical therapy in cholestatic liver
     disease. DHEW Publication No. (NIH) 79-1296, pp 277-282.

56. GARBUTT JT, KENNEY TJ: Effect of cholestyramine on bile acid
     metabolism in normal man. J Clin Invest 51: 2781-2789,
     1972.

57. ISENBERG JN, HANSON RF, WILLIAMS GC, ZAVORAL J, PAGE AR,
     SHARP HL: Immunodeficiency, xanthomas and obstructive
     liver disease. Am J Med 61: 393-400, 1976.

58. MILLER NE, NESTEL PJ: Altered bile acid metabolism during
     treatment with phenobarbitone. Clin Sci Mol Med 45:
     257-262, 1973.

59. REDINGER RN, SMALL DM: Primate biliary physiology VIII.
     The effect of phenobarbital upon bile salt synthesis
     and pool size, biliary lipid secretion, and bile
     composition. J Clin Invest 52: 161-172, 1973.

60. STIEHL A, THALER MM, ADMIRAND WH: Effects of phenobarbital
     on bile salt metabolism in cholestasis due to intrahepatic
     bile duct hypoplasia. Pediatrics 51: -92-997, 1973.

61. SHARP HL, KRIVIT W: Hereditary lymphedema and obstructive
     jaundice. J Pediatr 78: 491-496, 1971.

MICROFILAMENT DYSFUNCTION IN CHOLESTASIS: POSSIBLE INVOLVEMENT IN FAMILIAL PEDIATRIC CHOLESTATIC SYNDROMES

A. Weber, I. Yousef and B. Tuchweber

Départements de Pédiatrie, Pathologie et Nutrition
Université de Montréal, Montréal, Québec

INTRODUCTION

During the last decade, increased interest in cholestasis has developed, which can be explained by the recent advances made in the knowledge of factors involved in bile formation and/or secretion (1).   Recently the known concepts in muscle cell biology have been applied to the hepatocyte, drawing attention to the cytoskeleton, a highly elaborate system of proteins that regulates structure and motility, and probably participates in the dynamic process of bile flow (2).   A broader definition of cholestasis has also been proposed which is supposed to please physiologists, morphologists, clinical biochemists and clinicians.   Indeed cholestasis does no longer only imply jaundice, but, in the absence of extrahepatic biliary obstruction, it might be defined as a primary disturbance in hepatic bile formation (3).   This includes the conditions of "bilirubinostasis" as well as those associated with reduced bile flow where excretion of bile salts is primarily defective (4).

Several mechanisms have been implicated in clinical and experimental intrahepatic cholestasis, and at present no single mechanism appears to be selectively involved (1-4).   The search for a single defect responsible for cholestasis has been particularly intensive in the familial types of neonatal cholestasis, since in the presence of familial occurrence an inherited error of metabolism might be expected.   Abnormalities in bile acid metabolism have been documented and are discussed in another chapter of this volume.   The purpose of this paper is to review the role of microfilament dysfunction as a possible mechanism of cholestasis and to discuss its possible implication both in animals and in man, with special reference to pediatric cholestatic entities.

119

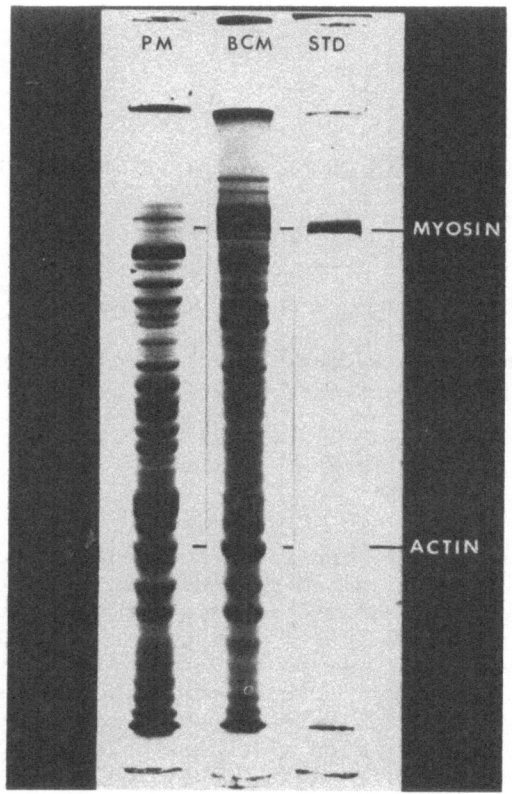

Fig 1   SDS - Polyacrylamide gel electrophoresis of liver cell
plasma membrane polypeptides showing increased content of
actin and myosin in a preparation rich in canalicular
membranes (BCM) as compared to the one containing mainly
sinusoidal membrane (PM).

HEPATOCYTIC MICROFILAMENT STRUCTURE AND FUNCTION AS POSTULATED FROM EXPERIMENTAL MODELS

In recent years several studies have emphasized the presence
of molecules with notable similarity to muscle actin and myosin in
different non-muscle cell systems (3,5).   In the liver these
proteins appear in association with the plasma membrane and are more
abundant at the canalicular face of the hepatocyte (Figure 1).
Actin probably comprises 1% to 2% of the cellular protein but in
hepatic cell plasma membrane fractions enriched in bile canaliculi

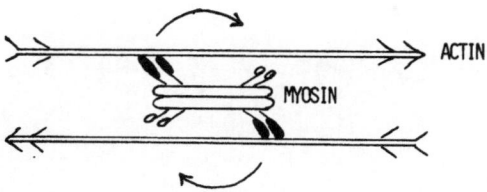

Fig. 2 *Suggested model for actomyosin interaction in BCM.*
In this model, one myosin filament is in association with
two oppositely oriented actin filaments. The arrows
indicate the direction of effective movement of the actin
filaments. Since the two sets of effective cross-bridges
are working against each other, myosin would be motionless
and the relative motion only would be in actin filaments.

it accounts for 20% of the total membrane polypeptides.   The mono-
meric form of actin (globular or G actin) through ionic interactions
polymerises to a filamentous form (F actin).   Myosin represents
about 10% of the canalicular membrane polypeptides and is immunologically similar to the one isolated from smooth muscle (6).   Its
interaction with actin has been extensively studied in muscle, and
by extrapolation a somewhat similar mechanism could be suggested
in the liver, as represented in Figure 2 (7).

TABLE I

DRUG-INDUCED MICROFILAMENT DYSFUNCTION IN

EXPERIMENTAL CHOLESTASIS

CHOLESTATIC AGENTS	MICROFILAMENT MODIFICATIONS
PHALLOIDIN	INCREASE IN ACTIN POLYMERIZATION DECREASE IN MYOSIN
CYTOCHALASIN B NORETHANDROLONE	DISSOCIATION FROM MEMBRANE BINDING SITES
CHLORPROMAZINE	SOLID GEL FORMATION DECREASE IN ACTIN POLYMERIZATION

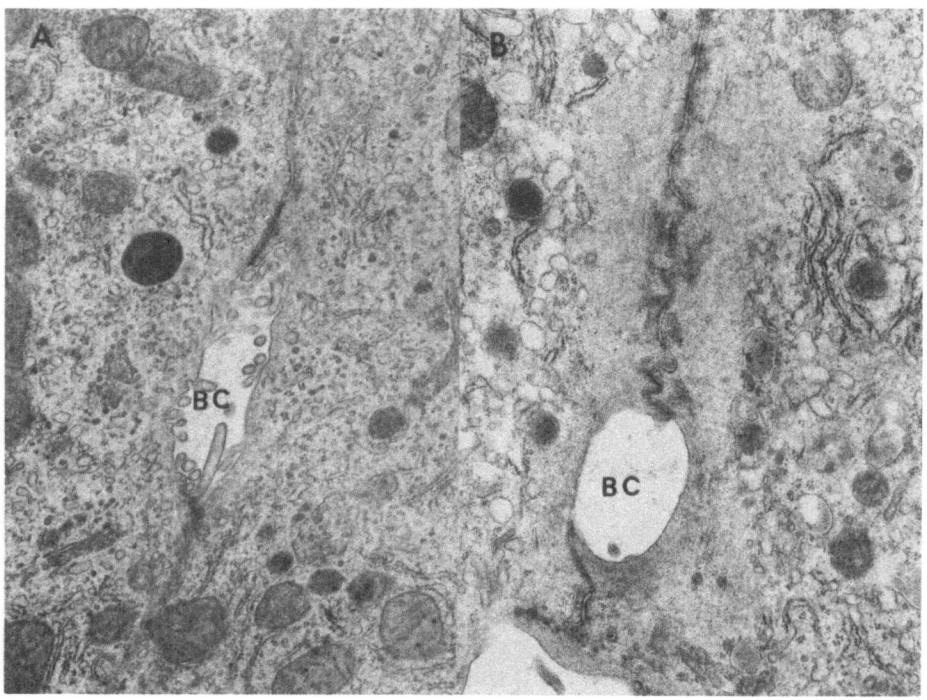

Fig. 3 *Ultrastructural appearance of a normal bile canaliculus in*
        rat liver (A) and after phalloïdin treatment (B).
        Disappearance of microvilli, dilatation of the lumen and
        striking thickening of the filamentous ectoplasm in the
        pericanalicular zone are noticed.   BC = bile canaliculus.

It is not suprprising that changes in canalicular cytoskeleton
proteins have been implicated in cholestasis because this face of
the membrane is almost always morphologically involved in this
process.   Microfilament dysfunction in the liver cell has been
induced in various experimental models (Table I) (8,9).   Phalloïdin
is a toxin isolated from the mushroom Amanita Phalloïdes.   In rats
this cholestatic toxin induced polymerisation of actin (Figure 3)
and decreased the myosin content of the hepatocyte plasma membrane.
However the attachment of microfilaments to the membrane was preserved (Figure 4).   In contrast, when the cholestatic agents
cytochalasin B or norethandrolone were used, a dissociation of
microfilaments was noted and their detachment from their membrane
binding sites was suggested (8).   Since in these experimental
models microfilament dysfunction was always associated with cholestasis, some role in the normal process of bile formation was postulated for the actin-myosin complex (Table II).   These cytoskeleton

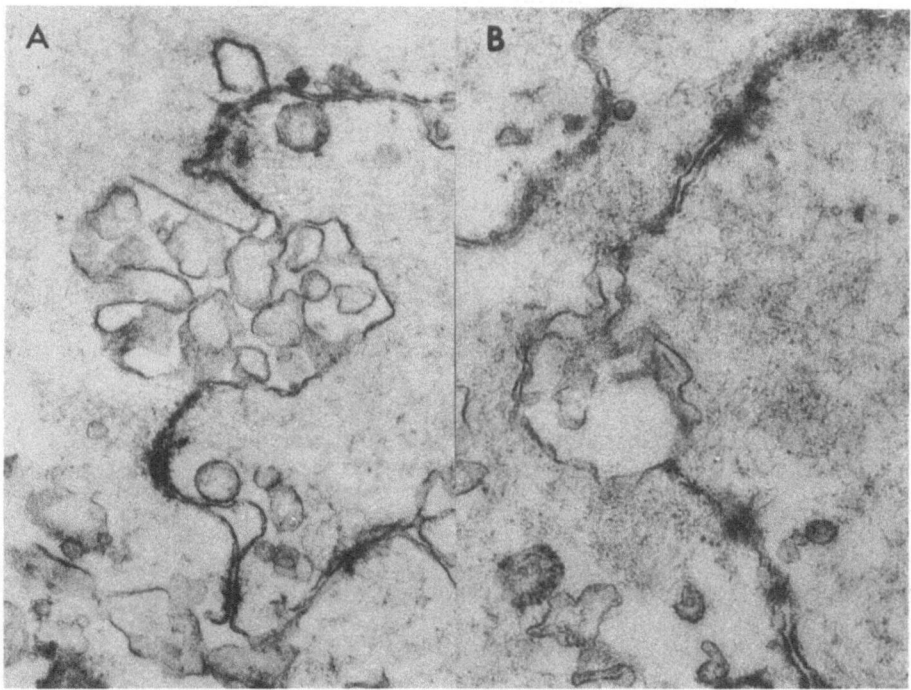

*Fig. 4 Ultrastructural appearance of a normal isolated bile
         canaliculus (A) and after phalloïdin treatment (B).
         The pericanalicular zone is enlarged and contains actin
         microfilaments associated with the membrane.*

proteins might provide a contractile force that facilitates canalicular bile flow and exocytotic transport process (10).   Transla-
tional mobility of the membrane components might be also regulated
by the microfilaments since they are attached to the integral
proteins (3).   Actin microfilaments might be necessary for the
regulation of certain membrane enzymes i.e. Mg^{++}-ATPase, Na^+K^+-ATPase.
Mg^{++}-ATPase activity has indeed been found to be reduced in the
cytochalasin B and chlorpromazine models (3,11).   More recently
Mg^{++}-ATPase activity was shown to be correlated to the amount of
membrane myosin (7).   This provided evidence for a role of this
enzyme in the mechanism of bile secretion.   Microfilaments are also
inserted into the junctional complexes and changes in permeability
have been attributed to their dysfunction.   It has been postulated
that by increasing the permeability of the paracellular pathway and
consequently dissipating the osmotic gradient, bile flow might be
reduced as shown in the phalloïdin model (12).

TABLE II

POSTULATED ROLE FOR MICROFILAMENTS IN LIVER CELL

POSTULATED ROLE IN CANALICULAR FUNCTION	TYPE OF DYSFUNCTION INDUCED IN EXPERIMENTAL MODELS
CONTROL OF CANALICULAR MEMBRANE FLOW	DECREASE IN EXOCYTOTIC TRANSPORT
PRESERVATION OF THE INTEGRITY OF MEMBRANE COMPONENTS	DECREASE IN MEMBRANE ENZYME ACTIVITY
REGULATION OF INTERCELLULAR JUNCTIONAL COMPLEXES	INCREASE IN CANALICULAR PERMEABILITY

MICROFILAMENT DYSFUNCTION IN HUMAN CHOLESTASIS

     The demonstration that agents which interfere with bile flow in experimental models also disturb the normal arrangement of the micro-filaments has led to the suggestion that filament dysfunction may be a mechanism of cholestasis in some human entities. However the role of cytoskeleton proteins in human cholestasis has not been extensively investigated and no human counterpart of the experimental models has yet been described.

     By electron microscopy, the findings in human intrahepatic cholestasis are not specific, and are virtually identical to those observed after extrahepatic obstruction (10,13,14). The ultra-structural hallmarks comprise changes roughly confined to the bile secretory apparatus of the liver cell, i.e. bile canaliculi, peri-canalicular ectoplasm and Golgi complex. These changes are summarized in Table III. Among them, widening of the pericanali-cular ectoplasm has been documented in various hepatic disorders associated with cholestasis (Table IV) (14-17). This feature has been described as a thickening of the pericanalicular microfilament-rich ectoplasm (10), and the exact nature of these microfilaments is not well defined. It must be pointed out that the enlargement of the pericanalicular region in the described cholestatic entities has always been moderate. But in a recent study of adult patients with cholestasis, it was claimed that microfilament thickening was comparable to that found in experimental models. However this statement is not fully corroborated by the electron-micrographs presented (15).

TABLE   III

ULTRASTRUCTURAL ASPECTS OF CHOLESTASIS

- DEPOSIT OF BILE PIGMENTS IN CANALICULI,
  HEPATOCYTES AND KUPFFER CELLS

- ENLARGEMENT OF THE GOLGI APPARATUS

- INCREASE IN LYSOSOMAL ACTIVITY AND IN
  SMOOTH ENDOPLASMIC RETICULUM

- CANALICULAR DILATATION AND ALTERATION
  OF MICROVILLI

- WIDENING OF PERICANALICULAR ECTOPLASM

TABLE   IV

THICKENING OF PERICANALICULAR ECTOPLASM

IN ADULT AND CHILDREN CHOLESTASIS

CHANGES IN ADULTS: MODERATE

- PRIMARY BILIARY CIRRHOSIS

- VIRAL HEPATITIS

- ERYTHROMYCIN ESTOLATE ASSOCIATED CHOLESTASIS

- ORAL CONTRACEPTIVES ASSOCIATED CHOLESTASIS

- ACUTE ALCOHOLIC LIVER DISEASE

- EXTRAHEPATIC BILIARY OBSTRUCTION

CHANGES IN CHILDREN: A) MODERATE

- EXTRAHEPATIC BILIARY ATRESIA

- INTRAHEPATIC DUCTULAR HYPOPLASIA

B) SEVERE

- BYLER'S DISEASE

- NORTH AMERICAN INDIAN CIRRHOSIS

In children the same ultrastructural findings have been found
in cholestasis associated with hypoplasia of intrahepatic bile
ducts (18) as well as in advanced stages of biliary atresia (Table
IV).   On the other hand, severe changes in the pericanalicular area
have been documented in Byler's disease, a fatal form of cholestasis
(19,20).   Here the thickening of the microfilamentous ectoplasm
was so striking that it was compared to the hepatic lesion produced
in animals by chronic phalloïdin administration (14).   The question
was raised as to whether the abnormality in Byler's disease was
a microfilament disorder.   More recently we were able to demonstrate
similar pericanalicular changes in a group of North American Indian
children with a familial "non structural type" of cholestasis (21).
Furthermore we showed by immunofluorescence studies (22) the actin
content of these microfilaments.   The presence of canalicular microvilli until the late stages of the disease was at variance with the
findings in Byler's disease (Figure 5).   This observation, along

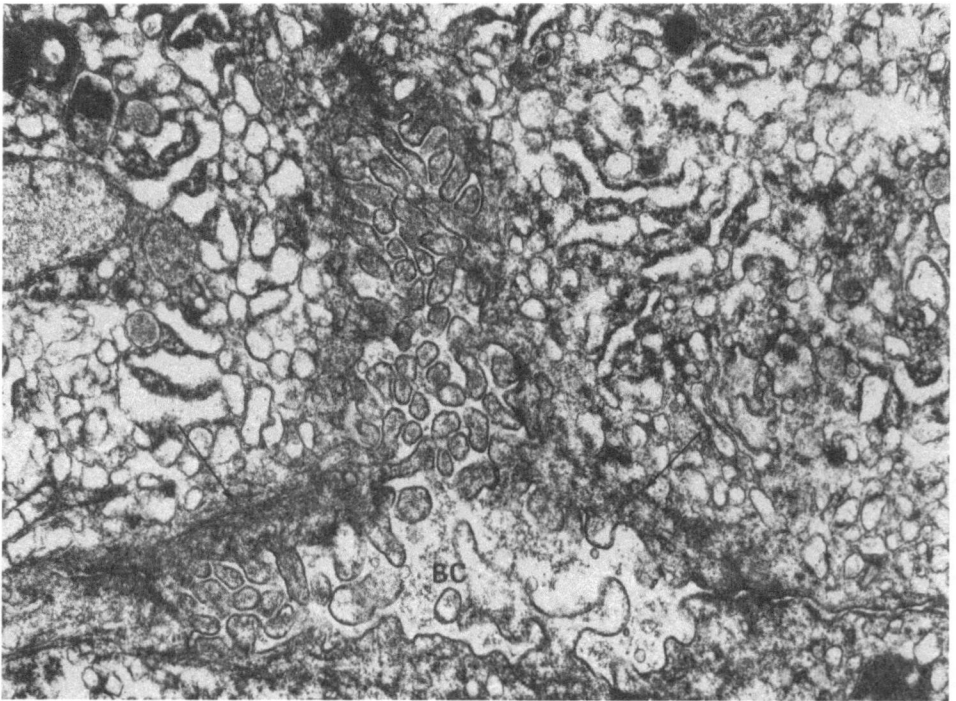

*Fig. 5   Electron microscopic appearance of the liver in a North
         American Indian child with severe cholestasis.   Thickening
         of the pericanalicular ectoplasm is noted.
         BC = bile canaliculus.*

with some particular clinical features, suggested that these two
entities might be different (23).   Furthermore, we still do not
know the exact nature of the filamentous material found in Byler's
disease.

It is too early to speculate on the possible cause and/or role
of microfilament dysfunction in children's cholestasis.   Examination of liver tissue by the methods described above are only beginning.   We propose that detection and characterization of such
abnormal filamentous deposits in the hepatocyte be used as a new
marker, in the hope to elucidate further these entities.   Since
in biliary cirrhosis associated with cystic fibrosis or biliary
atresia we did not find the electron microscopic and immunofluores-
cent changes described in Indian children, it is suggested that
microfilament dysfunction might be only involved in the familial
form of severe cholestasis in children.   Further studies on the
role of the submembranous cytoskeleton network in the regulation
of the chemical structure of the bile canalicular membrane might
help in the understanding of the pathogenesis of human familial
cholestasis.

SUMMARY

In hepatocytes, actin microfilaments appear in association
with the plasma membrane.   They are more abundant at the canalicular face which is morphologically almost always affected in
cholestasis.   In various experimental conditions, microfilament
dysfunction has been associated with cholestasis.   In rats,
phalloïdin-induced cholestasis is characterized by increased polymerisation of actin and a marked reduction in myosin.   On the other
hand, in the cholestatic models induced by cytochalasin B and norethandrolone, dissociation of microfilaments from their binding
sites has been observed.   Recently, it was shown that chlorpromazine
also interacts with actin.

Some thickening of the pericanalicular ectoplasm, consisting
of amorphous and microfilamental material, has been described in
adult patients with various liver diseases.   However, in all cases
the immunological reactivity of actin in the material has not been
documented.   In children with Byler's disease, this filamentous
zone has been found to be wider than in any other condition reported
in human liver.   More recently, by means of electron microscopy
and immunofluorescence techniques on liver cells, we documented
heavy accumulation of actin-containing microfilaments in a group
of North American Indian children with familial cholestasis, but
not in patients with biliary cirrhosis associated with extrahepatic
biliary atresia or cystic fibrosis.   This suggests that, at least
in children, microfilament accumulation and possible dysfunction
might only be found in the familial type of cholestatic syndromes.

REFERENCES

1. BOYER JL: New concepts of mechanisms of hepatocyte bile
       formation. Physiol Rev 60: 303-326, 1980.

2. FISHER MM, PHILLIPS MJ: Cytoskeleton of the hepatocyte.
       In Progress in Liver Diseases, volume VI. H Popper,
       F Schaffner (eds). Grune & Stratton, N.Y. 1978. pp 105-121.

3. ·ELIAS E, BOYER JL: Mechanisms of intrahepatic cholestasis.
       In Progress in Liver Diseases, volume VI. H Popper,
       F Schaffner (eds). Grune & Stratton, N.Y. 1978. pp 457-470.

4. DESMET VJ: Morphological features of intrahepatic cholestasis.
       In Problems in Intrahepatic Cholestasis. P Gentilini,
       H Popper, S Sherlock, U Teodori (eds). S. Karger, Basel.
       1979. pp. 11-18.

5. YOUSEF IM, MURRAY RK: Studies on the preparation of rat liver
       plasma membrane fractions and on their polypeptide patterns.
       Can J Biochem 56: 713-721, 1978.

6. TOYO-OKA T, OKAMOTO J, TANAKA T, MASSAKI T: Presence of
       smooth muscle myosin-like protein in liver cells.
       J Biochem (Tokyo) 87: 675-678, 1980.

7. YOUSEF IM, VONK RJ, TUCHWEBER B: Role of myosin-like protein
       in the cytoskeleton proteins of the hepatocyte.
       Gastroenterology 78: 1327, 1980.

8. PHILLIPS MJ, ODA M, YOUSEF IM, FUNATSU K: Effects of cyto-
       chalasin B on membrane-associated microfilaments in a
       cell free system. J Cell Biol (in press).

9. TUCHWEBER B, GABBIANI G: Phalloïdin-induced hyperplasia of
       actin filaments in rat hepatocytes. In The Liver:
       Quantitative Aspects of Structure and Function. R. Preisig,
       J Bircher, G Paumgartner (eds). Cantor, Aulendorf, 1976.
       pp 84-90.

10. PHILLIPS MJ: Electron microscopic findings in intrahepatic
       cholestasis. In Problems in Intrahepatic Cholestasis.
       P Gentilini, H Popper, S Sherlock, U Teodori (eds).
       S Karger, Basel, 1979. pp 19-29.

11. ELIAS E, BOYER JL: Chlorpromazine and its metabolites alter
       polymerization and gelation of actin. Science 206:
       1404-1406, 1980.

12. ELIAS E, HRUBAN Z, WADE JB, BOYER JL: Phalloïdin-induced

cholestasis: a microfilament-mediated change in junctional complex permeability. Proc Natl Aca Sci USA 77: 2229-2233, 1980.

13. DESMET VJ: Morphologic and histochemical aspects of chole-
    stasis. In Progress in Liver Diseases, volume IV.
    H Popper, F Schaffner (eds), Grune & Stratton, N.Y.
    1972, pp 97-132.

14. PHILLIPS MJ, ODA M, FUNATSU K: Cholestasis, its ultrastructural
    aspects. In Toxic Injury of the Liver. E Farber,
    MM Fisher (eds). M Dekker Inc., N.Y. 1979, pp 333-383.

15. ADLER M, CHUNG KW, SCHAFFNER F: Pericanalicular hepatocytic
    and bile ductular microfilaments in cholestasis in man.
    Am J Pathol 98: 603-610, 1980.

16. PHILLIPS MJ: Recent advances in the electron microscopic
    evaluation of the liver in cholestasis. In Neonatal
    Hepatitis and Biliary Atresia. NB Javitt (ed).
    DHEW, NIH, Bethesda, Md., 1979. pp 323-330.

17. BALAZS M: Comparative electron microscopic studies of benign
    hepatoma and icterus in patients on oral contraceptives.
    Virchows Arch (Path Anat) 381: 97-109, 1978.

18. SHARP HL, CAREY JB, WHITE JG, KRIVIT W: Cholestyramine therapy
    in patients with a paucity of intrahepatic bile ducts.
    J Pediatr 71: 723-736, 1967.

19. CLAYTON RJ, IBER FL, RUEBNER BH, McKUSICK VA: Byler Disease.
    Fatal familial intrahepatic cholestasis in an Amish
    Kindred. Amer J Dis Child 117: 112-124, 1969.

20. DE VOS R, DE WOLFE-PEETERS C, DESMET V, EGGERMONT E, VAN ACKER K:
    Progressive intrahepatic cholestasis (Byler's disease):
    case report. Gut 16: 943-950, 1975.

21. WEBER AM, TUCHWEBER B, ROY CC, et al: Neonatal intrahepatic
    cholestasis in North American Indians: a new entity?
    Gastroenterology 77: A46, 1979.

22. GABBIANI G, RYAN GB, LAMELIN JP et al: Human smooth muscle
    autoantibody: its identification as antiactin antibody
    and a study of its binding to nonmuscular cells.
    Am J Pathol 72: 473-488, 1973.

23. WEBER AM, TUCHWEBER B, YOUSEF I et al: Severe familial chole-
    stasis in North American Indian children: a clinical model
    of microfilament dysfunction? Gastroent 81: 653-662, 1981.

DISCUSSION

CHAIRMAN: J.L. WEBER

THALER: Dr. Weber, have you had the opportunity to study other
     forms of chronic liver disease?

A.M. WEBER: Not yet.

ISSENMAN: Marasmic infants studied in Chile had similar ultra-
     structural changes in microfilaments.   Might the changes
     be due to malnutrition?

A.M. WEBER: I didn't know that microfilament changes had been
     described in marasmus.   The subjects of our study were
     thriving normally and not malnourished at all.   The problem
     is quite different from Byler's disease where one finds
     growth and mental retardation.

RIELY: Is it possible that the EM changes and the results of the
     immunofluorescence studies are secondary?   This is a severe
     cholestatic syndrome and you would think that if these
     changes were the cause of the disease they would be there
     initially.

A.M. WEBER: I agree.   We can't tell if the changes are primary
     or secondary.   But in terms of a metabolic disease it is
     reasonable to postulate that it would take a few months or
     years before the accumulation is found in the biopsies.

130

EXTRAHEPATIC BILIARY ATRESIA: CLINICAL ASPECTS

Daniel Alagille

Unité de Recherche d'Hépatologie Infantile, INSERM U 56
& Clinique de Pédiatrie, Université Paris-Sud
Hôpital d'Enfants, Bicêtre, France

INTRODUCTION

The early diagnosis between intra- and extra-hepatic
cholestasis is essential since the latter can be treated surgically.
Until a few years ago, there were arguments against such an approach:
these included the "non correctability" of extrahepatic biliary
atresia, the rare occurrence of other forms of extrahepatic cholestasis and the adverse effects of surgery in patients with intrahepatic cholestasis.   Surgery was performed only in cases of
unresolved cholestasis after several months of evolution.   This
attitude has been challenged recently because surgical treatment
of extrahepatic biliary atresia is available and positive results
of surgical therapy are related to early intervention.

Between 1964 and 1978 (1), 331 cases of cholestasis in neonates
and infants were admitted at the Hôpital d'Enfants de Bicêtre:
177 patients with extrahepatic and 154 patients with intrahepatic
cholestasis.

COMMON CLINICAL SIGNS OF EXTRA-, AND INTRA-HEPATIC CHOLESTASIS

Clinical Signs

Jaundice is accompanied by dark urine and acholic stools.
The daily variation in stool colour is so important that it should
be described on the infant's hospital chart by experienced personnel
with the help of coloured disks.   There is no pruritus before
four to five months of age.   The liver size is always increased.

131

Laboratory Tests

Mixed hyperbilirubinemia is associated with an increase in total serum lipid levels, particularly of cholesterol. Serum alkaline phosphatase and 5'-nucleotidase levels are usually increased.

STATISTICAL STUDY

Clinical signs

Thirty-one clinical features obtained in 162 infants with cholestasis were subjected to computer analysis (2). The four following criteria appeared very useful to the pediatrician: 1) the colour of the stools during 10 consecutive days; 2) birth weight; 3) age at the beginning of stool discoloration; 4) the clinical features of hepatomegaly. With these criteria, intra-hepatic cholestasis could be differentiated from extrahepatic cholestasis in 82% of 162 patients studied. No other clinical or laboratory criterion increased this percentage. Normal birth weight, early stool discoloration which becomes permanent and complete, firm even hard hepatomegaly and signs of increasing cholestasis are more in favour of extrahepatic bile duct obstruction. However, prolonged periods of observation may be detrimental to patients with surgically correctable extrahepatic cholestasis.

Histologic signs

Patients underwent a needle biopsy of the liver within three weeks following admission. The histologic data were computerized. The most significant histologic criteria were: 1) ductular pro-liferation; 2) bile thrombi in portal areas; 3) significant portal fibrosis; 4) focal necrosis of the hepatic cells.

The four significant histologic findings were then added to the preceding four discriminant variables: the resulting eight variables were programmed by the computer as follows: 1) bile ductular proliferation; 2) stool colour within 10 days after admission; 3) birth weight; 4) age at onset of acholic stools; 5) focal liver cell necrosis; 6) intraportal bile thrombi; 7) clinical features of liver involvement; 8) portal fibrosis. These eight observations permitted accurate identification of extrahepatic and intrahepatic cholestasis in 85% of the patients tested.

BIOLOGICAL FINDINGS

The following laboratory tests have all been used in the differential diagnosis of intra- and extra-hepatic cholestasis, but none is unequivocally diagnostic. The red cell hydrogen

peroxide hemolysis test and the vitamin E absorption test have
recently been advocated (3).   Serum alpha-fetoprotein is increased
in neonatal hepatitis (4).   However, when radioimmunoassay techniques are used, there is an overlap between neonatal hepatitis
and extrahepatic cholestasis values (5).   Serum lipoprotein-X is
present in all cases of severe intra- or extra-hepatic cholestasis
(6).   A decrease in serum levels following cholestyramine therapy
has been suggested as an argument against a diagnosis of extrahepatic biliary atresia.   The increased serum concentration of bile
acids in extrahepatic biliary atresia is not significant (7) and
the chenodeoxycholate/cholate ratio is not discriminatory either (8).
Serum 5'-nucleotidases are secreted by the biliary epithelium;
since neoductular proliferation is characteristic of extrahepatic
biliary atresia, an increase in serum 5'-nucleotidase may be in
favour of this diagnosis (9).   Finally, ^{14}C-cholate stool excretion
is extremely low in patients with extrahepatic biliary atresia (10).
Some of these tests are difficult to perform and their discriminating
value is apparently not any better than that of the ^{131}I rose bengal
test.   In this test, an intestinal excretion of less than 10% of
the injected dose after 72 hours is consistent with complete
cholestasis.   When more than 20% of the injected dose is excreted,
the extrahepatic biliary tract is not completely obstructed.
Interpretation is difficult when excretion is between 10 and 20% of
the injected dose (11,12).   The classical ^{131}I rose bengal test
is an excellent investigation tool when surgical indications are
doubtful (Table I).   In our experience, combination of clinical
history, physical examination, percutaneous liver biopsy and ^{131}I
rose bengal test allows the right diagnosis in 95% of cases.

TABLE I

ROSE BENGAL TEST IN NEONATAL CHOLESTASIS

DIAGNOSIS	NO. OF TESTS	RANGE (%)	MEAN (%)	REMARKS
Extrahepatic biliary atresia	64	1.4-14.0	4.58	1 test > 10%
Neonatal hepatitis	24	3.2-91.0	31.0	3 tests < 10% (12.5% of patients)
Syndromatic paucity of interlobular bile ducts	13	3.0-64.0	19.8	4 tests < 10% (30.8% of patients)
Alpha-1-antitrypsin deficiency	7	4.6-13.7	8.8	5 tests < 10% (71.4% of patients)

RADIOLOGIC EXAMINATION

Extrahepatic biliary atresia is the most common but not the
only congenital abnormality of the extrahepatic biliary tract:
choledochal cysts and diffuse dilatation of the biliary tract are
not rare in infants (13). This is why biliary ultrasonography
should be performed as soon as possible in infants with complete
cholestasis. This leads quickly to the right diagnosis and to a
decision concerning surgery (14,15,16,17).

There is no single specific test for either intra- or extrahepatic cholestasis. Intravenous cholangiography is never
performed in patients with complete cholestasis (18).

ASSOCIATED ABNORMALITIES

The association of multiple abnormalities can help make the
diagnosis of extrahepatic biliary atresia. In Ivemark asplenia
syndrome, extrahepatic biliary atresia is never observed. On the
contrary, extrahepatic biliary atresia is common in the polysplenia
syndrome. Scintigraphy is helpful to assess the presence or
absence of the spleen.

CONCLUSION

Extrahepatic cholestasis in infants is usually easy to
distinguish from intrahepatic cholestasis. When complete and
permanent cholestasis is diagnosed, surgery should be performed as
soon as possible during the first few weeks of life: most of the
time radioisotopic examinations and percutaneous liver biopsy are
not necessary. Cases with early incomplete cholestasis may be
submitted to phenobarbital and cholestyramine therapy for one or
two weeks. If no clinical improvement occurs, they should be
explored surgically. Surgery should be done before three months
of age. At that age, the diagnosis is evident but the long-term
prognosis is poor. Surgical exploration is contra-indicated when,
in spite of intravenous vitamin K injection, blood clotting factors
remain below 50% of normal levels.

SUMMARY

The differential diagnosis between intra- and extra-hepatic
cholestasis is essential since the latter can be treated surgically.
Thirty-one clinical and histologic features obtained in 288 infants
with cholestasis were subjected to computer analysis. The resulting
8 variables were programmed by the computer as follows: 1) bile
ductular proliferation; 2) stool colour within 10 days after
admission; 3) birth weight; 4) age at onset of acholic stools;
5) focal liver cell necrosis; 6) intraportal bile thrombi; 7)
clinical features of liver involvement; 8) portal fibrosis.

These 8 criteria permitted accurate identification of extrahepatic
and intrahepatic cholestasis in 85% of the patients tested.   The
classical ^{131}I rose bengal test is an excellent investigation tool
when surgical indications are doubtful.   Its results, combined
with the former eight, allow the right diagnosis in 95% of the
cases.   Ultrasonography, performed as soon as possible in infants
with complete cholestasis, leads quickly to the right diagnosis and
to a decision concerning surgery.   The association of multiple
abnormalities can help in the diagnosis of extrahepatic biliary
atresia.

REFERENCES

1. ALAGILLE D, ODIEVRE M: Liver and Biliary Tract Disease in
        Children. Wiley and Sons, New York, 1979. pp. 68-93.

2. ALAGILLE D: Cholestasis in the first 3 months of life. In
        Progress in Liver Diseases, volume VI. H Popper,
        F Schaffner (eds). Grune & Stratton, N.Y. 1979. pp 471-485.

3. MELHORN DK, GROSS S, IZANT RJ: The red cell hydrogen peroxide
        hemolysis test and vitamin E absorption in the differential
        diagnosis of jaundice in infancy. J Pediatr 81: 1082-
        1087, 1972.

4. ZELTZER PM, FONKALSRUD EW, NEERHOUT RC, STIEHM ER: Differentia-
        tion between neonatal hepatitis and biliary atresia by
        measuring serum alpha-fetoprotein. Lancet 1: 373-375, 1974.

5. JOHNSTON DI, MOWAT AP, ORR H, KOHN J: Serum alpha-fetoprotein
        levels in extrahepatic biliary atresia, idiopathic neo-
        natal hepatitis and alpha-1-antitrypsin deficiency (PiZ).
        Acta Paediatr Scand 65: 623-629, 1974.

6. CAMPBELL DP, POLEY JR, ALAUPOVIC P, SMITH EI: The differential
        diagnosis of neonatal hepatitis and biliary atresia.
        J Pediatr Surg 9: 699-705, 1974.

7. JAVITT NB, MORRISSEY KP, SIEGEL E, GOLDBERG H, GARTNER LM,
        HOLLANDER M, KOK E: Cholestatic syndromes in infancy:
        diagnostic value of serum bile acid pattern and chole-
        styramine administration. Pediatr Res 7: 119-125, 1973.

8. JAVITT NB, KEATING JP, GRAND RJ, HARRIS RC: Serum bile acid
        patterns in neonatal hepatitis and extrahepatic biliary
        atresia. J Pediatr 90: 736-739, 1977.

9. YEUNG CY: Serum 5'-nucleotidase in neonatal hepatitis and
        biliary atresia. Pediatrics 50: 812-820, 1972.

10. NORMAN A, STRANDVIK B: Excretion of bile acids in extrahepatic
       biliary atresia and intrahepatic cholestasis of infancy.
       Acta Paediatr Scand 62: 253-263, 1973.

11. DESBUQUOIS B, TRON P, ALAGILLE D: Etude de l'excretion fécale
       et urinaire du Rose Bengale marqué par l'iode radioactif
       au cours des ictères obstructifs du nouveau-né et du
       nourrisson. Arch Fr Pediatr 25: 379-391, 1968.

12. SHARP HL, KRIVIT W, LOWMAN JT: The diagnosis of complete
       extrahepatic obstruction by Rose Bengal I^{131}. J Pediatr
       70: 46-53, 1967.

13. MIYANO T, SURUGA K, SUDA K: Abnormal choledocho-pancreatico
       ductal junction related to the etiology of infantile
       obstructive jaundice diseases. J Pediatr Surg 14: 16-26,
       1979.

14. TAYLOR KJW, ROSENFIELD AT: Grey-scale ultrasonography in the
       differential diagnosis of jaundice. Arch Surg 112:
       820-825, 1977.

15. LAPSIS JL, ORLANDO RC, MITTELSTAEDT CA, STAAB EV: Ultrasono-
       graphy in the diagnosis of obstructive jaundice. Ann
       Intern Med 89: 61-63, 1979.

16. DEWBURY KC, JOSEPH AEA, HAYES S, MURRAY C: Ultrasound in the
       evaluation and diagnosis of jaundice. Br J Radiol 52:
       276-280, 1979.

17. Editorial: Noninvasive methods for diagnosis of jaundice.
       Lancet 2: 18-20, 1979.

18. CHAUMONT P, FORTIER-BEAULIEU M, GUBERT JP, SAVARY M,
       SILVERSTOFF S: Indications des explorations vasculaires
       hépatiques et spléniques chez l'enfant. J Radio Electrol
       51: 696-705, 1970.

PATHOLOGY AND PATHOGENESIS OF EXTRAHEPATIC BILIARY ATRESIA

C.L. Witzleben

Professor of Pathology, University of Pennsylvania
School of Medicine and Director, Anatomic and Clinical
Pathology, Children's Hospital of Philadelphia

To discuss the pathology and pathogenesis of extrahepatic
biliary atresia (EHBA) is not a simple task, since we have no
current evidence incriminating any particular pathogenesis, and
since the pathology is, like all qualitative morphologic data,
somewhat subjective.

I shall first of all review certain specific aspects of the
pathology of EHBA as I have personally seen them.   Then I shall
attempt to formulate a description or characterization of the
pathogenetic process or processes we are seeking, based on these
pathologic findings and on certain clinical features as we currently
know them.   I shall conclude by briefly examining how well a
recently-proposed pathogenesis fits this characterization or
description.

A discussion of the pathology of EHBA naturally concentrates
on the duct system.   However, I should point out that although
duct pathology is an obvious focal point in a study of the pathogenesis of EHBA, there are several reasons why this pathology may
not be as critically revealing as we might hope.   One reason is
that we are at present observing and describing the duct changes
relatively late in their chronologic evolution, namely, when
complete obstruction has developed and been present for some period
of time.   Another reason is that in focussing on the bile duct
changes we may be looking at a phenomenon which is downstream,
literally and/or figuratively, in a pathologic sequence, and which
may be relatively remote from the pathogenetic springhead.   The
third reason is that we are required to interpret the fine (and
possibly critical) pathologic details largely without good control
material.   Despite these detractions from the value of our current

137

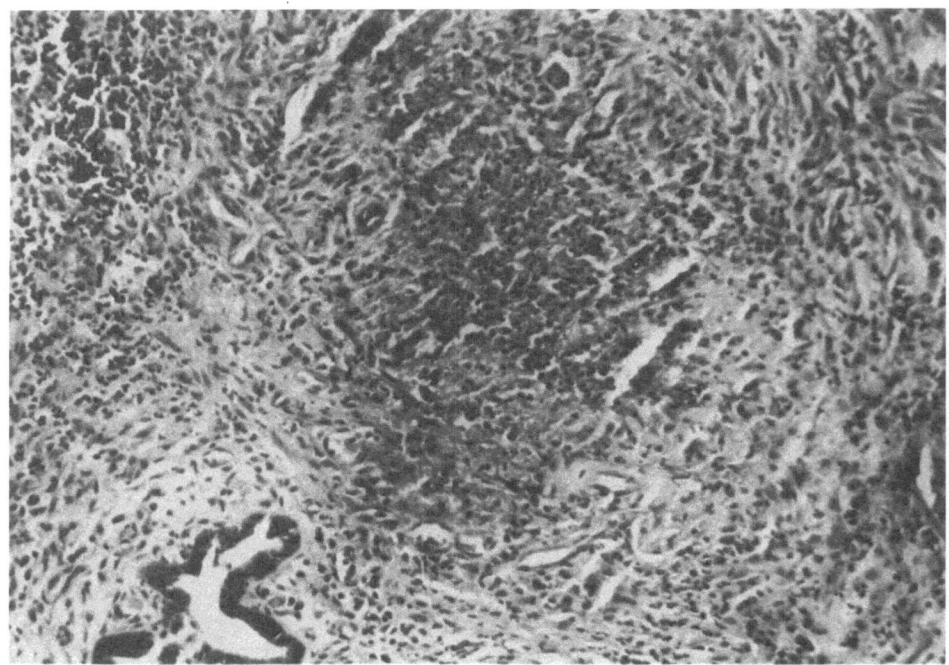

*Fig. 1   Light micrograph of porta hepatis from patient with EHBA.
An area of necrosis and acute inflammation in the center
of the field.   This is assumed to be a focus of recent
duct destruction.   A small duct element is present at
lower left.   Original magnification 10X, hematoxylin
and eosin.*

morphologic impressions of the pathology of the duct system, it
nevertheless seems appropriate to describe and analyze the duct
pathology as thoroughly as possible, since this may yield important
information in understanding the pathogenesis of this disorder.

     We now know that at the time hepatoportoenterostomy (HPE) is
usually done (6-8 weeks of age) the extrahepatic tree is the site
of active pathology (1,2,3).   This pathology includes a "classical"
pattern or spectrum of lesions, ranging from necrosis of the duct
epithelium and acute inflammation through chronic inflammation and
epithelial regeneration, and extending to scarring (Figures 1-5).
With the possible exception of so-called "primary" sclerosing
cholangitis (4), this pattern of lesions seems unique to the perinatal age group.   All areas of the extrahepatic tree have been
demonstrated to be involved with the inflammation and scarring.
Active epithelial injury or necrosis in the gallbladder seems only

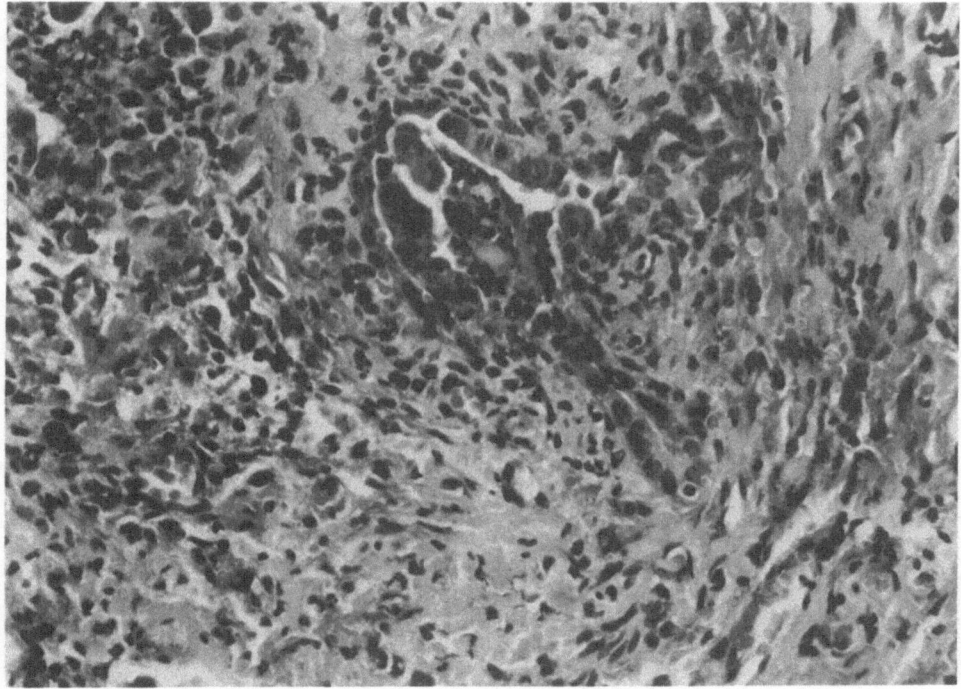

*Fig. 2 Light micrograph of duct from porta hepatis from patient
with EHBA, showing active necrosis of duct epithelium.
Original magnification 20X, hematoxylin and eosin.*

rarely observed.   But frequently the gallbladder is only a fibrous
remnant in cases of biliary atresia, so the opportunity to study
the gallbladder epithelium has been somewhat limited.   It is
important to recognize that the ducts which can be identified in
the extrahepatic tree in these patients are abnormally small.
This fact suggests either that the active pathology develops in
(is due to?) a malformed/hypoplastic duct system, or that the
destructive processes have been active sufficiently long so that
normal ducts have been previously destroyed and have been replaced
by smaller duct elements (in which the pathologic processes are
continuing).   The "stage" of the lesion (ranging from acute injury
to scarring) varies from patient to patient and from area to area
in an individual patient.   In individual patients there appears
to be a propensity for the lesions to be more active or acute in
the more proximal areas, particularly the porta.   This latter
finding could mean either a) that the distal areas are the first
affected by some primary process, or b) that a primary process
persists longer in the proximal ducts, or c) that the proximal
areas are the site of some additional or secondary process.

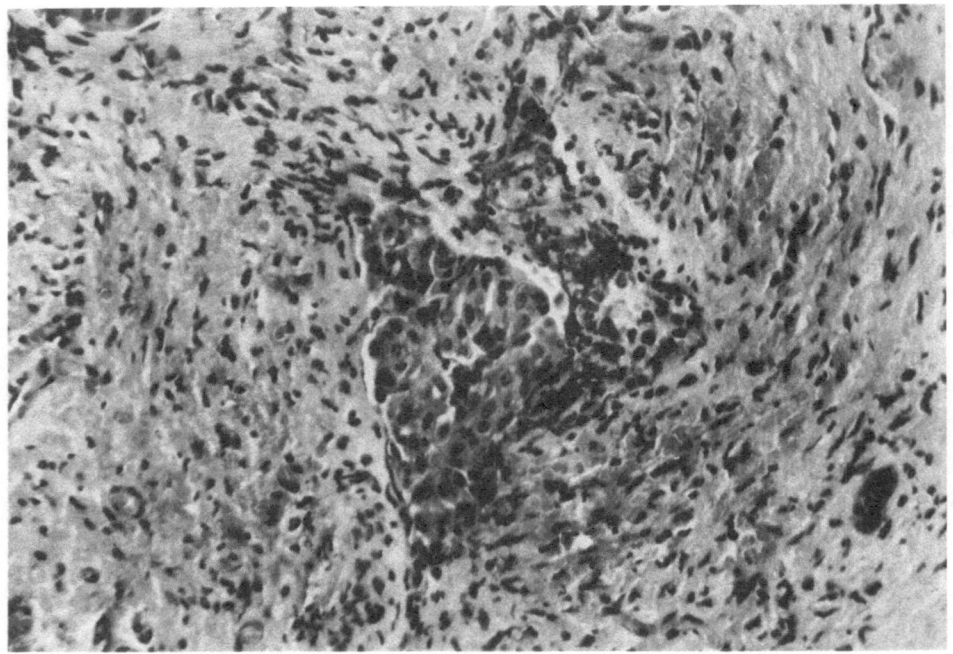

Fig. 3 *Light micrograph of small duct from porta hepatis. There has been proliferation of epithelial cells, indicative of a regenerative response. Original magnification 20X, hematoxylin and eosin.*

The demonstration of epithelial necrosis does not necessarily prove that this necrosis is the originating cause for the luminal obliteration which defines biliary atresia. If we were observing such necrosis in ducts of normal size, this would perhaps be the only reasonable assumption. Since, however, we are observing it in abnormally small ducts located proximally in an occluded system, we cannot eliminate the possibility that the epithelial injury is due to the small size and/or lack of patency of the duct system (i.e. is caused by bile secretory pressure in a small or occluded system). In other words, we do not know if the ducts are necrotic because they are small, or if they are small because the normal large ducts have been previously necrosed. If damage is due to bile secretory pressure in a small or obstructed system, one might anticipate finding bile pigment in and around the injured ducts. Generally speaking, bile pigment is uncommon in the areas of duct injury. Whether or not this disproves this possibility is problematic.

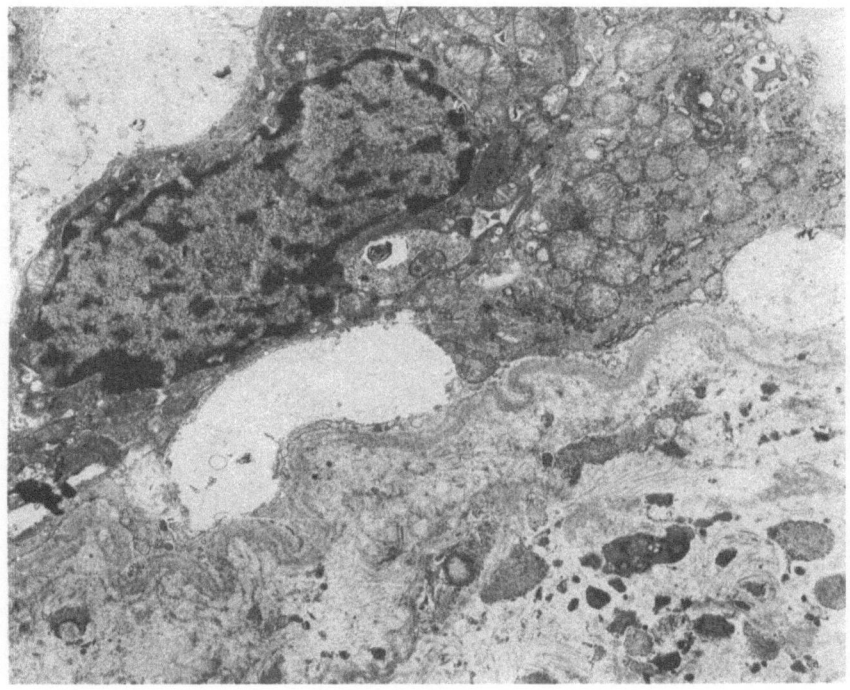

*Fig. 4   Electron micrograph of duct epithelium from porta hepatis.
Although the epithelial cells are relatively intact,
there is mitochondrial swelling in the cell on the right,
and large vacuoles are present in or immediately beneath
the base of the cells.   Original magnification 1500X.*

The frequent end-stage status (scarring, little inflammation)
of the distal area of the duct system at 6-8 weeks suggests that
the lesion, in this area at least, is of considerable duration,
probably beginning near birth or perhaps in utero.   I have already
mentioned the possible explanations for the frequent differences
in appearance between the distal and proximal tree.

I shall not attempt to discuss possible etiologies, except to
observe that search for cytomegalic, hepatitis B, hepatitis A,
and EB viruses, on liver and/or porta tissue, or in the sera of
patients and their mothers (1), has so far revealed no evidence to
suggest that infection with any of these agents is a cause of EHBA.
Also to date no "toxic" biliary substance has been identified, and
experimental attempts to create atresia through vascular insufficiency have yielded results which are indeterminate at best.

It is potentially important also to consider the duct system

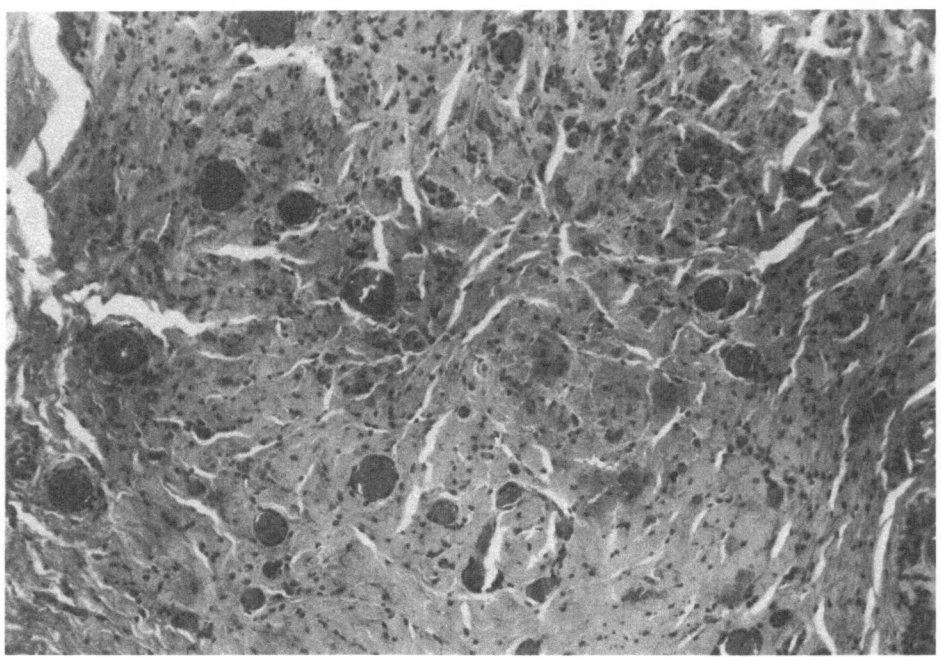

Fig. 5 Light micrograph of common duct area showing no duct lumen;
*   only well-vascularized fibrous tissue is present.   It*
*   appears likely that this represents an end-stage of the*
*   destructive process illustrated in Figures 1 and 2.*
*   Original magnification 10X, hematoxylin and eosin.*

within the liver.   Haas (3) has reported that there are necrotic
changes in the intrahepatic ducts essentially identical to those
which I have illustrated and discussed in the extrahepatic ducts.
In our material, the epithelial changes in the extrahepatic system
have been substantially more dramatic than in the intrahepatic
ducts and the presence of frank necrosis in the latter ducts has
been difficult to demonstrate.   Nor have we seen as dramatic an
inflammatory and reparative response in the portal tracts.   Possibly this difference in the two duct systems is similar or analogous
to that seen in the various areas of the extrahepatic tree.
Specifically, the intrahepatic duct changes may tend to be somewhat
"younger" than those seen in the extrahepatic tree.   During the
time period of which I have been speaking, the portal tracts show
quite marked inflammation and an increase in bile ductules.   The
acute inflammation in the portal tracts is largely found at their
periphery, in close relation to proliferating ductules.   The
ductular proliferation is the hepatic histologic hallmark of

extrahepatic obstruction and has traditionally been assumed to be
the result of the retention of bile components (presumably bile
acids), which are also held to be responsible for the acute inflammation.   As far as we are aware, the large portal tract bile ducts
in the liver periphery are present in normal numbers and have
normal diameters.

    There is, of course, an opportunity to observe the intrahepatic
duct changes over a longer period than the extrahepatic duct changes,
and this opportunity has yielded useful data in understanding
something about the disease process of extrahepatic atresia in its
entirety.   Haas (3) has reported persisting epithelial injury in
the intrahepatic ducts following "successful" HPE.   It has been
recognized for many years that with prolonged unrelieved atresia
the intrahepatic ducts tend to decrease in number ("disappearing
ducts" (5)).   Traditionally this has been attributed to "disuse
atrophy" of the ducts, but Landing (6) has raised the possibility
that it represents an extension in time and/or space of the obliterative process acting in the extrahepatic tree.   It is uncertain
which of these explanations is correct.   On the one hand there are
no data from other disorders establishing the occurrence of "disuse
atrophy" of bile ducts.   On the other hand, the "disappearance"
of ducts seems to be ameliorated by the establishment of bile
drainage by HPE.   Although the number and size of intrahepatic
ducts in patients with successful HPE have not been quantitatively
or even semi-quantitatively evaluated, it seems evident that neither
anatomic intrahepatic atresia nor severe cholestasis develops in
these patients.   This is despite the fact that portal fibrosis
can persist and perhaps even progress, and that portal hypertension
can develop (or at least become evident) after successful HPE (1).
The role (if any) of occult cholangitis in the persistent or progressive portal tract lesion is not known.   Despite the prolonged
persistence of portal tract lesions in patients with successful
HPE, the processes involved in the initiation and progression of
the liver disease eventually terminate in patients in whom the
complications of cholangitis can be managed.   It appears that the
basic processes in EHBA are in some sense "self-limited".

    I would like to digress and discuss EHBA as a congenital
anomaly.   Although EHBA was initially thought to be a developmental
defect, the recognition that it is rarely (if ever) seen in stillborns or neonates, and that the incidence of associated anomalies
is quite low, has led to the conclusion that EHBA is a post-natally
acquired disease.   This belief seemed to be strengthened by the
finding of active pathology in the specimens of the extrahepatic
biliary tree which became available from HPE.   There has, however,
been a growing recognition that in one congenital anomaly complex
there is an unusual incidence of EHBA.   This is the polysplenia
syndrome, in which it has been estimated that the incidence of
EHBA is in the range of 22% (7).   This observation suggests at

least two promising avenues of study: 1) attempts should be made
to compare the pathology of the extrahepatic tree in cases of EHBA
with and without polysplenia syndrome, and 2) methodical microscopic examination of the extrahepatic tree should be done in all
autopsied cases of polysplenia syndrome, especially those who die
in the first weeks of life.   The first of these studies could
throw light on the question of whether or not all cases of EHBA
are of malformative origin, and the second would reveal the earliest
post-natal stages of EHBA (of at least one "type").

If one assembles the pathologic features we have discussed,
and adds to them certain established clinical facts, it is possible
to sketch an outline of the pathogenic process involved in EHBA.
This process is sporadic in occurrence and tends to occur in females.
It may be particularly prone to develop in babies born to mothers
residing in Japan.   It is active in later intrauterine or early
neonatal life, does not reach its end-stage before that age period,
and does not occur at any older age.   It is self-limited (although
it may be prolonged), and is characterized morphologically by the
presence of excessive numbers of abnormally small extrahepatic ducts,
duct epithelial necrosis, inflammation, fibrosis, and complete loss
of duct lumens.

It is evident that this outline does not readily identify any
pathogenetic process for EHBA.   It may, however, be useful in
evaluating various pathogenetic possibilities, and in determining
which among these should be most vigorously pursued.   I would
like to conclude by demonstrating the possible use of this description in evaluating (and perhaps modifying) theories of the pathogenesis of EHBA.

It has recently been proposed (8) that EHBA may be the result
of inadequate L-proline synthesis in the early post-natal period.
This hypothesis is based on data indicating that L-proline is a
growth factor for bile duct epithelium in experimental animals,
and that in the blood of patients with EHBA (and certain other
possibly related neonatal liver disorders) there are increased
levels of L-glutamic acid (the major precursor of L-proline) and
low to low normal levels of L-proline.   The fact that L-proline is
a growth factor, presumably critical in the developmental period,
places this hypothesis in general accord with a major element in
our description of the pathogenetic process in EHBA.   However,
effects exerted specifically on the post-natal growth of the biliary
tree would appear to be relatively unimportant in the pathogenesis
of EHBA as described (since the extrahepatic ducts which can be
found in EHBA at 6-8 weeks are much smaller than those seen in the
normal neonate).   This objection, however, would require no more
than a modification of the L-proline theory to include the presence
and operation of such a deficiency in utero.   A more difficult
problem exists in explaining the role of L-proline deficiency in

creating the active pathology in the extrahepatic tree.   Such a
role would appear to depend upon either the ability of L-proline
deficiency to cause epithelial necrosis, or evidence that the
epithelial injury could reasonably be attributed to bile secretory
pressure in a small biliary tree.   On the basis of our profile
of the pathogenetic process involved in EHBA it would appear that
until one or the other of these latter effects can be established,
the hypothesis that L-proline causes EHBA is flawed.

REFERENCES

1. WITZLEBEN CL: Extrahepatic biliary atresia: concepts of
    cause, diagnoses and management. In Perspectives in
    Pediatric Pathology, Volume V.   H Rosenberg, R Bolande (eds)
    Masson, N.Y. 1979. pp. 41-62.

2. WITZLEBEN CL, BUCK BE, SCHNAUFER L, BROSZKO L: Studies on the
    pathogenesis of biliary atresia. Lab Invest 38: 525-531,
    1978.

3. HAAS J: Bile duct and liver pathology in biliary atresia.
    World J Surg 2: 561-569, 1978.

4. EDITORIAL: An unusual cholangitis. Brit Med J 2: 1090, 1976.

5. LANDING B, WELLS T, REED G, NARAYAN M: Disease of the bile
    ducts in children. In The Liver.   E Gall, F Mostofi (eds)
    Williams and Wilkens, 1973. pp 480-509.

6. LANDING B: Considerations on the pathogenesis of neonatal
    hepatitis, biliary atresia, and choledochal cyst - the
    concept of infantile obstructive cholangiopathy. In Progress
    in Pediatric Surgery, volume VI. AH Bill, M Kasai (eds).
    University Park Press, Baltimore, 1974.

7. MAKSEM J: Polysplenia syndrome and splenic hypoplasia associated
    with extrahepatic biliary atresia. Arch Pathol Lab Med
    104: 212-214, 1980.

8. VACANTI J, FOLKMAN J: Bile duct enlargement by infusion of
    L-proline: potential significance in biliary atresia.
    J Pediat Surg 14: 814-818, 1979.

THE SURGERY OF BILIARY ATRESIA: CURRENT INVESTIGATIONS

John R. Lilly and Christine M.L. Pau[§]

Department of Surgery
University of Colorado School of Medicine
Denver, Colorado

Until the past decade surgical attempts to correct biliary
atresia were uniformly unsuccessful.   In 1968 a new operation
was introduced by Dr. Morio Kasai (1) in which the extrahepatic
bile ducts were radically excised and replaced by an intestinal
conduit.   Dr. Kasai reported success in almost a quarter of his
cases.   The early American experience with the operation was dismal;
the initial reporting institution described not only outright
failure in every patient but a suspected shortened life expectancy
(2).   Because of the widely disparate results, an investigation
of Kasai's operation was instituted under the auspices of the
Children's Clinical Research Center in Denver beginning in 1974.

As of January 1980, 51 patients with biliary atresia were
treated by Kasai's operation.   Bile drainage was attained in 31
instances.   In nine patients, however, relief of biliary obstruction was insufficient to restore adequate liver function and all
died of complications of hepatic failure from 9 to 17 months after
operation.   In these patients, the quality and quantity of biliary
flow insidiously decreased several months after operation and, in
retrospect, was the first manifestation of the lethal prognosis.
In the remaining 22 patients, biliary drainage was sustained and
was coincident with a return toward good health and normal developmental landmarks (3).   The overall results and actuarial survival
analysis have been previously reported (4).   Despite relief of
biliary obstruction, multiple complications plagued almost all
patients.   In this communicaton we will concentrate on the special

[§]Visiting Assistant Professor of Surgery, C.H.U. Hôpital de la
Timone des Enfants, Boul. Jean-Molin, 13005 Marseille, France

therapeutic problems involved in the peri-operative care of patients
with biliary atresia.

INTRAOPERATIVE FACTORS

The extrahepatic biliary remnant.   The sine qua non for technical
success at operation is the identification of a true bile duct.
In reviewing our case material three basic types of microscopic
biliary structures at the porta hepatis were distinguished:
1) bile ducts, 2) collecting ductules of biliary glands, and 3)
biliary glands.   The latter two structures are normal morphological
components of the extrahepatic biliary system.   Neither communicates
with the intrahepatic bile ducts and consequently will not drain
into the juxtaposed bowel.   In the past both biliary glands and
collecting ductules of biliary glands were confused for true bile
ducts at operative histologic sectioning and an intestinal anastomosis
was done to the porta hepatis with no chance for success.   In our
series, postoperative drainage occurred only in patients in whom
a true bile duct was identified in the proximal portion of the
excised extrahepatic biliary system (5).   Currently, if such a
structure is not seen on immediate histologic section, re-excision
of the porta hepatis is carried out.

Biliary reconstruction.   Our early experience with the original
Kasai "closed" type of biliary reconstruction demonstrated conclu-
sively that exteriorization was essential to control postoperative
cholangitis.   Because of dissatisfaction with alternate types of
biliary reconstruction in use at the time, we evaluated a new
procedure beginning in 1974 which incorporated a Mikulicz exteriorized anastomosis in the bilio-enteric conduit (Figure 1).   The
reconstruction permitted an accurate assessment of bile flow during
the critical first weeks after operation, thus permitting early
reoperation if indicated (infra vide).   In addition, the double-
barreled exteriorization allowed handy refeeding of bile into the
"intestinal" stoma.   Absorption of fats and fat soluble vitamins
was thereby facilitated.   Employment of the gallbladder and distal
extrahepatic bile ducts, when patent, as the biliary conduit (Figure
2) was also evaluated (6).   Cholangitis never occurred under these
circumstances.   However, two of five children with the "gallbladder
Kasai" had to be converted to a standard intestinal conduit because
of subsequent loss of patency of the distal bile ducts.   Nevertheless, the absence of postoperative cholangitis, we believe, justifies
the risk of the procedure.

COMPONENTS OF BILE

    One of our first investigations was to document the components
of biliary drainage after operation.   This study demonstrated that
bile pigments and lipids were excreted in progressive amounts in
bile (Figure 3) and that previously elevated serum values returned

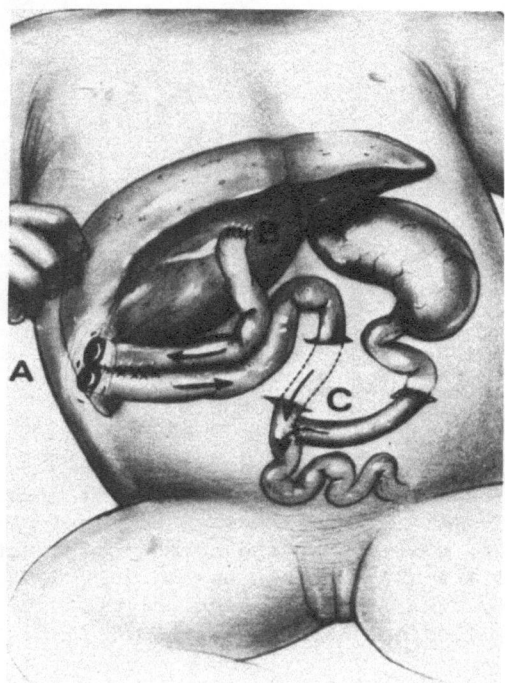

*Fig. 1 Drawing of the biliary reconstruction used in the Denver
          series of patients with biliary atresia. The bilio-
          enteric conduit is exteriorized as a Mikulicz enterostomy.
          Bile drainage from the liver is collected, an aliquot taken
          for analysis and then refed into the "intestinal" stoma.
          Exteriorization is now done in the left upper abdomen rather
          than in the right as shown because of encroachment by
          the liver.*

towards normal (7).   A parallel study involved postoperative
alterations in copper kinetics.   Analyses of hepatic copper were
carried out in patients before and at intervals after operation
and the results correlated with copper concentrations in postoperative bile.   An inverse linear relationship between biliary
copper excretion and hepatic copper deposition was established (8).
Thus, relief of biliary obstruction resulted in a return towards
normal metabolism of bile pigments, biliary lipids and copper.

RECURRENT CHOLANGITIS

    Our initial approach to the control of cholangitis was to treat
all infants with antibiotics for the first year after operation.
Qualitative and quantitative bacteriological studies of bile drainage,

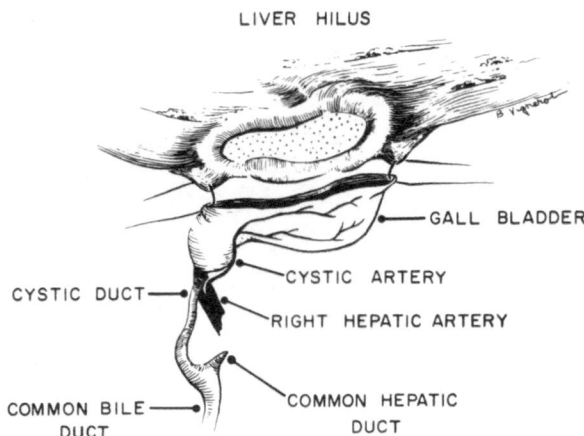

Fig. 2 "Gallbladder Kasai".   In the 10 to 15% of patients with
        biliary atresia in whom there is residual patency of the
        gallbladder, cystic duct and common bile duct, these
        structures are used for the new biliary conduit.
        (From Lilly, J.R.: Hepatic portocholecystostomy for biliary
        atresia. J Pediatr Surg, 14: 301, 1979. By permission.)

however, showed little correlation between the types and quantity
of bacteria and antibiotic administration (9).   Nor was there
bacteriological change or improvement in the frequency or severity
of cholangitis with the antibiotics tested.   Thus, our studies
did not support preventive antibiotic treatment.

        Since cholangitis is probably related to diminished bile flow,
an investigation of the effects of various choleretic agents on
postoperative bile drainage was undertaken.   Phenobarbital was
routinely prescribed to all patients for one year.   Other agents
evaluated were theophyllin, which did not improve bile flow enough
to justify side effects such as nervousness and vomiting; Zanchol[R]
which proved ineffective if not actually harmful; and decholin,
which was abandoned because of the sodium overload it often presented
to patients with liver disease.   A clinical trial of short term
steroid therapy is currently underway in patients with acute cholangitis.   The rationale for using this drug is that the infection
is probably precipitated by acute intraductal inflammation. Although
steroids have a mild choleretic effect they are perhaps more effective
in this context by decreasing periductal inflammation thereby
promoting bile flow and consequently aborting the infection.   Our
results with this regimen have been promising but greater patient
accrual is necessary.

        Thus far, the type of biliary reconstruction has proven to
be the single most important factor in the control of cholangitis.

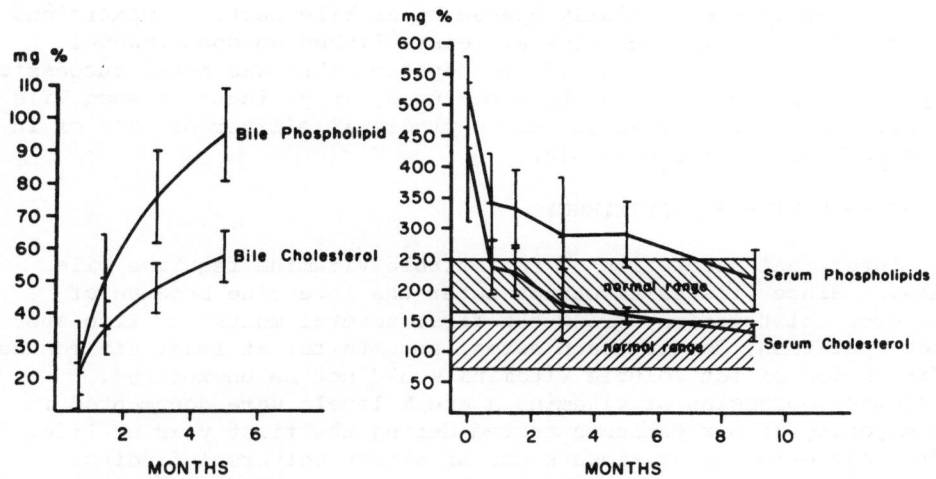

Fig. 3 *Serial levels of cholesterol and phospholipid in bile and serum.   Left, concentration of total cholesterol and phospholipid in biliary drainage after hepatic portoenterostomy.   Right, mean total serum cholesterol and phospholipid levels before and after hepatic portoenterostomy.   Standard errors of the means are in brackets. (From Lilly, JR and Javitt, NB: Biliary lipid excretion after hepatic portoenterostomy. Ann Surg 184: 369, 1976. By permission.)*

As alluded to earlier, infection has been conspicuously absent when the gallbladder was used for the biliary conduit.   In the absence of gallbladder patency, exteriorization of the bilio-intestinal conduit, as described above, appears to decrease the frequency and lessen the severity of cholangitis.   Exteriorization removes the biliary conduit from the vagaries of the gastrointestinal tract, a factor which has turned out to be of major importance in managing cholangitis.   Indeed, closure of the exteriorized conduit at one year precipitated cholangitis in four of nine patients. Cholangitis did not abate in the four patients until re-exteriorization was carried out.   Closure of the biliary conduit is now deferred for two or three years after operation.

REFIBROSIS OF THE HEPATIC ANASTOMOTIC SITE

In 12 patients bile drainage ceased following an episode of postoperative cholangitis during the first three postoperative months.   The complication was promptly detected and operation with re-excision of the hepatic hilus was carried out in all patients. Resumption of bile drainage occurred in eight infants.   Presumably the consequence of cholangitis in these patients was scar tissue

obliteration of the initially opened hilar bile duct.   Reexcision,
by removal of the fibrous tissue, reestablished an open channel.
Parenthetically, reexcision of the hepatic hilus was never successful
in patients without initial bile drainage, in patients in whom bile
drainage gradually decreased due to progressive liver disease or in
patients beyond six months old.

FAT SOLUBLE VITAMIN DEFICIENCY

    Intestinal absorption of fat soluble vitamins requires bile
salts.   Since bile salts cannot enter the intestine because of
bile duct obliteration during the first several months of life and,
after operation, do not reach normal amounts for at least six months,
deficiencies of fat soluble vitamins would not be unexpected.
Serologic depression of vitamins A and E levels were documented in
the majority of our patients tested during the first year of life.
Radiologic evidence of rickets was an almost universal finding.
Without treatment, radiographic rickets disappeared between the
second and fourth year after surgery suggesting vitamin D metabolism
became normal at this time.   Serial analysis of serum vitamin D
metabolites should verify this point.   Because of the background
of spontaneous improvement, we have treated only one patient with
special vitamin D supplementation, an infant with bilateral femoral
fractures, presumably ricketiform.   A study of the possible
relationship of depressed serum vitamin E levels and the transient
ataxia observed in some of our patients was begun last year.   There
is suggestive clinical evidence linking vitamin E deficiency and
ataxic neurologic disease (10).   Until more data are obtained we
have not prescribed special vitamin E supplementation.   In contrast,
vitamin A deficiency has been actively corrected.   Vitamin A has a
yet poorly defined role in infection (11).   Nevertheless, we are
giving supplemental vitamin A to all patients after operation and
will attempt to determine if achieving normal levels of the vitamin
reduces the incidence and severity of cholangitis.

ONGOING PARENCHYMAL DISEASE

    Several years ago we reported that progressive hepatic fibrosis
took place in the majority of our patients with successful bile
drainage during the first year after operation (12).   Since then,
we have noted usually stable and, in a few cases, improved liver
histology in liver biopsies taken two to three years after operation.
Similarly, intermittent ascites which occurred in several patients
with sustained biliary drainage resolved between the first and
second postoperative year.   Also, esophageal varices disappeared
from serial barium esophagograms between the third and fourth postoperative year.   This kind of information suggested that a dynamic
process is present in patients with biliary atresia, one which is
ongoing and self-limited to about one to two years after operation.

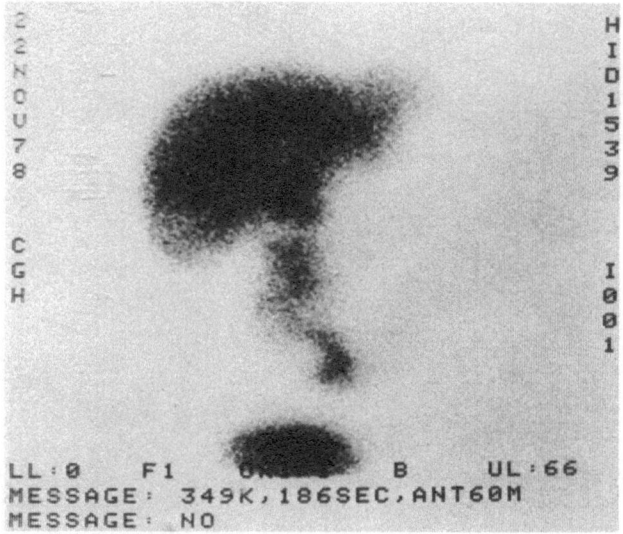

*Fig. 4   Diethyl-IDA (Tc-99m-N-(2,6-diethylacetanilide)-iminodiacetic
acid) scan in patient with biliary atresia following Kasai
hepatic portoenterostomy operation.   Hepatocyte clearance
of the isotope is used to evaluate the degree of residual
parenchymal disease.   The surgical bilio-enteric conduit
is clearly shown.*

Currently, rather than sequential liver biopsies we are using
diethyl-IDA scintography to evaluate long term hepatic recovery.
This new radiopharmaceutical, because of its greater molecular
weight and increased lipid solubility, has enhanced biliary excretion compared to standard radiopharmaceutical agents.   In infants
with successful operations for biliary atresia, scintigraphy has
clearly demonstrated the progress of the isotope through the liver
into the biliary conduit and thence into the distal intestine
(Figure 4).   Of equal importance has been the assessment of improvement of preexisting liver damage in chronic survivors.   Serial
analysis of the early hepatic phase of the study has provided
accurate information about the temporal changes in hepatocyte
function (13).

Finally, the spontaneous resolution of liver disease and,
as a consequence, of portal hypertension, has made us reluctant to
perform portosystemic shunts in patients with esophageal variceal
hemorrhage.   In the unusual occurrence of major variceal hemorrhage,
we have instead treated the child by endosclerosis.   In this
procedure esophageal varices are directly injected with sodium
morrhuate[R] (Figure 5).   Although experience is limited, bleeding
has thus far been controlled by this manoeuvre (14).

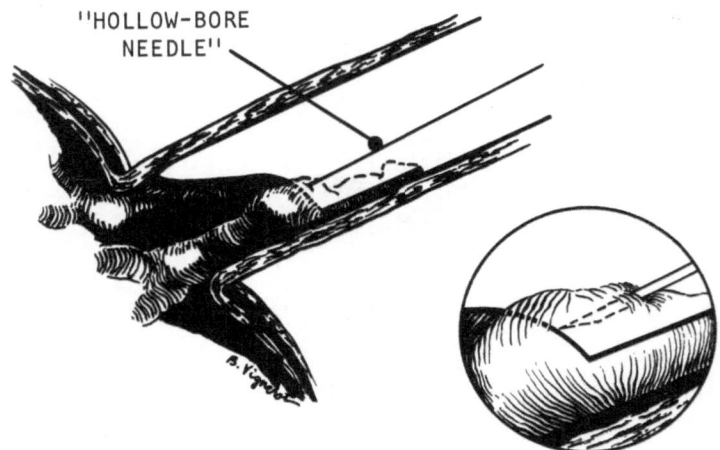

Fig. 5   *Endosclerosis of esophageal varices.   A specially slotted*
         rigid standard esophagoscope is advanced to the esophago-
         gastric junction.   The varices are injected with sodium
         morrhuate using a long hypodermic needle (inset).

SUMMARY

     There is no longer any question that relief of biliary
obstruction and consequent protracted survival can be achieved by
operation in a substantial number of patients with biliary atresia.
Surgical success is contingent upon the presence of a true bile
duct in the residual extrahepatic biliary tract at the porta hepatis.
Analysis of the components of bile drainage after surgery confirms
that biliary lipids, bile pigments and copper are secreted in
progressive amounts, coincident with a return towards their normal
values in the serum and liver.   Cholangitis is foremost among a
number of unresolved postoperative problems.   Thus far, the type
of surgical reconstruction has turned out to be the most important
factor in its control.   Unless the gallbladder is available, the
biliointestinal conduit should be exteriorized.   Fat soluble
vitamin deficiencies are present in most patients during the first
postoperative years but the deficiencies may be self-correctable.
Occasional esophageal variceal hemorrhage is treated by endosclerosis
since portal hypertension also appears to improve spontaneously.
As an alternative to liver biopsy, a new radiopharmaceutical,
diethyl-IDA, has been helpful in evaluating changes in residual
liver disease.

ACKNOWLEDGEMENT

This work was supported in part by the Biliary Atresia Fund and by grants RR-00051 and RR-00069 from the General Clinical Research Centers Program of the Division of Research Resources, National Institutes of Health.

REFERENCES

1. KASAI M, KIMURA S, ASAKURA Y, et al: Surgical treatment of biliary atresia. J Pediatr Surg 3: 665-671, 1968.

2. CAMPBELL DP, POLEY JR, BHATIA M, et al: Hepatic portoenterostomy - is it indicated in the treatment of biliary atresia? J Pediatr Surg 9: 329-335, 1974.

3. BARKIN RM, LILLY JR: Biliary atresia and the Kasai operation: continuing care. J Pediatr 96: 1015-1019, 1980.

4. HITCH DC, SHIKES RH, LILLY JR: Determinants of survival after Kasai's operation for biliary atresia using actuarial analysis. J Pediatr Surg 14: 310-314, 1979.

5. OHI R, SHIKES RH, LILLY JR: Bile duct remnants in biliary atresia. (Submitted for publication)

6. LILLY JR: Hepatic portocholecystostomy for biliary atresia. J Pediatr Surg 14: 301-304, 1979.

7. LILLY JR, JAVITT NB: Biliary lipid excretion after hepatic portoenterostomy. Ann Surg 184: 369-386, 1976.

8. OHI R, LILLY JR: Copper kinetics in infantile hepatobiliary disease. J Pediatr Surg 15: 509-512, 1980.

9. HITCH DC, LILLY JR: Identification, quantification, and significance of bacterial growth within the biliary tract after Kasai's operation. J Pediatr Surg 13: 563-569, 1978.

10. SUNG JH, STADLAN EM: Neuraxonal dystrophy in congenital biliary atresia. J Neuropath and Exp. Neurol. 25: 341-361, 1966.

11. COHEN BE, COHEN IK: Adjuvant and steroid antagonist in the immune response. J Immunol 111: 1376-1380, 1973.

12. ALTMAN RP, CHANDRA R, LILLY JR: Ongoing cirrhosis after successful porticoenterostomy in infants with biliary atresia. J Pediatr Surg 10: 685-691, 1975.

References (continued)

13. LILLY JR: Endosclerosis of esophageal varices in children.
        Surg Gynecol Obstet 152: 513-514, 1981.

14. OHI R, KLINGENSMITH WC, LILLY JR: Diethyl-IDA imaging in
        childhood hepatobiliary disease. (Submitted for
        publication)

DISCUSSION

            CHAIRMAN: B. SHANDLING

RAPPAPORT: In biliary atresia does one see an arterial supply
    frequently, less frequently or none at all?

WITZLEBEN: We have never been able to evaluate this.   The
    surgeons usually don't have time to check the vascular supply.
    Histologically there is so much scarring that it is really not
    possible to tell.

RAPPAPORT: Are there arterial branches in the tissues that you
    examine?

WITZLEBEN: There are small arteries of course.   But we are
    dealing with extremely diseased tissue and I cannot comment
    on the adequacy of the vasculature.   Angiography during life
    or even postmortem may be the best approach to this problem.

SHANDLING: As a surgeon I have the impression that the arterial
    supply is somewhat more generous than usual in patients with
    biliary atresia.

LILLY: I agree.   Grossly the arterial blood supply of the liver
    looks absolutely normal.   There seem to be more anomalies of
    the arterial inflow with branches taking off from the left
    gastric or superior mesenteric artery, but the blood vessels
    at the porta hepatis look absolutely normal.   It is also true
    that brisk bleeding occurs when the duct is transected in the
    younger patient.   However in older children, 3 or 4 months of
    age, there is very much less bleeding and the fibrous
    connective tissue contains hardly any blood vessels.

COHEN: It has been suggested that lymphatic drainage stimulates bile flow in some of these patients, even among some in whom anastomosis has failed.   Have you seen this?

LILLY: A theory from Switzerland claims that cholangitis secondary to interruption of the lymphatics at operation is responsible. We have done transhepatic cholangiograms postop on these patients and have seen the development of a rich network of lymphatics between the liver and intestines both in successful and nonsuccessful cases.

COHEN: Is the drainage bile or lymph?

LILLY: Measurement of the constituents of the drainage suggests that it is straight bile and not lymph.

ALAGILLE: What is the real efficacy of preventive jejunostomy against cholangitis?   When we don't use the gallbladder we always use a preventive jejunostomy and we have observed the same number of episodes of cholangitis.

LILLY: I cannot argue with that.   We have many attacks of cholangitis with the jejunostomy, the exteriorization procedure, but I think they are easier to control.   We have had a very bad experience with attempted closure of the jejunostomy in that cholangitis recurs and cannot be controlled until we re-exteriorize it.   Some of these patients I am afraid are permanently damaged, so I think there is a place for exterior-ization.   What I don't know is when it should be closed.

ALAGILLE: What do you think is the minimum period of time that it should be left?

LILLY: I said one year several years ago.   Dr. Kasai came by and said two years.   I am up to three years now.

PETERS: Do any of these people have normal portal pressures after they have been treated?

ALAGILLE: We have observed, almost constantly, high portal vein pressures during surgery, even in very young patients, say two months of age.   We haven't any explanation for this. Furthermore, the portal pressure does not fall after surgery.

LILLY: Dr. Kasai has found that the portal pressure does decrease about the same time as the liver histology improves.

ALAGILLE: That is not our experience in France.   When babies have portal hypertension, it remains even after restoration of bile flow and persists in those who are considered to be long-

term successes.   We have observed that esophageal varices
decrease or disappear and for this we have no explanation.

GARTNER: I have a strong opinion that biliary atresia can be a
viral disease and have been studying the model of Dr. Stanley
of Perth, Australia, in which biliary atresia is induced by
the injection of reovirus type III in weanling mice.
The interesting part of the model is that for about 8 days after
injection one can recover virus from the liver and biliary
tissue.   However biliary obstruction occurs after the period
of time in which virus is recoverable, usually 2-3 weeks after
inoculation.   We have cultured some 20 or 30 children and
have done electron microscopy but cannot find any evidence of
a virus in the biliary tree or liver.   This has led our
virologist to suggest that we are dealing with an incomplete
virion.   We have found two instances of biliary atresia with
a significant rise in antibody titres to reovirus type III
during the newborn period.   However the majority of infants
that have had titres done are negative for reo III and it is
probably not the major agent involved.   Perhaps we are dealing
with a multitude of viruses and with a unique susceptibility
on the part of certain infants.   But biliary atresia should
not be thought of as a single disease.   There may be several
different etiologic mechanisms, one viral, another perhaps
some type of embryologic malformation.

WITZLEBEN: I also think the possibility of a multifactorial etiology is a good one.   Does the virus destroy the epithelial
cells?

GARTNER: Yes.   In fact the histology of the region involved,
which in mice tends to be the distal common bile duct, is
indistinguishable from the histology that you showed.

PERRAULT: Would Dr. Alagille or Dr. Lilly consider using phenobarbital or any other bile flow stimulant, and would either
consider using steroids following the surgery to reduce
inflammation?

ALAGILLE: We used phenobarbital or cholestyramine after Kasai
surgery in a double blind study and did not observe any
effect with either drug.   I think steroid therapy is very
dangerous in these patients because they are very sensitive
to infections.

LILLY: We give phenobarbital routinely for the first year after
operation.   Whether it does any good or not I don't know.
Steroids we use on re-operations.   Occasionally we will see
a patient who will drain bile for a week or two and then get
an episode of cholangitis and stop.   We reoperate on these

patients and put them on steroids for a week or ten days, to
prevent the recurrence of cholangitis and obliteration of the
anastomosis.

SHANDLING: I wouldn't like everybody to leave here with the idea
that all is rosy in the field of biliary atresia. I was
recently in touch with children's hospitals in Philadelphia,
New York, Pittsburgh, Boston and Los Angeles. Most of these
places have appalling results, as do we at the Hospital for
Sick Children. We have operated on about 30 patients with
biliary atresia, and I think bile drainage was achieved in
eight. Various factors come into play but apart from a few
specialized centres such as Denver and Washington DC, etc,
results are poor.

LILLY: I don't think our results are so great. Only 40% of our
patients have sustained bile drainage, defined as bile drainage
for over a year, but this is no guarantee of survival. Of our
25 patients who drained bile for over a year, 4 have died of
progressive liver disease. Now there are some tricks to the
operation; you must have experience in the portal area.
Seventeen of our patients came from outside hospitals where
general surgeons who had never done the operation had taken
the first crack. Our results aren't as good in those patients.

ALAGILLE: Jacques Valayer has operated on about 120 patients with
biliary atresia and has had about the same success rate of
35% to 40%. Patients with temporary bile flow die 3 or 4 years
postoperatively while those without bile flow restoration die
two years after surgery.

COX: Alpha-1-antitrypsin deficiency in many respects mimics
biliary atresia and I wonder if alpha-1-antitrypsin deficiency
has always been excluded?

ALAGILLE: I don't think alpha-1-antitrypsin deficiency is an
etiologic process in extrahepatic biliary atresia. It is a
cause of intrahepatic cholestasis with secondary extrahepatic
hypoplasia.

COX: But is it safe to assume that all of the patients reported
as biliary atresia have had alpha-1-antitrypsin deficiency
excluded?

LILLY: No. We have had two patients who had Kasai operations
done at other hospitals who had alpha-1-antitrypsin deficiency.
Neither drained a drop of bile through the conduit. They
behaved as if they were totally obstructed.

COX: This certainly may affect the figures and could affect them either way since some do well and some don't.

LILLY: I don't think anybody confuses the two any more.

THALER: I would like to know what the American experience really is now that there are at least some patients with a 5-6 year follow-up.   How many patients live this long postoperatively and how well are they?

LILLY: The biliary atresia registry does not yet have the long-term survival figures, and I can't give you the data on the 20 patients we initially reported because Pete Altman has most of them.   But since I have been in Denver we have accumulated 10 patients who are 5 years or more postoperative, the longest being 7 years.   It looks like our experience is closer to that of the Japanese than to that of Professor Alagille.   As far as their health is concerned, I am optimistic in that ascites and portal hypertension have seemed to decrease, they are not jaundiced and they are in school.   But all have some problems with their social rehabilitation.   They have been in hospital so much that they should have special schools.   How long they will do this well I don't know.

VIRAL HEPATITIS TYPE A: REDEFINITION OF VIROLOGIC, CLINICAL AND EPIDEMIOLOGIC FEATURES

Jules L. Dienstag

Gastrointestinal Unit (Medical Services), Massachusetts
General Hospital and Department of Medicine, Harvard
Medical School, Boston, Massachusetts

VIROLOGY: FROM VISUALIZATION TO IN VITRO CULTIVATION

During the last decade, hepatitis A research has accelerated dramatically. Until the early 1970's, no practical serologic tests were available to identify hepatitis A infection, and investigative tools were limited. Still, painstaking epidemiologic observations and experimental transmission of the virus in volunteers (1,2) and marmoset monkeys (3-6) provided the foundations for the advances of recent years. Such studies had shown that hepatitis A virus (HAV) is excreted in feces during the late incubation period and early acute phase of illness and that convalescent serum (as well as immune serum globulin) contains neutralizing antibodies to HAV. Based on these studies, Feinstone et al (7) incubated convalescent serum, likely to contain antibody to HAV (anti-HAV), with filtrates of acute phase stool specimens, likely to contain HAV and, by electron microscopy, visualized HAV particles aggregated by antibody (immune electron microscopy). At the same time, almost a decade of work on experimental HAV infection in marmosets culminated in the detection by Provost et al (8) of virus-like particles morphologically similar to those described in human stools in homogenates and thin-section electron micrographs of liver and in concentrated serum of Saguinus mystax marmosets infected experimentally with the CR326 strain of HAV.

Hepatitis A virus, which had not been visualized until 1973, has now been characterized exhaustively. The virion has a mean diameter of 27 nm, has cubic capsid symmetry, and lacks a virus envelope or a complex internal substructure. Both complete (containing a genome) and incomplete (lacking a genome) virions can be visualized, but all HAV particles, whether complete or

incomplete, from human or nonhuman primate sources, regardless
of geographic origin and strain, are <u>immunologically</u> indistinguishable (9,10). Despite its uncharacteristic heat stability, small
genome (1.9 x 10^6 daltons), and multiplicity of buoyant densities,
HAV has biophysical-biochemical properties which most closely
resemble those of an enterovirus. These include a major buoyant
density of 1.34 g/cm^3 in cesium chloride, a sedimentation coefficient of 160S, a RNA genome, polypeptides similar to those of polio-
virus, stability to ether and acid, and cytoplasmic localization
(6,8,11-13).

Since the visualization of HAV, very sensitive in vitro serologic tests have been developed to identify HAV antigens and antibodies. The techniques of immune electron microscopy (7), complement fixation (14), immune adherence hemagglutination (15,16),
radioimmunoassay (17,18), and enzyme-linked immunosorbent assay
(19,20) were applied to serodiagnosis of HAV infection, and immuno-
fluorescence/immunoperoxidase staining techniques were developed
to demonstrate the presence of HAV within hepatocytes (21,22).
These assays have provided the tools to delineate the pattern of
virologic and immunologic events associated with acute HAV infection
both in man and in nonhuman primates. Such studies have shown
that the liver is the first site in which HAV can be localized,
as early as the first to second week after exposure to an infectious
inoculum (21). Hepatitis A virus particles can be detected within
cytoplasmic vesicles of hepatocytes and Kupffer cells, and the
presence of virus antigen in liver outlasts the brief period of
fecal HAV shedding and elevated serum aminotransferase activity.
Viremia, also an early event, is brief in duration and low in
concentration; it is most intense during the late incubation
period and lasts no more than a few days after the onset of jaundice.

Shedding of the virus in feces is one of the earliest virologic
events detectable with in vitro techniques in routinely available
clinical material (23,24). Detectable fecal excretion of HAV
coincides temporally with non-specific prodromal symptoms, such
as fatigue, malaise, and anorexia, and peaks in intensity several
days to more than a week before the onset of biochemical indicators
of acute hepatitis. Both infectivity and fecal shedding of HAV
diminish precipitously once jaundice appears. Obviously, then,
attempts to base a diagnosis of acute HAV infection on the detection
of HAV in liver, serum, or stool (or bile) are unlikely to be
productive. Viremia is too limited in duration and concentration,
and liver (as well as bile) is not a routinely available clinical
specimen. By the time a patient seeks medical attention, fecal
shedding of HAV is barely, if at all, detectable. Therefore,
for a diagnosis of type A hepatitis, we rely on serologic techniques
which demonstrate rising titers of antibody to HAV (anti-HAV)
between acute illness and convalescence or more conveniently the
presence of anti-HAV of the IgM class during acute illness (25).

Recently detection of copra antibody of the IgA class in stool
has been applied successfully to the diagnosis of acute HAV infection (26).   Both serum IgM anti-HAV and fecal IgA anti-HAV remain
detectable for several months after acute illness;   therefore,
both of these markers can be used to make a diagnosis retrospectively,
if the patient is seen for the first time late in the illness
or even during early convalescence.   Because of the relative
ease of working with serum and the availability of a commercial
radioimmunoassay for serum IgM anti-HAV (HAVAB-M, Abbott Laboratories,
North Chicago, Illinois), the method of choice for making a diagnosis
of acute type A hepatitis is the detection of IgM anti-HAV in
acute phase serum.

While these serologic tests were being developed, animal
models, which were being studied extensively, contributed enormously
to advances in hepatitis A research.   The susceptibility of marmosets, especially Saguinus mystax, to HAV infection had been established even before the virus was visualized.   Since serologic
tests for HAV infection became available, two additional nonhuman
primate models were discovered and evaluated, chimpanzees (27)
and another marmoset species, known alternatively as Saguinus
labiatus or Jacchus rufiventer (28).   The availability of serologic
techniques and animal models culminated at the end of the 1970's
in a remarkable, long-awaited breakthrough, the successful cultiva-
tion of HAV in vitro.   Provost and Hilleman (29) demonstrated
serial propagation of HAV in primary explant cultures of liver
from adult S. labiatus marmosets infected experimentally with
a multiply passaged HAV strain and even more efficiently in a
continuous fetal rhesus monkey kidney cell line, FRhK6.   Among
the factors contributing to this breakthrough were: (1) the use
of a HAV inoculum adapted by extensive serial passage in marmosets,
(2) the availability of sensitive immunoassays to detect HAV in
culture homogenates and supernatants, especially of an immunofluorescence assay to detect HAV in cover-slip cultures, which
permitted demonstration of infected cells despite the absence
of a cytopathic effect (a feature atypical of enteroviruses),
(3) the availability of hospitable cell lines and the marmoset
model, (4) the highly developed state of HAV technology, and (5)
almost a decade of unrelenting investigation.   Currently, efforts
to cultivate HAV in vitro are being expanded, and it is now possible
to cultivate HAV directly from clinical specimens and to propagate
it in a variety of epithelial cell lines.   An attenuated live
HAV vaccine is being developed and is not far from readiness for
immunogenicity and efficacy trials.

CLINICAL FEATURES

Viral hepatitis type A had been characterized in the past
as a relatively mild illness of limited duration, and recent
investigations corroborate this traditionally held view.   Although

children are more likely to develop mild or anicteric illnesses,
other factors besides age, including virus dose, host immune competence, and virus strain virulence, have been postulated to play
a role in determining severity.   Preliminary studies indicate
that certain HAV strains cause disease of shorter incubation period,
greater severity, and more prolonged shedding of virus in feces
than others.   In general, however, type A hepatitis is most
frequently a subclinical or unrecognized illness, a clinical observation supported by recent seroepidemiologic investigations (30).
Its relative mildness notwithstanding, HAV infection, in rare
instances, can be complicated by the development of acute fulminant
hepatitis (31,32).   Among 188 cases of acute fulminant hepatitis
characterized by the Acute Hepatic Failure Study Group, HAV alone
accounted for 2% and concurrent HAV and HBV for another 2% of
cases (33).   In a smaller study of 22 cases of fulminant hepatitis,
Mathiesen et al (34) documented HAV infection in 18% and concurrent
HAV and HBV infection in 5%, but the small number of cases renders
these figures less representative than those of the Acute Hepatic
Failure Study Group (35).   When all clinical and subclinical
cases of HAV infection are considered, however, the case fatality
rate for HAV infection must be very low.

Whereas HAV can, in rare instances, cause fulminant hepatitis,
there is considerable evidence that HAV infection is a self-limited
infection (1,31,35-39) that does not cause chronic hepatitis or
cirrhosis and that is unassociated with a chronic carrier state,
a feature that is characteristic of the enteroviruses.

To date typical, serologically bonafide hepatitis type A
has not been associated with such extrahepatic manifestations
of hepatitis as urticaria, arthritis, glomerulonephritis, and
polyarteritis.   Similarly, there is no evidence that HAV contributes to neonatal hepatitis, biliary atresia, or Indian childhood
cirrhosis (40,41).

EPIDEMIOLOGY

Modes of Transmission

Hepatitis A infection is transmitted in nature almost
exclusively by the fecal-oral route, a mode of spread enhanced
by poor personal or environmental hygiene and epidemiologic settings
favoring dissemination of enteric infections.   This is not to
say that HAV replicates in the gut, for attempts to demonstrate
intracellular localization of HAV in intestinal tissue of experimentally infected nonhuman primates have met with failure (42).
Most likely, the liver is the exclusive site for HAV replication,
and from the liver HAV gains access to the stool via the biliary
tree.   Thus, outbreaks of type A hepatitis have been attributed
to contaminated food, water, milk, and shellfish, and such enteric

spread occurs readily within families and institutionalized persons
and among contacts of infected nonhuman primates (43-45).   Because
types B and non-A, non-B hepatitis are not transmitted by the fecal-
oral route, the concept emerged that all enterically spread hepatitis
was type A hepatitis.   Recently, however, several classical water-
borne outbreaks of hepatitis have been re-evaluated with new serologic tools and in at least three such instances, HAV could not
be incriminated.   For example, in late 1955, there was an outbreak
of hepatitis related to contamination with sewage of the water
supply in Delhi, India (46,47).   Approximately 40 days after
this contamination was noted, 35,000 cases of acute hepatitis
(HBsAg-negative) (48) occurred in a population that by all standards
should have been largely immune to HAV.   Other unusual features
of this outbreak were the relatively old age, 20 to 40 years,
of those predominantly affected; the higher incidence in upper
than lower socioeconomic groups; the high mortality (1%), especially
among pregnant women (10%) (46,47); and the unusual frequency
and degree of cholestasis observed during morphologic examination
of liver biopsies (49).   Recently, stored serum samples from
that outbreak were evaluated with current serologic techniques,
but in these cases, serologic criteria for acute HAV infection
were not met.   Similar water-borne non-A hepatitis outbreaks
have occurred more recently in Burma (Tin, K.M., Khim, M.M., personal
communication) and Kashmir (50).   In short, there appears to
be a non-A, non-B hepatitis agent similar to HAV and epidemio-
logically distinct from the non-A, non-B agent(s) associated with
transfusion and other categories of percutaneous spread.

Hepatitis A virus also accounts for 20% to 40% of sporadic
hepatitis cases, that is, those occurring in the absence of a
well-defined epidemiologic setting (51).   Although type A hepatitis
can be transmitted experimentally by percutaneous inoculation,
HAV plays no role in transfusion-associated hepatitis (52,53).
In contrast with exposure to HBV, exposure to HAV is not increased
among hemodialysis patients and staff (54), multiply transfused
persons (55,56), health care personnel (57), or those who self-
administer illicit drugs intravenously (55).   Nor does vertical
transmission of HAV infection occur readily from mother to fetus
(58).   In male homosexuals, especially those who engage in oral-
anal sexual activity, fecal-oral spread of infectious agents is
facilitated, but a preliminary survey of anti-HAV prevalence in
this group failed to distinguish between the anti-HAV prevalences
of heterosexual and homosexual males (30).   This early study
involved a small number of homosexual men whose anti-HAV prevalences
were not stratified as a function of age.   When larger numbers
of homosexual males were studied, a subtle increase in HAV exposure
among them was noted.   Whereas their overall prevalence of anti-
HAV was not dramatically high, their exposure occurred earlier,
that is, at an earlier age than in a heterosexual population.   In
a recently published study, both prevalence of past infection and

yearly incidence of new HAV infections were increased dramatically
in a group of homosexual men attending a venereal disease clinic
(59).   Therefore, homosexual men are at an enhanced risk of developing not only HBV infections but also HAV infections.

Distribution of Exposure

Since the introduction of serological assays to detect anti-HAV,
seroepidemiologic studies have shown that exposure to HAV is widely
distributed and increases as a function of increasing age and
decreasing socioeconomic status (30,60).   Reflecting exposure to
HAV, the prevalence of serum anti-HAV in populations varies considerably among geographic locales largely as a function of environmental and personal standards of hygiene.   Higher prevalences of
anti-HAV among older persons in modern urban populations appear to
reflect more universal exposure of this older cohort when they were
younger, before improvements in hygienic conditions were introduced.
This cohort effect is compatible with the overall decrease in the
incidence of HAV infection (61,62) and is reflected in falling
prevalences of HAV exposure observed in these modern urban societies
(63).   Perpetuation of HAV in nature depends not on the presence
of chronic viremic or intestinal virus carriers, against the existence of which there is substantial evidence (60), but on a reservoir
of non-epidemic, inapparent cases, which outweigh heavily the number
of apparent, reported cases.   The importance of non-epidemic spread
is supported by the substantial contribution of HAV to sporadic
hepatitis in urban adults (51).

PROPHYLAXIS

     The efficacy of immune serum globulin (ISG) in the prophylaxis
of acute HAV infection had been well established even before current
seroepidemiologic techniques were developed.   Studies in the past
had shown that administration of ISG within two weeks after exposure
to HAV is effective in either preventing HAV infection or ameliorating
the illness and in conferring passive-active immunity (2,64);
however, recent serologic re-evaluation has shown that passive
immunization with ISG, while ameliorating illness in some and
inducing passive-active immunity, more frequently prevents both
illness and infection (65,66).   Contrary to popular opinion, then,
passive-active immunity after ISG prophylaxis for type A hepatitis
is uncommon;   instead, complete protection is more likely to occur
(67).

     All commercial preparations of ISG have appreciable levels
of anti-HAV.   Prophylaxis is recommended at a dose of 0.02 ml/kg
body weight for close personal contacts (e.g. household and institu-
tional but not casual contacts at work or school) of patients with
type A hepatitis and for travelers to endemic areas (68).   Higher
doses (0.05 ml/kg) are recommended for prolonged (>3 months)

exposures in endemic areas.   Until active immunization with a
vaccine is available, passive immunization with ISG is our only
alternative; however, work is in progress to develop a live
attenuated HAV vaccine.

SUMMARY

     Since the visualization of HAV in 1973, rapid progress has
been made in the study of the properties, the host immune response
to, and the epidemiology of HAV.   Hepatitis A virus is a RNA virus
with a mean diameter of 27 nm and biochemical-biophysical properties
similar to those of an enterovirus.   Sensitive, specific serological
techniques have been developed with which to identify HAV and anti-
HAV, and animal models (chimpanzees and marmosets) have been
studied extensively.   Emanating from these studies, in vitro culti-
vation of HAV has finally been accomplished, and a commercial radioimmunoassay for IgM anti-HAV has been developed for rapid diagnosis
of HAV infection during acute illness.   Clinically, the illness
caused by HAV is relatively mild - often subclinical - and of limited
duration and does not progress to chronic liver disease; however,
rarely HAV can cause fulminant hepatitis.   Type A hepatitis is
transmitted almost exclusively by the fecal-oral route, and its
spread is enhanced by poor personal and environmental hygiene and
by epidemiologic settings favoring dissemination of enteric infections.   Hepatitis A virus does not contribute to transfusion-
associated hepatitis.   Exposure to the virus increases as a function
of age and decreasing socioeconomic class, but the incidence of
HAV infection in urbanized societies is decreasing.   There is no
evidence for the existence of chronic HAV carriage; natural perpetuation of HAV in urban communities appears to depend on a reservoir
of non-epidemic, clinically inapparent cases.   Prevention of HAV
infection depends on maintenance of high standards of environmental
and personal hygiene and on timely administration of immune serum
globulin.   Such prophylaxis may confer passive-active immunity
but more frequently prevents infection entirely.

ACKNOWLEDGEMENTS

Dr. Dienstag is supported in part by Research Grant AM-25553 and
Contract HB-9-2919 from the National Institutes of Health, United
States Public Health Service.

REFERENCES

1. KRUGMAN S, WARD R, GILES JP: The natural history of infectious
        hepatitis.   Am J Med 32: 717-728, 1962.

2. HAVENS WP Jr, PAUL JR: Infectious hepatitis and serum hepatitis.
        In Viral and Rickettsial Infections of Man. I. Tamm, F.L.
        Horsfall (eds). J.B. Lippincott Co. Pa,1965. pp. 965-993.

3. DEINHARDT F, HOLMES AW, CAPPS RB, POPPER H: Studies on the transmission of human viral hepatitis to marmoset monkeys. I. Transmission of disease, serial passages and description of liver lesions. J Exp Med 125: 673-688, 1967.

4. HOLMES AW, WOLFE L, ROSENBLATE H, DEINHARDT F: Hepatitis in marmosets: induction of disease with coded specimens from a human volunteer study. Science 165: 816-817, 1969.

5. MASCOLI CC, ITTENSOHN OL, VILLAREJOS VM, ARGUEDAS JA, PROVOST PJ, HILLEMAN MR: Recovery of hepatitis agents in the marmoset from human cases occurring in Costa Rica. Proc Soc Exp Biol Med 142: 276-282, 1973.

6. PROVOST PJ, ITTENSOHN OL, VILLAREJOS VM, ARGUEDAS JA, HILLEMAN MR: Etiologic relationship of marmoset-propagated CR326 hepatitis A virus to hepatitis in man. Proc Soc Exp Biol Med 142: 1257-1267, 1973.

7. FEINSTONE SM, KAPIKIAN AZ, PURCELL RH: Hepatitis A: Detection by immune electron microscopy of a virus-like antigen associated with acute illness. Science 182: 1026-1028, 1973.

8. PROVOST PJ, WOLANSKI BS, MILLER WJ, ITTENSOHN OL, MCALEER WJ, HILLEMAN MR: Physical, chemical and morphologic dimensions of human hepatitis A virus strain CR326. Proc Soc Exp Biol Med 148: 532-539, 1975.

9. DIENSTAG JL, ROUTENBERG JA, PURCELL RH, HOOPER RR, HARRISON WO: Foodhandler-associated outbreak of hepatitis type A: An immune electron microscopic study. Ann Intern Med 83: 647-650, 1975.

10. DIENSTAG JL, SCHULMAN AN, GERETY RJ, HOOFNAGLE JH, LORENZ DE, PURCELL RH, BARKER LF: Hepatitis A antigen isolated from liver and stool: Immunologic comparison of antisera prepared in guinea pigs. J Immunol 117: 876-881, 1976.

11. SIEGL G, FRÖSNER GG: Characterization and classification of virus particles associated with hepatitis A. I. Size, density, and sedimentation. J Virol 26: 48-53, 1978.

12. SIEGL G, FRÖSNER GG: Characterization and classification of virus particles associated with hepatitis A. II. Type and configuration of nucleic acid. J Virol 26: 48-53, 1978.

13. COULEPIS AG, LOCARNINI SA, FERRIS AA, LEHMANN NI, GUST ID: The polypeptides of hepatitis A virus. Intervirol 10: 24-31, 1978.

14. PROVOST PJ, ITTENSOHN OL, VILLAREJOS VM, HILLEMAN MR: A
    specific complement-fixation test for human hepatitis A
    employing CR326 virus antigen: diagnosis and epidemiology.
    Proc Soc Exp Biol Med 148: 962-969, 1975.

15. MILLER WJ, PROVOST PJ, MCALEER WJ, ITTENSOHN OL, VILLAREJOS VM,
    HILLEMAN MR: Specific immune adherence assay for human
    hepatitis A antibody. Application to diagnostic and epi-
    demiologic investigations. Proc Soc Exp Biol Med 149:
    254-261, 1975.

16. MORITSUGU Y, DIENSTAG JL, VALDESUSO J, WONG DC, WAGNER J,
    ROUTENBERG JA, PURCELL RH: Purification of hepatitis A
    antigen from feces and detection of antigen and antibody by
    immune adherence hemagglutination. Infect Immun 13: 898-
    908, 1976.

17. HOLLINGER FB, BRADLEY DW, MAYNARD JE, DREESMAN GR, MELNICK JL:
    Detection of hepatitis A viral antigen by radioimmunoassay.
    J Immunol 115: 1464-1466, 1975.

18. PURCELL RH, WONG DC, MORITSUGU Y, DIENSTAG JL, ROUTENBERG JA,
    BOGGS JD: A microtiter solid-phase radioimmunoassay for
    hepatitis A antigen and antibody. J Immunol 116: 349-
    356, 1976.

19. MATHIESEN LR, FEINSTONE SM, WONG DC, SKINHOEJ P, PURCELL RH:
    Enzyme-linked immunosorbent assay for detection of hepatitis
    A antigen in stool and antibody to hepatitis A antigen in
    sera: Comparison with solid-phase radio-immunoassay, immune
    electron microscopy and immune adherence hemagglutination
    assay. J Clin Microbiol 7: 184-193, 1978.

20. LOCARNINI SA, GARLAND SM, LEHMANN NI, PRINGLE RC, GUST ID:
    Solid-phase enzyme-linked immunosorbent assay for detection
    of hepatitis A virus. J Clin Microbiol 8: 277-282, 1978.

21. MATHIESEN LR, FEINSTONE SM, PURCELL RH, WAGNER J: Detection
    of hepatitis A antigen by immunofluorescence. Infect
    Immun 18: 524-530, 1977.

22. SHIMIZU YK, MATHIESEN LR, LORENZ D, DRUCKER J, FEINSTONE SM,
    WAGNER J, PURCELL RH: Localization of hepatitis A antigen
    in liver tissue by peroxidase-conjugated antibody method:
    Light and electron microscopic studies. J Immunol 121:
    1671-1679, 1978.

23. DIENSTAG JL, FEINSTONE SM, KAPIKIAN AZ, PURCELL RH, BOGGS JD,
    CONRAD ME: Fecal shedding of hepatitis A antigen.
    Lancet 1: 765-767, 1975.

24. RAKELA J, MOSLEY JW: Fecal excretion of hepatitis A virus
     in humans. J Infect Dis 135: 933-938, 1977.

25. FEINSTONE SM, PURCELL RH: New methods for the serodiagnosis
     of hepatitis A. Gastroenterol 78: 1092-1094, 1980.

26. YOSHIZAWA H, ITOH Y, IWAKIRI S, TSUDA F, NAKANO S, MIYAKAWA Y,
     MAYUMI M: Diagnosis of type A hepatitis by fecal IgA
     antibody against hepatitis A antigen. Gastroenterol 78:
     114-118, 1980.

27. DIENSTAG JL, FEINSTONE SM, PURCELL RH, HOOFNAGLE JH, BARKER LF,
     LONDON WT, POPPER H, PETERSON JM, KAPIKIAN AZ: Experimental
     infection of chimpanzees with hepatitis A virus. J Infect
     Dis 132: 532-545, 1975.

28. PROVOST PJ, VILLAREJOS VM, HILLEMAN MR: Suitability of the
     rufiventer marmoset as a host animal for human hepatitis A
     virus. Proc Soc Exp Biol Med 155: 283-286, 1977.

29. PROVOST PJ, HILLEMAN MR: Propagation of human hepatitis
     virus in cell culture in vitro. Proc Soc Exp Biol Med
     160: 213-221, 1979.

30. SZMUNESS W, DIENSTAG JL, PURCELL RH, HARLEY EJ, STEVENS CE,
     WONG DC: Distribution of antibody to hepatitis A antigen
     in urban adult populations. N Engl J Med 295: 755-759,
     1976.

31. RAKELA J, REDEKER AG, EDWARDS VM, DECKER R, OVERBY LR, MOSLEY
     JW: Hepatitis A virus infection in fulminant hepatitis
     and chronic active hepatitis. Gastroenterology 74: 879-
     882, 1978.

32. MATHIESEN LR, LINGLÖF T, MØLLER AM, TUFVESSON B, JOHNSSON T,
     NORDBRING F: Case report: fulminant hepatitis A.
     Scand J Infect Dis 11: 303-305, 1979.

33. ACUTE HEPATIC FAILURE STUDY GROUP: Etiology and prognosis in
     fulminant hepatitis. Gastroenterol 77: 33A, 1979.

34. MATHIESEN LR, SKINOJ P, NIELSEN JO, PURCELL RH, WONG DC,
     RANEK L: Hepatitis type A, B, and non-A, non-B in
     fulminant hepatitis. Gut 21: 72-77, 1980.

35. LINDBERG J, FRÖSNER G, HANSSON BG, HERMODSON S, IWARSON S:
     Serologic markers of hepatitis A and B in chronic active
     hepatitis. Scand J Gastroenterol 13: 525-527, 1978.

36. NORKRANS G: Clinical epidemiological and prognostic aspects
      of hepatitis A, B, and "non-A, non-B". Scand J Infect Dis
      Suppl 17: 1-44, 1978.

37. MÜLLER R, WILLERS H, FREISE J, HÖPKEN W: Chronic hepatitis as
      sequela of acute viral hepatitis A and hepatitis non-A,
      non-B. Zeitschrift für Gastroenterologie 16: 760-767,
      1978.

38. RENNER F, HORAK W, GRABNER G, DITTRICH H: Aetiology of chronic
      active hepatitis in Vienna. Zeitschrift für Gastroentero-
      logie 17: 106-109, 1979.

39. ROUTENBERG JA, DIENSTAG JL, HARRISON WO, KILPATRICK ME,
      HOOPER RR, CHISARI FV, PURCELL RH, FORNES MF: Foodborne
      outbreak of hepatitis A: Clinical and laboratory features
      of acute and protracted illness. Am J Med Sci 278: 123-
      137, 1979.

40. BALISTRERI W, TABOR E, DRUCKER J, GERETY R: Serologic markers
      of hepatitis A (HAV) and B (HBV) in biliary atresia (BA)
      and neonatal hepatitis (NH). Pediatric Res 12: 429
      (abstract), 1978.

41. AGARWAL S, LAHORI UC, MEHTA SK, BAJPAI PC, WERNER B, BRADLEY
      DW: Hepatitis A and Indian childhood cirrhosis. Arch Dis
      Child 54: 901-903, 1979.

42. MATHIESEN LR, DRUCKER J, LORENZ D, WAGNER J, GERETY RJ, PURCELL
      RH: Localization of hepatitis A antigen in marmoset organs
      during acute infection with hepatitis A virus. J Infect
      Dis 138: 369-377, 1978.

43. PURCELL RH, DIENSTAG JL, FEINSTONE SM, KAPIKIAN AZ: Relation-
      ship of hepatitis A antigen to viral hepatitis. Am J Med
      Sci 270: 61-71, 1975.

44. DIENSTAG JL, GUST ID, LUCAS CR, WONG DC, PURCELL RH: Mussel-
      associated viral hepatitis, type A: Serologic confirmation.
      Lancet 1: 561-564, 1976.

45. DIENSTAG JL, DAVENPORT FM, MCCOLLUM RW, HENNESSY AV, KLATSKIN G,
      PURCELL RH: Nonhuman primate-associated viral hepatitis
      type A: Serologic evidence of hepatitis A virus infection.
      JAMA 236: 462-464, 1976.

46. MELNICK JL: A water-borne urban epidemic of hepatitis. In
      Hepatitis Frontiers. FW Hartman, G LoGrippo, JG Mateer,
      J Barron (eds). Little Brown & Co. Boston 1957,
      pp 211-225.

47. MELNICK JL, BOGGS JD: Human volunteer and tissue culture
     studies of viral hepatitis. Canad Med Assoc J 106:
     461-467, 1972

48. PAVRI KM, NIPHADKAR KB, SHEIKH BH: Retrospective studies on
     Australia antigen in sera collected during the epidemic of
     viral hepatitis at Delhi in 1965. Indian J Med Res 60:
     1575-1578, 1972.

49. SMETANA HF: Pathologic anatomy of early stages of viral
     hepatitis. In Hepatitis Frontiers. FW Hartman, G LoGrippo,
     JG Mateer, J Barron (eds). Little Brown and Co., Boston
     1957, pp 77-111.

50. KHUROO MS: Study of an epidemic of non-A, non-B hepatitis:
     Possibility of another human hepatitis virus distinct from
     post-transfusion non-A, non-B type. Amer J Med 68: 818-
     824, 1980.

51. DIENSTAG JL, ALAAMA A, MOSLEY JW, REDEKER AG, PURCELL RH:
     Etiology of sporadic hepatitis B surface antigen-negative
     hepatitis. Ann Intern Med 87: 1-6, 1977.

52. FEINSTONE SM, KAPIKIAN AZ, PURCELL RH, ALTER HJ, HOLLAND PV:
     Transfusion-associated hepatitis not due to viral hepatitis
     type A or B. N Engl J Med 292: 767-770, 1975.

53. DIENSTAG JL, FEINSTONE SM, PURCELL RH, WONG DC, ALTER HJ,
     HOLLAND PV: Non-A, non-B post-transfusion hepatitis.
     Lancet 1: 560-562, 1977.

54. SZMUNESS W, DIENSTAG JL, PURCELL RH, PRINCE AM, STEVENS CE,
     LEVINE RW: Hepatitis type A and hemodialysis: A sero-
     epidemiologic study in 15 U.S. centers. Ann Intern Med
     87: 8-12, 1977.

55. GUST ID, LEHMANN NI, LUCAS CR, FERRIS AA, LOCARNINI SA:
     Studies on the epidemiology of hepatitis A in Melbourne.
     In Viral Hepatitis. GN Vyas, SN Cohen, R Schmid (eds).
     Franklin Institute Press, Philadelphia 1978. pp 105-112.

56. STEVENS CE, SILBERT JA, MILLER DR, DIENSTAG JL, PURCELL RH,
     SZMUNESS W: Serologic evaluation of hepatitis A and B
     virus infections in thalassemia patients: A retrospective
     study. Transfusion 18: 356-360, 1978.

57. MAYNARD JE: Viral hepatitis as an occupational hazard in the
     health care profession. In Viral Hepatitis. GN Vyas,
     SN Cohen, R Schmid (eds). Franklin Institute Press,
     Philadelphia 1978. pp. 321-331.

58. TONG MJ, RAKELA J, MCPEAK CM, THURSBY MW, EDWARDS VM, MOSLEY JW:
     Studies in infants born to mothers with type A hepatitis and
     acute non-A, non-B hepatitis during pregnancy. Gastroent
     75: 991 (abstract), 1978.

59. COREY L, HOLMES KK: Sexual transmission of hepatitis A in
     homosexual men: incidence and mechanism. N Engl J Med
     302: 435-438, 1980.

60. DIENSTAG JL, SZMUNESS W, STEVENS CE, PURCELL RH: Hepatitis
     A virus infection: New insights from seroepidemiologic
     studies. J Infect Dis 137: 328-340, 1978.

61. MOSLEY JW: Epidemiologic implications of changing trends in
     type A and type B hepatitis. In Hepatitis and Blood Trans-
     fusion. GN Vyas, HA Perkins, R Schmid (eds). Grune &
     Stratton, N.Y. 1972. pp 23-26.

62. SKINHØJ P, MIKKELSEN F, HOLLINGER FB: Hepatitits A in Greenland:
     Importance of specific antibody testing in epidemiologic
     surveillance. Am J Epidemiol 105: 140-147, 1977.

63. GUST ID, LEHMANN NI, LUCAS CR: Relationship between prevalence
     of anti-HAV and age - a cohort effect? J Infect Dis 138:
     425-426, 1978.

64. KRUGMAN S, WARD R, GILES JP, JACOBS AM: Infectious hepatitis:
     Studies on the effect of gamma globulin and on the
     incidence of inapparent infection. JAMA 174: 823-830, 1960.

65. KRUGMAN S: Effect of human immune serum globulin on infectivity
     of hepatitis A virus. J Infect Dis 134: 70-74, 1976.

66. HALL WT, MADDEN DL, MUNDON FK, BRANDT DEL, CLARKE NA: Protec-
     tive effect of immune serum globulin (ISG) against hepatitis
     A infection in a natural epidemic. Amer J Epidem 106:
     72-75, 1977.

67. MOSLEY JW: Epdiemiology of HAV infection. In Viral Hepatitis.
     GN Vyas, SN Cohen, R Schmid (eds). Franklin Institute
     Press, Philadelphia 1978. pp 85-104.

68. PUBLIC HEALTH SERVICE ADVISORY COMMITTEE ON IMMUNIZATION
     PRACTICES:: Immune globulins for protection against viral
     hepatitis. Morbid Mortal Weekly Report 26: 425-428, 1977.

DISCUSSION

CHAIRMAN: D.H. CARVER

PERRAULT: Have you measured hepatitis A antigen or antibody in neonatal hepatitis?

DIENSTAG: No, but it has been done by a number of investigators. There doesn't seem to be any relationship between hepatitis A virus and neonatal hepatitis, biliary atresia or Indian childhood cirrhosis.

ROY: What do you think about the eventual usefulness of hepatitis A vaccine, since hepatitis A doesn't seem to contribute to chronic liver disease and since only 2% of cases of fulminant hepatitis can be attributed to hepatitis A?

DIENSTAG: It probably will not be distributed widely, but it will be important in areas where there is sufficient spread. It will be important in male homosexuals and in institutions such as those for the mentally retarded, the military and perhaps the convicted.

VIRAL HEPATITIS, TYPE B

Saul Krugman and Wolf Szmuness

Department of Pediatrics, New York University Medical
Center and The Lindsley F. Kimball Research Institute
of the New York Blood Center, New York, N.Y.

The disease that is recognized as type B hepatitis today was
first described in 1885 by Lürman (1). He observed an outbreak
of jaundice among shipyard workers who were inoculated with
smallpox vaccine two months previously. Later it became clear
that the human lymph component of the vaccine was obtained from a
donor who undoubtedly was a hepatitis B carrier. Although type B
hepatitis was first recognized during this past century, it is
likely that it existed as an unrecognized disease for many hundreds
of past generations.

The discovery of Australia antigen (2) and its association
with type B hepatitis (3) provided the technology needed to identify
and characterize the causative agent, to clarify further the
natural history of the disease, to expand knowledge of its epidemiology and to enhance prospects for prevention by passive and active
immunization.

The Agent

Electronmicrographic studies of serum specimens obtained from
patients with acute type B hepatitis or from those with a chronic
carrier state have revealed the presence of virus-like particles.
These particles exist in three morphological forms: (1) spherical
particles that are 22 nm in diameter, (2) tubular and filamentous
forms of the same diameter and 200 nm or more in length, and (3)
more complex larger particles, 42 nm in diameter, with an outer
surface of envelope and an inner core measuring 27 nm in diameter
(Figure 1).

The 42 nm particle, described by Dane and his colleagues (4),

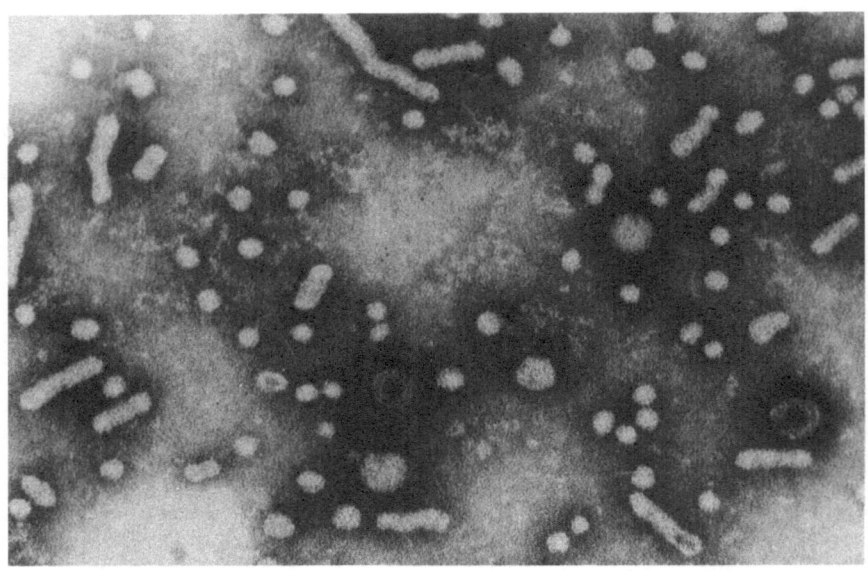

Fig. 1 *Electronmicrograph of Hepatitis B Virus (HBV) Particles*
Note 42 nm HBV (Dane) particles and 20 nm spherical and
filamentous hepatitis B surface antigen (HBsAg) particles

is now known to be the hepatitis B virus.   Its outer surface, the
hepatitis B surface antigen (HBsAg), is immunologically distinct
from its core component, the hepatitis B core antigen (HBcAg).
Another antigen, the hepatitis B e antigen (HBeAg) has been
identified as a component of the core particle.   DNA polymerase
activity and endogenous DNA template consisting of double-stranded
DNA have been shown to be associated with the core.   The technology
is now available to detect the following antibodies induced by the
hepatitis B antigens: anti-HBs, anti-HBc and anti-HBe.

The 22 nm spherical and filamentous particles are biochemically
and immunologically identical to the surface component of the HBV.
These HBsAg particles probably represent excess surface material
unused during synthesis of the HBV.   As indicated in Figure 2,
the core component (HBcAg) is synthesized in the nucleus of the
hepatocyte, and the surface component (HBsAg) in the cytoplasm.
The hepatitis B virion is formed when the core that traverses from
the nucleus to the cytoplasm is coated by HBsAg.   Finally, the
HBV particles and the enormous number of excess HBsAg particles
leave the cytoplasm and enter the circulation.   It has been
estimated that 1 ml of blood may contain about 10^{12} HBsAg particles.

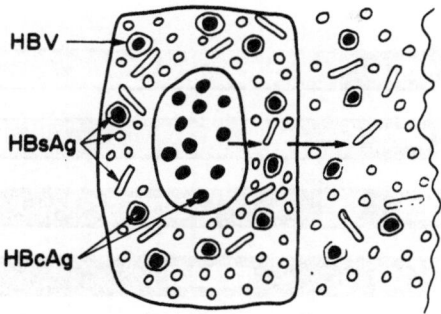

Fig. 2 Schematic Diagram of the Synthesis of Hepatitis B Virus
        (HBV) in a Hepatocyte. Note synthesis of (1) the core
        component (HBcAg) in the nucleus, and (2) the surface
        component (HBsAg) in the cytoplasm. The HBV is formed
        when the HBsAg particles coat the HBcAg particles. The
        42 nm HBV particles and the excess spherical and filament-
        ous HBsAg particles leave the cytoplasm and enter the
        circulation.

Purified preparations of HBsAg have been found to contain
four polypeptides and four glycoproteins with molecular weights
ranging between 68,000 and 22,000.   All HBsAg particles have a
common antigenic specificity that has been designated a.   Two
sets of mutually exclusive determinants d or y and w or r have
been identified.   Thus, the four principal subtypes of HBsAg are
adw, ayw, adr and ayr.   The production of monoclonal antibodies
to HBsAg by somatic cell hybrids (5) will provide improved diagnostic reagents for both the detection of antigen and subtyping of
HBsAg.

During the past two years several investigators have demonstrated that DNA extracted from HBV particles can be successfully
cloned in bacteria using a plasmid vector (6).   The possible
production of large quantitites of HBV DNA may provide antigen
for vaccine production.

CLINICAL ASPECTS

The availability of specific markers has made it possible to
follow the course of hepatitis B infection from the time of
exposure to onset of disease and for many months and years thereafter.   Most patients recover completely.   In about 10 per cent
of cases, chronic active hepatitis may occur.

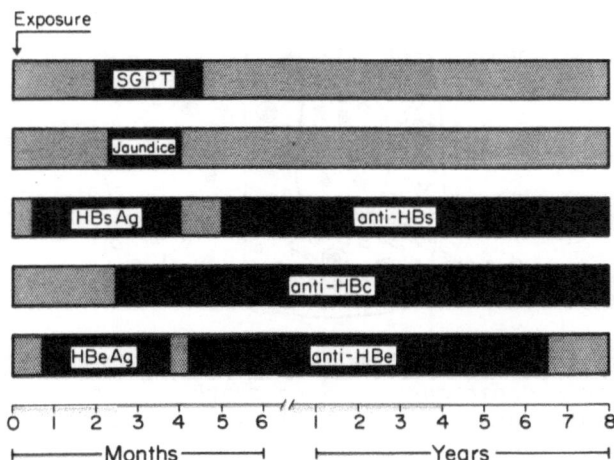

Fig. 3 *Acute Type B Hepatitis with Recovery.* *Note (1) onset of
hepatitis with jaundice 2 months after exposure; (2) detection of hepatitis B surface antigen (HBsAg) about 2 weeks
after exposure, followed by appearance of its antibody
(anti-HBs) about 2 to 4 weeks after HBsAg is no longer
detectable; (3) detection of hepatitis B core antibody
(anti-HBc) at the time of onset of disease about 2 months
after exposure; (4) detection of hepatitis B e antigen
(HBeAg) shortly after appearance of HBsAg and its disappearance shortly before HBsAg disappears, followed by the
appearance of antibody to HBeAg (anti-HBe) that persists
for 2 to 7 years.*

Acute type B hepatitis with recovery

The sequence of events in a patient who recovers from acute
type B hepatitis is shown in Figure 3.   Evidence of abnormal
serum glutamic pyruvic transaminase (SGPT) activity and jaundice
is usually detected about two months after exposure.   The first
detectable marker of infection is HBsAg; it may appear as early
as one to three weeks after exposure and it disappears after a
variable period ranging from three weeks to three months.   Antibody to HBsAg (anti-HBs) becomes detectable about two weeks to two
months after HBsAg disappears; it persists for many years in most
patients.   HBcAg is not detectable in the blood but its antibody
(anti-HBc) is detected at the time of onset of disease, usually
about two months after exposure.   Anti-HBc, like anti-HBs, usually
persists indefinitely in most patients.   HBeAg is detected shortly
after HBsAg, it disappears before HBsAg, and it is followed by the
appearance of anti-HBe.

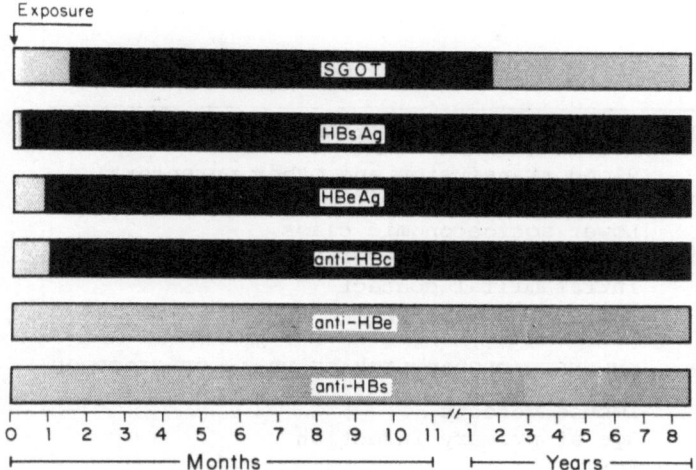

Fig. 4   *Chronic Active Type B Hepatitis.*
          Note (1) prolonged period of abnormal serum transaminase
          (SGOT) levels;   (2) persistence of HBsAg and HBeAg;   and
          (3) no detectable anti-HBe and anti-HBs.

Chronic active hepatitis

The prolonged period of abnormal serum transaminase activity
is shown in Figure 4.   It may be associated with persistence of
HBsAg, HBeAg, and anti-HBc.   In some patients the carrier state
is characterized by the disappearance of HBeAg and the appearance
of anti-HBe.   Chronic infection may occur in the presence or
absence of HBeAg.   The available evidence indicates that HBeAg
is not a marker of chronic infection.   On the other hand, HBeAg
is an excellent marker of infectivity.   HBsAg-positive and HBeAg-
positive blood is highly infectious while HBsAg-positive, anti-
HBe-positive blood is minimally infectious.

EPIDEMIOLOGICAL ASPECTS

The various risk factors that have been associated with
hepatitis B infection are listed in Table I.   These factors may
enhance the probability of exposure and/or the probability of
HBsAg persistence.   Geography, age and sex may have a profound
effect on the epidemiology of hepatitis B virus infections.

Geographic distribution

The striking geographic distribution of HBV infection associated with HBsAg-carrier rate is shown in Figure 5.   The prevalence
of HBsAg varies between less than 0.5% in the United States and

TABLE   I

RISK FACTORS IN HBV INFECTIONS

A.   ENHANCED PROBABILITY OF EXPOSURE

Blood transfusion and other parenteral
  procedures
Lower socioeconomic class
Sexual promiscuity
Intrafamilial contact
Medical profession

B.   ENHANCED PROBABILITY OF HBsAg PERSISTENCE

Immune defects
Age at primary infection
Sex
Race (?)
Genetic (?)

C.   BOTH ENHANCED EXPOSURE AND PERSISTENCE

Birth to carrier-mothers
Maintenance hemodialysis
Institutionalization due to Mongolism

From Szmuness et al (7)

Europe, one to two per cent in South America and Southern Europe,
three per cent in North Africa and many parts of the U.S.S.R. and
six to ten per cent and higher in other parts of Africa and Southeast Asia.

Striking variations in the prevalence of HBsAg may be observed
within each geographic area.   For example, in the United States,
evidence of past infection (HBsAg and/or anti-HBc, and/or anti-HBs)
may range between about 10 per cent in normal blood donors to about
70 per cent in male homosexuals.

Age distribution

The age distribution of HBV infection is dependent, in great
part, upon the prevalence of the infection in a particular area,
socioeconomic class, sexual promiscuity or exposure to blood or
blood products.   Seroepidemiological surveys of anti-HBs indicate
that prevalence increases gradually with age and then it stabilizes.
The age at which this plateau is reached varies considerably;   it
is about 45 years of age or older in American donors as compared
with 10 to 19 years in Taiwanese.

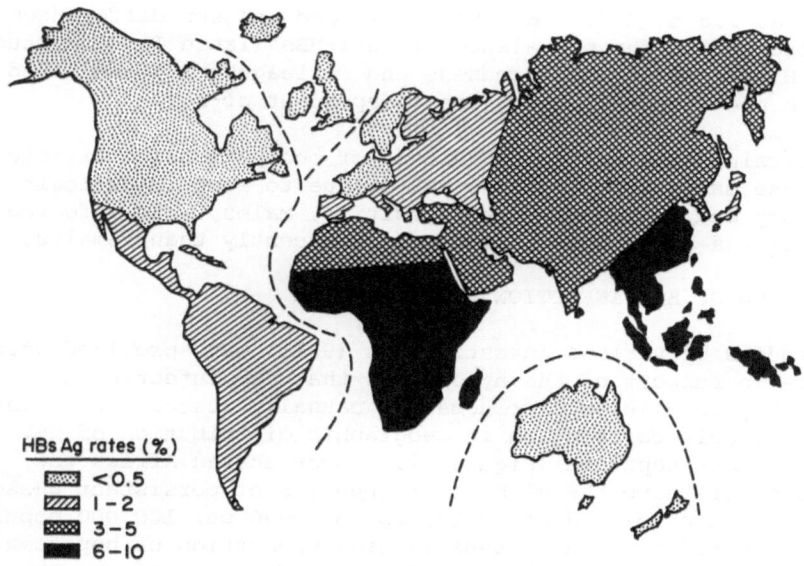

*Fig. 5 Schematic Map of the Worldwide Distribution of HBsAg
        Carriers*

The age distribution of HBsAg-positive carriers is different
from those who have detectable anti-HBs.   In developed areas of
the world, HBsAg is very rarely detected in infants and small
children.   By contrast, in Senegal and in Taiwan, extraordinarily
high HBsAg-positive carrier rates are detected in infants and young
children.   After peak levels of HBsAg carrier rates occur in all
population groups, there is a progressive decline in prevalence
with increasing age.   For example, studies by Szmuness and
colleagues in Chinese-Americans revealed the HBsAg prevalence to
be zero in persons 70 years of age or older as compared with 10 to
15 per cent in younger persons.   These findings suggest that the
HBsAg-carrier state may be self-limited in certain persons.   A
decrease in HBeAg reactivity has also been observed in older
carriers but it appears to be related to the "age" of the carrier
state rather than the age of the person.

Sex distribution

When both sexes are exposed equally there is little difference
in the incidence of acute hepatitis between males and females.
However, a study of hepatitis B marker prevalence and incidence of
acute hepatitis in open populations reveals various differences (7).
For example, HBsAg is detected more frequently among males than
among females in all populations studied, with male/female ratios

as high as 2.5 to 2.7.   On the other hand, no sex differences
were observed in the prevalence of anti-HBs (Table I).   A study
of 749 HBsAg carriers by Szmuness and colleagues (8) indicated
that the prevalence of HBeAg was independent of sex.

Certain sex-specific behavioral or occupational activities
may expose males more often to HBV or due to some immunologic
deficiency and/or genetic predisposition, males, when infected,
may develop a chronic infection more frequently than females.

ASSOCIATION OF HBV INFECTION WITH HEPATOMA

Studies by various investigators (9-11) have provided strong
evidence in support of the hypothesis that HBV infection and
primary hepatocellular carcinoma are causally associated.   There
is a remarkable correlation in geographic distribution of HBV
infections and hepatoma (Figure 5).   Sub-Saharan Africa and
Southeast Asia have the highest frequencies of persistent HBsAg
(8-15%) and hepatoma (death rates up to 10-40 per 100,000 population).   In addition, an unusually high proportion of hepatoma
patients are positive either for HBsAg and/or anti-HBc.   The
cumulative percentage of hepatoma patients positive for these
markers ranges between 50 and 90 per cent, or 10-50 times higher
than the rate in healthy people or those with other types of
cancer.

PROPHYLACTIC ASPECTS

The routine testing of all blood donors since 1972 has been
associated with a striking reduction in the incidence of type B
post-transfusion hepatitis.   In addition, the availability of
hepatitis B immune serum globulin (HBIG) has provided a passive
immunizing preparation for post-exposure prophylaxis of type B
hepatitis.   However, the ultimate control of hepatitis B in high
risk population groups will depend upon the development of a safe
and effective hepatitis B vaccine.   Studies that have been in
progress since 1971 indicate that this objective should be achieved
by 1981.

The demonstration in 1971 and 1973 that heat-inactivated serum
containing HBV and HBsAg was not infectious but was immunogenic and
partially protective indicated that it should be possible to develop
an inactivated hepatitis B vaccine (12).   By 1975 Hilleman and
colleagues (13) and Purcell and Gerin (14) had prepared formalin-
inactivated hepatitis B vaccines from purified HBsAg particles.
A similar vaccine was prepared by Maupas and his colleagues in
France (15).   These vaccines proved to be non infectious, immunogenic and protective when tested in susceptible chimpanzees.

Subsequent studies in susceptible adult volunteers confirmed

the safety and immunogenicity of various preparations when prepared
with an aluminum hydroxide adjuvant.   Our studies with one lot
of Merck inactivated hepatitis B vaccine (No. 751) revealed that
the anti-HBs response was about 85% after two inoculations at a
one month interval; it was greater than 95% after a third inoculation given either two months or six months after the first
inoculation.

Studies to evaluate the efficacy of inactivated hepatitis B
vaccine are currently in progress in New York (15) and in France
and Senegal (16).   The results of these efficacy trials should be
available by 1981.   If the results of these studies confirm the
efficacy of the vaccine, it should qualify for licensure in 1981.

REFERENCES

1. LÜRMAN A: Eine icterusepidemie.   Berlin Klin Wochschr 22:
        20-23, 1885

2. BLUMBERG BS, ALTER HJ, VISNICH S: A "new" antigen in leukemia
        sera.   JAMA 191: 541-546, 1965

3. PRINCE AM: An antigen detected in the blood during the
        incubation period of serum hepatitis.   Proc Natl Acad
        Sci USA 60: 814-821, 1968.

4. DANE DS, CAMERON CH, BRIGGS M: Virus-like particles in serum
        of patients with Australia-antigen-associated hepatitis.
        Lancet 1: 695-698, 1970.

5. SHIH JWK, COTE PJ Jr, GERIN JL: Production of monoclonal
        antibodies against hepatitis B surface antigen by somatic
        cell hybrids.   J Virol Methods, in press.

6. SNISKY JJ, SIDDIQUI A, ROBINSON WS: Cloning and endonuclease
        mapping of the hepatitis B viral genome.   Nature 279:
        346-348, 1979.

7. SZMUNESS W, HARLEY EJ, IKRAM H, et al: Sociodemographic
        aspects of the epidemiology of hepatitis B.   In Viral
        Hepatitis.   GN Vyas, SN Cohen, R Schmid (eds).   The
        Franklin Institute Press, Philadelphia, pp. 297-320.

8. SZMUNESS W, NEURATH AR, STEVENS CE, et al: Prevalence of
        hepatitis B "e" antigen and its antibody in various

9. SIMONS MJ, YAP EH, YU M, et al: Australia antigen in Singa-
    pore Chinese patients with hepatocellular carcinoma and
    comparison groups: influence of technique on differential
    frequencies. Int J Cancer 10: 320-325, 1972

10. TONG MJ, SUN SC, SCHAEFFER BT, et al: Hepatitis-associated
    antigen in hepatocellular carcinoma in Taiwan. Ann Int
    Med 75: 687-691, 1971.

11. SZMUNESS W, STEVENS CE, IKRAM H, et al: Prevalence of hepatitis
    B virus infection and hepatocellular carcinoma in Chinese
    Americans. J Infect Dis 137: 822-829, 1978.

12. KRUGMAN S, GILES JP, HAMMOND J: Viral hepatitis, type B
    (MS-2 strain): Studies on active immunization.
    JAMA 217: 41-45, 1971.

13. HILLEMAN MR, BUYNAK EG, ROEHM RR, et al: Purified and
    inactivated hepatitis B vaccine: A progress report.
    Am J Med Sci 270: 401-404, 1975.

14. PURCELL RH, GERIN JL: Hepatitis B subunit vaccine: A prelim-
    inary report of safety and efficacy tests in chimpanzees.
    Am J Med Sci 270: 395-399, 1975.

15. SZMUNESS W: Large-scale efficacy trials of hepatitis B
    vaccines in the USA: Baseline data and protocols.
    J Med Virol 4: 327-340, 1979.

16. MAUPAS P, GOUDEAU A, COURSAGET P et al: Immunization against
    hepatitis B in man. Lancet 1: 1367-1370, 1976.

HEPATITIS NON A NON B: A NEWLY RECOGNIZED OLD DISEASE

Harvey J. Alter

Immunology Section, Blood Bank Department, Clinical
Center, National Institutes of Health
Bethesda, Maryland

INTRODUCTION

Viral hepatitis represented a major public health problem
during World War II and the number of soldiers incapacitated by
this disease called forth an intensive effort to elucidate the
routes of transmission and potential means of prevention.   Studies
of epidemic hepatitis among soldiers in the Middle East and Africa
and of hepatitis traced to yellow fever vaccine clearly distinguished
two epidemiologic forms which came to be known as infectious (type
A) and serum (type B) hepatitis.   The former was an explosive,
epidemic disease found to be transmitted by the fecal-oral route
and the latter a more indolently transmitted disease borne primarily
by parenteral inoculation of virus.   The distinction of these two
clinical entities was further established by epidemiologic studies
at the Willowbrook State School (1).   A patient, "M.S.", developed
two sequential episodes of hepatitis, one having a short incubation
period similar to infectious hepatitis (MS-1) and the other, a long
incubation period similar to serum hepatitis (MS-2).   MS-1 serum
consistently produced short incubation disease and MS-2, long
incubation disease, when administered to volunteers.   Later,
following discovery of the Australia antigen (2), it could be shown
that MS-1 disease and natural epidemics of infectious hepatitis
were consistently Australia antigen-negative, whereas MS-2 disease
and many cases of parenterally induced hepatitis were Australia
antigen-positive (3).   The distinction of two forms of human viral
hepatitis was thus unequivocal on clinical, epidemiologic and
serologic grounds.

Many years were to pass before serologic breakthroughs
established the presence of one or more additional human hepatitis

viruses, now designated non-A, non-B (NANB). Suspicion that there might be a third human hepatitis virus actually emanated from the earlier observation that, among the general population, the incubation periods of human viral hepatitis did not describe the bimodal curve that would be predicted by two entities with the diverse incubation periods of hepatitis A and B (4). It was thus suggested that there might be a disease with an intermediate incubation period accounting for the unimodal curve which was observed. As was later established, the mean incubation period of NANB hepatitis is indeed intermediate between that of hepatitis A and hepatitis B.

. In essence, the existence of NANB hepatitis as a clinical entity was established when cases of post-transfusion hepatitis were shown to be serologically distinct from hepatitis A and from hepatitis B; it can not as yet be established by a specific serologic test for the agent(s) of NANB. Thus, in the presence of elevated serum transaminase, the diagnosis of NANB hepatitis is based upon the serologic exclusion of hepatitis A and B and upon the clinical exclusion of other causes of hepatocellular injury. The terminology "non-A, non-B", though awkward, is retained in this manuscript because it allows for the possibility of more than one agent or groups of agents and because it does not presume etiologic relationships which are as yet unknown. When specific and proven serologic tests become available, then specific designations such as hepatitis C, D, etc., can be applied.

RELATION TO POST-TRANSFUSION HEPATITIS

Most of what is currently known about NANB hepatitis has derived from prospective studies of post-transfusion hepatitis (PTH). In seeking the causes of PTH, such studies first demonstrated the inordinate hepatitis risk of commercial donor blood (5,6). With rare exception in specific population areas, every prospective study which has compared volunteer and commercial blood sources has demonstrated the extraordinarily high risk of paid-donor blood. Similarly, the adoption of an all-volunteer program by blood banks previously dependent on commercial donors has resulted in dramatic decreases in PTH (7). Presently there is no serologic test, no specific blood product (including frozen red cells), and no donor screening measure which can so profoundly effect the incidence of PTH as can exclusion of the paid blood donor. This is because paid donors are 3-5 times more likely than volunteer donors to be carriers of both hepatitis B and hepatitis NANB viruses. Also, because paid donors often come from derelict populations dependent on the income derived from blood donation, they tend to donate as frequently as possible and by using assumed names they may donate more frequently than is permitted by FDA regulations. A single asymptomatic hepatitis carrier might thus transmit hepatitis to as many as 6-10 recipients per year, especially if their blood is divided into specific components.

The discovery of the Australia antigen (hepatitis B surface antigen, HBsAg) and its eventual association with type B hepatitis (8) provided another means to exclude high-risk donors. Prospective studies (9,10) clearly demonstrated the hepatitis risk of HBsAg-positive blood and the combined exclusion of paid and HBsAg-positive donors was shown to effect an 85% reduction in PTH (7). Despite this dramatic reduction and despite the exclusion of these two major risk factors, it was shown that approximately 10% of prospectively followed, multiply-transfused patients continued to develop either icteric or anicteric hepatitis. The initial assumption was that many of these residual cases were due to transmission of the hepatitis B virus (HBV) by donors who carried this virus at levels which could not be detected by the relatively insensitive screening methods employed in the early 1970's. Indeed, such a mechanism did account and continues to account for some cases of PTH, but the number of such cases is exceedingly small. The introduction of very sensitive radioimmunoassays for HBsAg in the mid and late 1970's reduced the incidence of type B hepatitis to almost negligible levels, but did not markedly affect the overall incidence of PTH. Hence it became clear that most PTH was due to an agent or agents distinct from HBV (11). Parenthetically, by testing stored sera by radioimmunoassay it could be shown that, even prior to HBsAg screening of donors, no more than 25-30% of PTH was due to HBV (9,12). Hence, from its inception the major portion of PTH was really due to a virus other than the "serum" hepatitis virus i.e., was "Non-B". With these observations in mind, it was then assumed that a large proportion of PTH was due to the hepatitis A virus (HAV). This, however, was inconsistent with several facts. First, studies performed in World War II and thereafter had shown that the period of infectivity in hepatitis A was relatively brief and that persons were seldom infectious for more than 2-3 weeks after the onset of clinical hepatitis; a chronic carrier state for the hepatitis A virus had never been established. Second, the epidemiology of PTH was markedly different from that of hepatitis A in that the incubation period was considerably longer and in that there was no evidence for fecal-oral transmission from patients with PTH to their families or other close personal contacts (13). These epidemiologic inconsistencies were clarified when Feinstone, Kapikian and Purcell (14) developed a reliable test (immune electronmicroscopy) to establish recent exposure to the HAV. Applying this test to paired sera from patients who had developed PTH demonstrated that none of 22 such patients had been exposed to HAV in temporal relation to the development of PTH (15). Expansion of these and other techniques for detecting immune responses to HAV to hundreds of cases of PTH have now clearly demonstrated that the hepatitis A virus is rarely, if ever, responsible for PTH. The reasons for this are twofold. First, and most important, there does not appear to be a chronic carrier state for HAV as there is for HBV and, as will be shown later, for NANB virus(es). Second, many people are exposed to

HAV in early life and already have immunity to this virus by the
time they are transfused.   The transmission of hepatitis A by a
blood donor would thus depend on their presentation during the late
incubation period of hepatitis A infection and the transfusion of
their blood to a susceptible recipient.   This combination of events
must be an extremely rare occurrence.

By employing sensitive serologic markers for hepatitis A and
hepatitis B virus exposure, between 86 and 94 percent of PTH is
now classified as non-A, non-B (16-18).   In essence, virtually no
PTH is due to HAV and, when employing an HBsAg-screened, volunteer-
donor population, a vanishingly small number of cases are due to
HBV.   In a prospective study of over 600-multiply transfused
recipients at the National Institutes of Health, there has not been
one single case of type B PTH in the past three years.   Serologic
studies have also shown that PTH is unrelated to the Epstein-Barr
virus.   The role of the cytomegalovirus (CMV) in PTH is harder to
ascertain because of the peculiar serologic qualities of this virus
and because it tends to be reactivated in patients whether or not
they are transfused.   Since CMV antibody seroconversion occurs
with almost equal frequency among transfused patients who do and
do not develop hepatitis, it is difficult to establish an etiologic
relationship of this virus to the ensuing hepatitis.   Our recent
observations (17) suggest that a subset of non-A, non-B hepatitis
cases may represent CMV infection.   This subset is characterized
by a short incubation period (mean - five weeks), anicteric disease,
minimal transaminase elevation (less than 200 IU/L), brief duration
(less than four weeks), occasional fever and anti-CMV seroconversion.
Approximately 15% of our non-A, non-B cases fulfill these criteria
and may be due to CMV.   The remaining cases cannot be attributed
to any known virus and hence represent a newly recognized etiologic
agent which currently accounts for approximately 90% of post-
transfusion hepatitis.

TRANSMISSION BY ROUTES OTHER THAN BLOOD

Although most NANB hepatitis has been recognized in the setting
of recent blood transfusion, it has become increasingly apparent
that this virus must also be transmitted by non-parenteral routes.
In 1975, Villarejos (19) reported that of 103 non-transfused
patients with hepatitis in an endemic zone of Costa Rica, 12
demonstrated no serologic evidence for infection related to HAV,
HBV or EBV.   Only one case might have been related to CMV, leaving
at least 11 cases of NANB hepatitis unrelated to blood transfusion.
Dienstag and co-workers (20) studied 40 patients hospitalized for
sporadic acute hepatitis serologically unrelated to HBV.   Of these,
half represented type A hepatitis and half were NANB.   Of the 20
patients with NANB hepatitis, ten gave a history of blood transfusion or illicit self-injection in the preceding six months, but
in the remaining ten there was no known percutaneous exposure.

The full extent of non-parenteral transmission of NANB cannot
be ascertained until reliable serologic markers are identified.
Only then can populations be screened for silent carriers and for
evidence of past exposure as assessed by the presence of specific
antibody.   It is anticipated that when such markers are available
the spread of NANB will be found to parallel that of HBV with
transmission occurring not only by percutaneous inoculation, but
also by sexual contact, by transmission from mother to fetus and
perhaps by other routes associated with close personal contact.
As with hepatitis B, there is no evidence for fecal-oral transmission or common source epidemics.   Increasingly, blood donors
and other individuals are being found with persistently elevated
serum transaminase and no history of overt hepatitis, blood transfusion or illicit drug usage.   It is probable that these represent
cases of anicteric NANB hepatitis which have evolved into clinically
inapparent chronic liver disease.

EVIDENCE FOR A TRANSMISSIBLE AGENT

Although prospective studies of PTH strongly implicated a
transmissible agent in NANB hepatitis, direct proof was lacking in
that no virus particle was observed and no serologic marker was
identified.   Could the transaminase elevations in these blood
recipients have actually been coincidental to the transfusion?
Could they represent a toxic reaction to anesthesia, to medication
or to some other element in the hospital or home environment?
That the transaminase elevations were due to the transfusion was
shown by the introduction of a non-transfused control population
which had undergone similar surgical procedures (18).   Although
there were some controls with abnormal transaminase, this number
was markedly lower than among transfused patients, clearly implica-
ting the transfusion itself as the vehicle for a transmissible
agent.   Further, the fact that paid donors were 3 to 5 times
as likely to transmit NANB as volunteer donors clearly indicated
that this form of hepatitis was a donor-related event rather than
some idiosyncratic host response.   This evidence for spread from
donor to recipient via transfusion strongly implies an infectious
transmissible agent.   More direct evidence for a transmissible
agent came from studies in chimpanzees.   These studies (21,22)
not only demonstrated that the human NANB hepatitis agent could be
transmitted to chimpanzees, but also proved the existence of a
chronic carrier state for NANB.   The latter was demonstrated when
plasma, derived from both patients with chronic hepatitis and
implicated blood donors, was able to infect chimpanzees when volumes
as low as 0.1 ml were parenterally inoculated.   Although a chronic
carrier state for NANB was highly suspect from the large number of
hepatitis cases occurring after transfusion from presumably healthy
donors, these studies in chimpanzees were necessary to unequivocally
establish this important epidemiologic occurrence.   Thus, NANB is
identical to hepatitis B in the existence of chronic asymptomatic

carriers and in the prolonged presence of virus during the course
of chronic hepatitis.   An asymptomatic carrier state in excess of
three years has been documented and it is anticipated that some
persons will be lifelong carriers of this agent.

     Further evidence for the existence of a transmissible agent
came from a retrospective serologic analysis of human hepatitis
transmission studies performed in the early 1950's (23).   In this
study, serum from three HBsAg-negative donors previously implicated
in the transmission of icteric PTH was inoculated into three groups
of human volunteers.   Serum from one donor caused hepatitis in 7
of 15 (47%) recipients, whereas serum from each of the other two
donors caused hepatitis in 1 of 10 (10%) recipients.   Hepatitis
in each of the recipients was classified as non-A, non-B.   Serum
from these donors was obtained 149 to 385 days after the implicated
blood donation.   The infectivity of these sera thus attests not
only to the transmissibility of NANB hepatitis but also to the
existence of a chronic carrier state, findings identical to those
obtained in the above noted chimpanzee transmission studies.

     Although the transmissible agent in NANB is presumed to be a
virus, its viral nature has not been proved.   We do, however,
know that the agent can be filtered and is in the size range of
other established viruses, and that the histologic changes induced
in human and chimpanzee liver are typical of that of viral hepatitis.
Final proof of its viral nature will have to await the confirmed
demonstration of an associated virus particle and particularly the
demonstration of viral nucleic acid or nucleic acid polymerase.

EVIDENCE FOR MULTIPLE NANB AGENTS

     No sooner had the concept of a third major human hepatitis
virus been accepted, than the spectre of still additional human
hepatitis viruses was raised.   Indeed, it was the possibility of
multiple agents that led to the adoption of the term non-A, non-B,
rather than a more specific terminology such as hepatitis C.
Evidence for the possible existence of more than one NANB agent
comes from three sources.   First, it was observed that occasional
patients had multiple histologically documented episodes of acute
hepatitis, at least two of which could be classified as non-A, non-B
(24,25).   This apparent lack of cross-immunity suggests that within
the broad classification of NANB there may be at least two serologically distinct agents.   Second, wide divergence in incubation
periods also suggests the possibility of multiple NANB agents.
While most post-transfusion hepatitis is associated with an incubation period ranging between 5 and 13 weeks (mean 7-8 weeks), some
cases have a prolonged incubation period (20-26 weeks) and some
have a distinctly shorter incubation period.   The short incubation
disease has been particularly striking and has been associated with
the administration of coagulation factor concentrates (26) and with

a hepatitis outbreak in an oncology unit (27).   In the first
instance, six hemophiliac children developed NANB hepatitis with
an incubation period of only 4 to 19 days from the time of receipt
of factor VIII concentrate to the onset of clinical illness (26).
In this regard, Zuckerman and co-workers (28) have reported that
a chimp previously infected with NANB hepatitis developed fatal
fulminant hepatitis less than two weeks after the administration
of commercial factor IX concentrate.   In a serologic re-evaluation
of a hepatitis epidemic in an oncology unit, cases originally
thought to represent hepatitis A because of their short incubation
period were actually found to be NANB (27).   The mean incubation
period in these cases was 27 days with a range of 22 to 37 days.

Still further indirect evidence for more than one NANB agent
derives from electronmicroscopic (EM) studies by Shimizu et al (29).
These investigators demonstrated two distinct ultrastructural
abnormalities in chimpanzees developing NANB hepatitis following
inoculation of human blood.   The majority of animals developed
characteristic cytoplasmic changes, most notably in the endoplasmic
reticulum.   Other chimpanzees developed well defined nuclear
inclusions.   The striking feature was that each chimpanzee developed
one or the other of these morphologic changes, but not both.   Thus,
while these EM changes did not represent viral particles per se,
they did represent distinct ultrastructural abnormalities which
appeared to "breed true" on serial passage and which could apparently
distinguish two classes of human inocula and, by inference, two
NANB agents.   Since these initial observations, there have been
two instances where an inoculum which generally produced nuclear
changes instead resulted in cytoplasmic change.   This could mean
that the morphologic changes observed do not actually indicate
separate infectious agents, or it could mean that the inoculum
contained both agents.   Studies are now in progress to sort this
out.

In lieu of direct observation of the virus and in lieu of
specific serologic tests, attempts to provide evidence for multiple
NANB agents have centred on cross-challenge studies in chimpanzees.
The presumption of these studies is that a second episode of acute
hepatitis is due to an agent serologically distinct from that
causing the first episode.   Thus far, most laboratories performing
these experiments have failed to demonstrate a successful cross-
challenge.   Studies at Baylor University, however, do suggest a
successful cross-challenge and provide additional evidence for two
NANB agents (30).

VIRUS DETECTION

Most laboratories performing EM studies of serum and liver
derived from humans or chimpanzees with acute or chronic hepatitis
have not observed a characteristic particle associated with NANB.

These studies are difficult because there are many structures in human sera and tissue which can simulate viruses, and because the lack of a confirmed anti-NANB reagent restricts the ability to determine specificity by immune-electronmicroscopy (IEM).   Several candidate NANB particles have, however, been reported.   In 1979 Bradley and co-workers at the Center for Disease Control (31) reported that two lots of factor VIII concentrate implicated in human hepatitis transmission also induced hepatitis in experimental chimpanzees.   Virus-like particles, 27 nm in diameter, were observed by IEM in a homogenate prepared from a wedge liver biopsy from the factor VIII-infused chimp that had developed the most severe disease.   Both empty and full particles were aggregated by convalescent serum derived from a hemophiliac patient that had originally been infected by the same factor VIII concentrate. These particles were purified on a cesium chloride gradient and then inoculated into two additional chimpanzees, both of which developed hepatitis.   Thus, not only were particles observed, but they appeared to be infectious.   A different particle recovered from serum and urine of renal dialysis patients with NANB hepatitis has also been briefly reported (32).   This particle was 60 nm in diameter and had a 40 nm core.   IEM was not attempted.

In a provocative study, Hantz et al (33) have recently reported hepatitis B-like virus particles occurring in the sera of patients with NANB hepatitis.   These particles included small spheres and filaments 15-25 nm in diameter and 35-40 nm Dane-like particles. Studied under code, such particles were detected transiently in 3 of 4 acute and 7 of 8 chronic cases of NANB hepatitis-associated with a positive serologic test for NANB antigen.   These particles were not observed in cases of drug-induced hepatitis, obstructive jaundice, or type A hepatitis and were only rarely seen in very small numbers in type B hepatitis.   The particles did not express hepatitis B surface antigen or NANB antigen on their surface but they were associated in three patients with endogenous DNA poly- merase activity.   Lastly, particles similar to the core of HBV were recovered from the liver homogenate of a patient who died with NANB hepatitis.   The investigators concluded that the NANB hepatitis virion appears as a hepatitis B-like virus, though the exact kinship between these two agents is presently unknown.   This important study must be confirmed, but if verified would suggest that NANB and hepatitis B are closely related agents and that together they represent a new class of human virus.   Their morphologic similarity would fit well with the similarity of their clinical and epidemio- logic patterns.

Just as interpretation of observed particles has been difficult, so too has interpretation of NANB tests.   Prince et al (34) reported a radioimmunoassay test for NANB in 1978, but subsequently these investigators have been unable to reproduce this result and have retracted their initial claim.   In 1978, Shirachi et al (35)

reported an agar gel diffusion (AGD) test for non-A, non-B.   This
test has been reproducible in the investigators' laboratory and
has unofficially been confirmed in other laboratories, but scarcity
of reagents has made wide-scale confirmation and usage of this test
difficult.   Shirachi et al divided their NANB post-transfusion
hepatitis cases into two types based on the pattern and duration of
transaminase (ALT) elevation.   Type-1 (monophasic) hepatitis cases
had a rapid rise and then sharp fall in serum ALT; the mean incubation period was relatively short (5.7 weeks) and the mean duration
of abnormal ALT was only 5.8 weeks.   The NANB antigen (designated
"HC" antigen in the publication) was detected in only 4 of 10
type-1 hepatitis cases and the corresponding antibody could not be
found in the convalescent sera from any of these patients.   Type-2
(biphasic) hepatitis was characterized by a rapid increase and
decrease in ALT similar to the monophasic type-1, but this was
followed by another increase and then gradual decrease in serum ALT.
The mean incubation period in these cases was 7.2 weeks and abnormal
ALT persisted for eight to 24 weeks.   HC antigen was universal in
this group, occurring in 13 of 13 acute phase sera.   HC antibody
was also more common in this group than in type-1, but still
relatively uncommon, occurring in only four of the 13 patients
during convalescence from their disease.   Typically HC antigen
appeared one to five weeks after transfusion and hence before the
onset of transaminase abnormality or clinical illness.   HC antigen
was not found in 25 patients with alcoholic hepatitis, but was
found in two of nine patients with acute type B hepatitis unrelated
to transfusion.   Neither HC nor anti-HC was found in any of 60
blood donors.   Subsequent studies from this laboratory (U.S. -
Japan Symposium, unpublished data) indicate that the HC system is
more complex than originally proposed.   There appear now to be two,
and possibly three "NANB" antigens and the relationship to transfusion hepatitis is not as clear, in that many patients already
have the antigen prior to transfusion.   Lastly, biophysical studies
indicate that HC antigen is not associated with a particle, but
rather is of low molecular weight having sedimentation characteristics more like a serum protein than like other virus particle-
associated antigens.

Using convalescent serum obtained from an experimentally
infected chimpanzee, Tabor et al (36) detected an antigen by
counterelectrophoresis in the acute phase sera of six or seven
chimpanzees with experimentally induced NANB hepatitis.   Although
the antigen was found in these animals, its relationship to serum
transaminase was very inconstant, sometimes appearing before and
sometimes weeks to months after the first transaminase elevation.
This antigen was not found in pre-inoculation serum samples or in
chimpanzees that had developed type A or type B hepatitis.   The
antigen was also detected in the sera of three humans with chronic
NANB hepatitis whose blood had transmitted NANB to other humans
and to chimpanzees.   In addition, the antigen was detected in the

serum of 11 of 31 blood donors previously implicated because they
were the only donor to patients who developed NANB post-transfusion
hepatitis.   Lastly, utilizing indirect immunofluorescence and
convalescent chimpanzee and human antibody, this laboratory (37)
demonstrated nuclear fluorescence in the livers of some infected
chimpanzees, but not in the livers of uninfected animals.   The
relationship of the antigen detected by CEP and immunofluorescence
to the HC antigen detected by AGD is not completely clear, but there
does appear to be some serologic identity (38).

     NANB-related precipitin lines have also been detected by agar
gel diffusion by Vitvitski and co-workers in France (39).   Using
sera from repeatedly transfused or NANB convalescent patients they
detected antigen in 12 of 14 patients during the early acute phase
of NANB hepatitis, but did not find the antigen in 17 patients with
drug-induced hepatitis, or hepatitis due to hepatitis viruses A or
B, nor in 50 normal blood donors.   In the 12 patients with antigen
after transfusion, the antigen became detectable 2-4 weeks before
a significant rise in ALT in five, and within four weeks of the
peak ALT in the others.   Antigenemia was transient in two cases
(less than 12 weeks) and persistent for as long as two and a half
years in the other cases.   NANB antibody developed in 5 of the 14
cases, all of whom had cleared antigen previously.   In those who
developed NANB antibody, the serum transaminase returned to normal,
whereas ALT returned to normal in only one of five patients with
persistent antigenemia.   Of interest, the NANB antigen was also
demonstrated in liver extracts from patients with chronic hepatitis
and chronic NANB antigenemia and specific hepatic nuclear fluorescence was demonstrated by direct immunofluorescence.

     In composite, these studies suggesting a specific NANB antigen
or antigens are very encouraging.   However, caution must still be
expressed because the exact relation among the various described
antigens is not yet known and because the specificity of these
reactions for NANB has not been unequivocally demonstrated.   Because
of these uncertainties, a coded panel of suspected NANB antigens
and of sera known to transmit NANB hepatitis has been distributed
to 15 laboratories actively engaged in this area of research.   The
code will be broken at a NANB workshop to be held in Vienna soon
after completion of this manuscript.   Hopefully this workshop will
determine if the described antigens are indeed specific for NANB,
will determine the number of distinct NANB antigens, and will
identify an antibody which is available in sufficient quantity to
take these tests out of the research laboratory and into the area
of practical application.

CLINICAL SPECTRUM

     Data on the clinical manifestations of NANB are accumulating
rapidly and a pattern, albeit diverse, is beginning to emerge.

Most of these data have derived from prospective studies of PTH, although sporadic cases where the transmission pattern is unknown seem to be clinically similar.

As mentioned previously, the incubation period of NANB tends to be intermediate between that of type A and type B hepatitis. Cases generally occur between five and 13 weeks post-transfusion with a mean incubation of approximately 8 weeks. However, cases with incubation periods under three weeks and over 20 weeks have also been described. Although the mean incubation periods of type A, type B and NANB hepatitis differ, the range of incubation periods is so broad that these cases overlap considerably; in individual cases the time of onset of disease cannot be reliably used to determine the virus etiology.

A striking feature of NANB is the relatively benign acute illness. The number of icteric cases in PTH studies (13,17,18,40) has varied from 18-39%; a general approximation is that 75% of cases are anicteric. ALT values tend to parallel the severity indicated by the serum bilirubin. In one study of 26 cases of NANB PTH (17), 65% had maximal ALT values less than 800 IU/L, 27% had maximal values between 800 and 2,000 IU/L and 8% had ALT values in excess of 2,000 IU/L. In general, type B hepatitis tends to be more acutely severe than NANB and more frequently requires hospitalization; indeed the need for hospitalization during the more acute phase of NANB hepatitis is extremely unusual. Despite the trend of NANB to be clinically mild, individual cases may be severe and thus, as with incubation period, clinical and biochemical severity cannot be used to reliably distinguish NANB hepatitis from that caused by HAV or HBV.

Another characteristic, but not pathognomonic feature of NANB is the tendency for ALT values to fluctuate markedly over relatively brief intervals. This is particularly true in chronic NANB hepatitis where the ALT may fluctuate from normal to markedly abnormal in a period of days to weeks and where this cycle may be repeated many times over the course of months to years. Another unusual finding, both in humans and chimpanzees developing NANB hepatitis, is the sometimes biphasic nature of the initial transaminase elevations. In prospectively followed cases, one may see rises in ALT to from 1 to 1.5 times the upper limit of normal occurring at 3-4 weeks after inoculation. The transaminase then tends to return toward baseline only to rise more dramatically with the true onset of a more severe and prolonged episode of hepatitis. The reasons for this early transaminase rise and for the subsequent widely fluctuating ALT levels are unknown.

Perhaps the most significant aspect of NANB hepatitis is its tendency to progress to chronic liver disease. In a prospective study at NIH (41), 46% of 26 cases still had abnormal transaminase

values one year after the onset of their disease.   In this study
and in others (16,18,40,42) the majority (approximately 70%) of
biopsied patients had chronic active hepatitis;   most of the
remainder had chronic persistent hepatitis and some had cirrhosis.
Some of the patients with CAH also had elements of cirrhosis
suggesting progression to this end stage lesion.   The percentage
of patients with acute NANB hepatitis who rapidly and fully recover
from the acute episode is unknown.   It would appear from the above
that almost half the patients do not recover within the first year
as assessed by persistent or fluctuating enzyme abnormalities and
then by biopsy confirmation.   In addition to this large group,
there are other patients who make an apparent sustained full recovery
only to have abnormal ALT values reappear six months to a year later.
Lastly, it is probable that, as in type B hepatitis, there are other
patients who become chronic carriers of the NANB virus despite
normalization of serum transaminase.

Fortunately, the chronic hepatitis in NANB infection tends to
be clinically and histologically less severe than would be indicated
by the biopsy classification of chronic active hepatitis.   While
there is no doubt the biopsies fulfill the histologic criteria for
chronic active hepatitis (43), bridging necrosis is rarely seen
and, in the few cases where serial biopsy has been performed, the
histologic lesion seems to be stable or resolving rather than progressive.   On the other hand, there are clearly some cases that do
progress to cirrhosis and indeed this may be one of the major etiologies of what had been termed cryptogenic cirrhosis.

Most patients with chronic NANB hepatitis are relatively
asymptomatic and in others, the only symptom is easy fatigibility;
most patients are able to continue full time employment and some,
despite severe persistent enzyme abnormalities, are totally asymptomatic.   Even those with biopsy proven cirrhosis do not present
with the signs and symptoms generally associated with cirrhosis.
Hepatomegaly and sometimes splenomegaly are observed, but ascites,
gastrointestinal bleeding, esophageal varices and other evidences
of abnormal collateral circulation are not seen and no prospectively
followed patient has yet been reported to have died from hepatic
coma and end-stage liver disease.   One must caution, however, that
NANB is still a newly recognized disease and that an insufficient
number of patients has been followed for a long enough period to
assess the long term sequelae.   There is hope however, based on
the gradual downward trend of serum transaminase and on the observed
histologic resolution in some cases, that chronic NANB hepatitis
might, in most cases, be a slowly resolving disease rather than
one which is rapidly and insidiously progressive.

PREVENTION AND TREATMENT

Obviously the most significant preventive measure in terms of

NANB post-transfusion hepatitis will be the development of a
practical test to detect silent virus carriers at the time of blood
donation.   As noted above, such a test may be imminent, but caution
dictates that the reported tests be confirmed in independent laboratories and that reagents be exchanged to determine the total number
of NANB antigens which must be screened.   Unfortunately, practical
tests for NANB will not be as easy to develop as they were for type
B hepatitis.   There are two major reasons for this.   First, the
circumstances for detection of the type B virus were fortuitous in
that this virus produces an enormous excess of free antigen which
never gets incorporated into a true virus particle.   Thus, in
type B hepatitis, there are approximately 1,000-2,000 antigenic
particles for every complete virus particle.   Whether this serves
a teleologic function to protect the virion from host attack or
whether it merely represents inefficient virus production and
assembly is not known.   Whatever the explanation, it results in
extremely high levels of circulating antigen and allows for viral
detection by relatively insensitive techniques such as agar gel
diffusion.   If in NANB hepatitis, the ratio of viral antigen to
whole virus particles more closely approaches unity, then this
virus will be proportionately harder to detect.

        Another problem in NANB testing is the scarcity of reagent
antibody.   If indeed 50% of NANB hepatitis cases fail to resolve
as judged by persistent transaminase elevation and if an additional
group of patients initially appears to resolve but later exacerbates
(see above) and if there is a chronic asymptomatic carrier state
with normal transaminase levels, then perhaps as little as 25% of
cases truly resolve and develop convalescent antibody.   Certainly
one of the limiting steps at present, even in attempting to confirm
reported antigens, is the lack of reagent antibody.   If such can
be identified in quantity, then commercially available assays can
be developed and the frequency of NANB PTH will diminish just as
did the frequency of type B PTH.   Still one other caveat in this
equation relates to the number of non-A, non-B agents that exist.
If this number is small (two or less), then the likelihood of
developing "broad spectrum" screening reagents is increased.   If
the number of such agents is three or more, then significant inroads
into the prevention of PTH may be greatly delayed.   In summary, at
the present time, there are multiple unknowns, including the specificity of reported tests, the amount of circulating antigen, the
availability of specific antibody and the total number of agents
which must be screened.   It is difficult to predict at present how
this equation will resolve, but the field is moving rapidly and a
large number of investigators are dedicated to the problem.   Hence
many of these answers may soon be at hand.

        As an interim measure to the development of a specific test
for NANB, it has been suggested that measuring donor ALT might
detect those donors who are chronic carriers of NANB and have a

concomitant chronic hepatitis.   A positive correlation between
donor ALT and recipient hepatitis was first reported by the
Transfusion Transmitted Virus (TTV) Study Group (18).   Of 353
recipients given volunteer units with normal ALT activity, 12 (3.4%)
developed NANB PTH.   In contrast, of 36 recipients given at least
one unit with an elevated ALT, 14 or 39% developed NANB hepatitis
(p < 0.05).   Indeed, discriminant analysis showed that donor ALT
was a far more important determinant in the occurrence of PTH than
the number of units transfused.   Analysis of this relationship in
our NIH study is not complete, but preliminary data also suggests
a significant relationship between abnormal donor ALT and recipient
hepatitis.   If this association is confirmed, then blood banks will
have to weigh the obvious advantage of hepatitis reduction against
the increased expense and time of donor screening and particularly
against the potential loss of donors who have elevated ALT levels
for reasons other than viral hepatitis.   In one study (44), 5.7%
of over 4,000 volunteer donors were found to have an abnormal ALT.
Overall it is anticipated that 3-5% of donors will have an elevated
ALT.   If such donors were routinely excluded, this would result
in the loss of roughly 300,000 to 500,000 blood units per year in
the United States alone.   Such a loss would have considerable
impact on blood delivery systems.   This loss might be tolerated
if it was unequivocally demonstrated that ALT screening would
prevent most cases of PTH.   Unfortunately, in the TTV study, 55%
of those who developed NANB hepatitis received blood only from
donors with a normal serum ALT.   Thus while ALT screening may
prevent many cases of NANB hepatitis, it will also fail to prevent
an equal or greater number.   Whether this degree of hepatitis
prevention warrants the significant depletion of donor resources
cited above is a difficult question to answer, but one which soon
will have to be faced by both blood consumer and blood supplier.
If in the interim, practical, specific tests for the NANB virus
are developed, then the decision regarding ALT testing will become
moot.

The role of gamma globulin for prophylaxis against PTH, in
general, and NANB hepatitis, in particular, represents another area
of considerable uncertainty.   There has been a large number of
publications relating to the efficacy or non-efficacy of immune
serum globulin (ISG) in the prevention of PTH (45).   As a rule,
the better controlled studies have not demonstrated efficacy and
at present neither ISG nor hepatitis B immune globulin (HBIG) is
recommended for the prophylaxis of PTH.

There have been three studies which specifically examined the
effect of gamma globulin on NANB hepatitis.   In a VA cooperative
study (40), it appeared that ISG reduced the incidence of icteric
non-B PTH, but did not significantly affect the total number of
non-B hepatitis cases observed.   Interpretation of this study was
hampered because of the large number of commercial blood donors

utilized at that time.   The paid donor was such a significant
deleterious variable in that study that it was difficult to assess
independently any other variable having a lesser impact such as
might be the case for ISG.   Knodell and coworkers (16) compared
ISG with an albumin placebo in patients undergoing open heart surgery
and found a significant decrease in both total and icteric hepatitis
among recipients of ISG.   In addition, they found that recipients
of ISG were less likely to develop chronic hepatitis.   These
provocative findings have not been confirmed and, in fact, are
partially contradicted by a later study (46) which showed no protective effect of ISG against non-B hepatitis developing in the
transfusion setting.   Thus while the role of ISG in PTH has not
been fully resolved, there is no compelling reason to advocate
its usage.

A perhaps more relevant question relates to the use of ISG
following accidental needlestick contaminated by blood from a
patient with NANB hepatitis.   Unfortunately, there have been no
published studies in this regard and I am not aware of any that are
in progress.   The use of ISG in this setting is thus empirical,
but probably indicated because of the small virus inoculum and the
extremely low risk of this product.

The use of steroids in the treatment of NANB hepatitis is yet
another unresolved issue.   Indeed, although steroids have shown
significant benefit in the treatment of "auto-immune" hepatitis,
their efficacy in any form of viral hepatitis is unproved.   Their
use in NANB hepatitis is even more difficult to evaluate because
of the generally benign clinical course, because of the naturally
occurring wide fluctuations in serum transaminase, because of the
trend toward slow spontaneous improvement and because of the lack
of proven serologic markers of virus infection.   There is thus
little way to assess the effect of therapy except perhaps by serial
liver biopsy.   There is a definite need for a placebo-controlled,
prospective study of the role of steroids in the treatment of
asymptomatic or mildly symptomatic chronic viral hepatitis.   Until
such data are forthcoming, I do not feel that steroids are generally
indicated in the treatment of chronic NANB hepatitis.   Clinically
and histologically severe cases will have to be evaluated individually to assess the risk-benefit ratio of such treatment.

The ultimate hope for NANB is the development of a specific
vaccine similar to that currently being evaluated for type B
hepatitis.   Such a vaccine is obviously far off and will have to
await the identification and purification of specific viral antigens.
Based on the similarities between this form of hepatitis and type B
hepatitis and based on the rapidity with which a type B vaccine has
evolved following the discovery of Australia antigen, it is optimistic, but not unrealistic to assume that NANB research and development will proceed along a similar pathway.

SUMMARY

The development of sensitive tests for the detection of
hepatitis A (HAV) and hepatitis B (HBV) viruses unmasked the presence
of an additional human hepatitis virus(es) tentatively designated
non-A, non-B (NANB).   Blood borne transmission of NANB from human
to human and from human to chimpanzee is now unequivocally established.   In addition, there is increasing evidence for spread by
routes other than percutaneous inoculation; the mechanism of such
transmission is currently unknown.   There is also indirect evidence
for more than one NANB agent.

NANB hepatitis is characterized by: 1) an incubation period
intermediate between hepatitis A and B; 2) anicteric disease (75%
of cases); 3) an acute phase which is generally milder than either
type A or type B hepatitis, but which cannot be distinguished from
A or B in individual cases; 4) widely fluctuating transaminase
values; 5) a very high predisposition to chronic hepatitis with
some cases progressing to cirrhosis while others seem to resolve
spontaneously.

Further progress in the elucidation and prevention of this
disease will depend on the development of specific and practical
serologic tests.   Some serologic tests have been reported, but are
at present unconfirmed.   In the interim, transaminase screening
of donors may serve to reduce the incidence of NANB post-transfusion
hepatitis.

REFERENCES

1   KRUGMAN S, GILES JP, HAMMOND J: Infectious hepatitis: evidence
          for two distinctive clinical, epidemiological and immuno-
          logical types of infection.   J Amer Med Assoc 200: 365-
          372, 1967.

2.   BLUMBERG BS, ALTER HJ, VISNICH S: A "new" antigen in leukemia
          sera.   J Amer Med Assoc 191: 541-546, 1965.

3.   GILES JP, McCOLLUM RW, BERNDTSON LW, KRUGMAN S: Viral
          hepatitis: relation of Australia/SH antigen to the
          Willowbrook MS-2 strain.   New Eng J Med 281: 119-122,
          1969.

4.   MOSLEY JW: The epidemiology of viral hepatitis: an overview.
          Amer J Med Sci 270: 253-270, 1975.

5.   WALSH JH, PURCELL RH, MORROW AG, CHANOCK RM, SCHMIDT PJ: Post-
          transfusion hepatitis after open-heart operations:
          incidence after the administration of blood from

commercial and volunteer donor populations. *J Amer Med Assoc* 211: 261-265, 1970.

6. SEEF LB, ZIMMERMAN HJ, WRIGHT EC, FINKLESTEIN JD, GARCIA-PONT P, GREENLEE HB, DIETZ AA, LEEVY CM, TAMBURRO CH, SCHIFF ER, SCHIMMEL EM, ZEMEL R, ZIMMON DS, McCOLLUM RW: A randomized double blind controlled trial of the efficacy of immune serum globulin for the prevention of post-transfusion hepatitis. *Gastroenterology 72*: 111-121,1977.

7. ALTER HJ, HOLLAND PV, PURCELL RH, LANDER JJ, FEINSTONE SM, MORROW AG, SCHMIDT PJ: Post-transfusion hepatitis after exclusion of commercial and hepatitis B antigen positive donors. *Ann Intern Med 77*: 691-699, 1972.

8. PRINCE AM: An antigen detected in the blood during the incubation period of serum hepatitis. *Proc Nat Acad Sci 60*: 814-821, 1968.

9. GOCKE VJ, GREENBERG HB, KAVEY NB: Correlation of Australia antigen with post-transfusion hepatitis. *J Amer Med Assoc 212*: 877-879, 1970.

10. HOLLAND PV, ALTER HJ, PURCELL RH, WALSH JJ, MORROW AG, SCHMIDT PJ: The infectivity of blood containing the Australia antigen. In: *Australia Antigen*. JE Prior, H Friedman (eds). University Park Press, Baltimore, 1973. pp 191-203.

11. ALTER HJ, PURCELL RH, HOLLAND PV, FEINSTONE SM, MORROW AG, MORITSUGU Y: Clinical and serological analysis of transfusion associated hepatitis. *Lancet 2*: 838-848, 1975.

12. PURCELL RH, WALSH JH, HOLLAND PV, MORROW AG, WOOD S, CHANOCK RM: Seroepidemiological studies of transfusion-associated hepatitis. *J Inf Dis 123*: 406-413, 1971.

13. PRINCE AM, BROTMAN B, GRADY GF, KUHNS MH, HAZZI C, LEVINE RW, MILLIAM SJ: Long-incubation post-transfusion hepatitis without serological evidence of exposure to hepatitis-B virus. *Lancet 2*: 241-246, 1974.

14. FEINSTONE SM, KAPIKIAN AZ, PURCELL RH: Hepatitis A: detection by immune electron microscopy of a virus-like antigen associated with acute illness. *Science 182*: 1026-1028, 1973.

15. FEINSTONE SM, KAPIKIAN AZ, PURCELL RH, ALTER HJ, HOLLAND PV: Transfusion associated hepatitis not due to viral hepatitis

type A or B. New Eng J Med 292:   767-770, 1975.

16.   KNODELL RG, CONRAD ME, GINSBERG AL, BALL CJ, FLANNERY EP:
       Efficacy of prophylactic gamma globulin in preventing
       non-A, non-B post-transfusion hepatitis. Lancet 1:
       557-561, 1976.

17.   ALTER HJ, PURCELL RH, FEINSTONE SM, HOLLAND PV, MORROW AG:
       Non-A, non-B hepatitis: a review and interim report of
       an ongoing prospective study.   In: Viral Hepatitis.
       GN Vyas, SN Cohen, R Schmid (eds). Franklin Institute
       Press, Philadelphia, 1978. pp. 359-369.

18.   AACH RD, LANDER JJ, SHERMAN LA, MILLER WV, KAHN RA, GITNICK GL,
       HOLLINGER FB, WERCH J, SZMUNESS W, STEVENS CE, KELLNER A,
       WEINER JM, MOSLEY JW: Transfusion-transmitted viruses:
       interim analysis of hepatitis among transfused and non-
       transfused patients.   In: Viral Hepatitis. GN Vyas,
       SN Cohen, R Schmid (eds). Franklin Institute Press,
       Philadelphia, 1978. pp. 359-369.

19.   VILLAREJOS VM, VISONA KA, EDUARTE CA, PROVOST PJ, HILLEMAN MR:
       Evidence for viral hepatitis other than type A or type B
       among persons in Costa Rica. New Engl J Med 293: 1350-
       1352, 1975.

20.   DIENSTAG JL, ALAAMA A, MOSLEY JW, REDEKER AG, PURCELL RH:
       Etiology of sporadic hepatitis B surface antigen-negative
       hepatitis.   Ann Int Med 87: 1-6, 1977.

21.   ALTER HJ, PURCELL RH, HOLLAND PV, POPPER H: Evidence for a
       transmissible agent in non-A, non-B hepatitis. Lancet 1:
       459-463, 1978.

22.   TABOR E, GERETY RJ, DRUCKER JA, SEEF LB, HOOFNAGLE JH,
       JACKSON DR, APRIL M, BARKER LF, PINEDA-TAMONDONG G:
       Transmission of non-A, non-B hepatitis from man to
       chimpanzee. Lancet 1: 463-465, 1978.

23.   HOOFNAGLE JH, GERETY RJ, TABOR E, FEINSTONE SM, BARKER LF,
       PURCELL RH: Transmission of non-A, non-B hepatitis.
       Ann Int Med 87: 14-20, 1977.

24.   MOSLEY JW, REDEKER AG, FEINSTONE SM, PURCELL RH: Multiple
       hepatitis viruses in multiple attacks of acute viral
       hepatitis. New Engl J Med 296: 75-78, 1977.

25.   NORKRANS G: Clinical epidemiological and prognostic aspects
       of hepatitis A, B and non-A, non-B. Scand J Inf Dis
       Suppl 17, 1978.

26.   HRUBY MA, SCHAUF V: Transfusion-related short-incubation
      hepatitis in hemophiliac patients. J Amer Med Assoc
      240: 1355-1359, 1978.

27.   MEYERS JD, DIENSTAG JL, PURCELL RH, THOMAS ED, HOLMES KK:
      Parenterally transmitted non-A, non-B hepatitis: an
      epidemic reassessed. Ann Int Med 87: 57-59, 1977.

28.   TSIQUAYE KN, BIRD RG, TOBEY G, WYKE RJ, WILLIAMS R,
      ZUCKERMAN AJ: Further evidence of cellular changes
      associated with non-A, non-B hepatitis.   J Med Virol 5:
      63-71, 1980.

29.   SHIMIZU YK, FEINSTONE SM, ALTER HJ, PURCELL RH: Non-A, non-B
      hepatitis: ultrastructural alterations associated with
      acute illness in livers of experimentally infected
      chimpanzees. Science 205: 197-200, 1979.

30.   HOLLINGER B: Personal communication.

31.   BRADLEY DW, COOK EH, MAYNARD JE, McCAUSTLAND KA, EBERT JW,
      DOLANA GH, PETZEL RA, KANTOR RH, HEILBRUNN A, FIELDS HA,
      MURPHY BL: Experimental infection of chimpanzees with
      antihemophiliac (factor VIII) materials: recovery of
      virus-like particles associated with non-A, non-B hepa-
      titis. J Med Virology 3: 253-269, 1979.

32.   CORSAGET P, MAUPAS PH, LEVIN P, BAREN F: Virus-like particles
      associated with non-A, non-B hepatitis.   Lancet 2: 92,
      1979.

33.   HANTZ O, VITVITSKI L, TREPO C: Non-A, non-B hepatitis:
      identification of hepatitis B-like virus particles in
      serum and liver.   J Med Virology 5: 73-86, 1980.

34.   PRINCE AM, BROTMAN B, VAN DEN ENDE MA, RICHARDSON L, KELLNER A:
      Non-A, non-B hepatitis: identification of a virus-
      specific antigen and antibody. A preliminary report.
      In: Viral Hepatitis. GN Vyas, SN Cohen, R Schmid (eds)
      Franklin Institute Press, Philadelphia, 1978. pp. 633-640.

35.   SHIRACHI R, SHIRAISHI H, TATEDA A, KIKUCHI K, ISHIDA N:
      Hepatitis "C" antigen in non-A, non-B post-transfusion
      hepatitis. Lancet 2: 853-856, 1978.

36.   TABOR E, MITCHELL FD, GOUDEAU AM, GERETY RJ: Detection of an
      antigen-antibody system in serum associated with human
      non-A, non-B hepatitis. J Med Virology 4: 161-169, 1979.

37.   KABIRI M, TABOR E, GERETY RJ: Antigen-antibody system

associated with non-A, non-B hepatitis detected by indirect
immunofluorescence. Lancet 2: 221-224, 1979.

38. TABOR E: Personal communication.

39. VITVITSKI L, TREPO C, PRINCE AM, BROTMAN B: Detection of
virus-associated antigen in serum and liver of patients
with non-A, non-B hepatitis. Lancet 2: 1263 - 1267,
1979.

40. SEEF LB, WRIGHT EC, ZIMMERMAN HJ, HOOFNAGLE JH, DIETZ AA,
FELSHER BF, GARCIA-PONT PH, GERETY RJ, GREENLEE HB,
KIERNAN T, LEEVY CM, NATH N, SCHIFF EG, SCHWARTZ C,
TABOR E, TAMBURRO C, VLAHCEVIC Z, ZEMEL R, ZIMMON DS:
Post-transfusion hepatitis, 1973-1975: a Veterans Admin-
istration cooperative study. In: Viral Hepatitis.
GN Vyas, SN Cohen, R Schmid (eds). Franklin Institute
Press, Philadelphia, 1978. pp. 371-381.

41. BERMAN M, ALTER HJ, ISHAK KG, PURCELL RH, JONES EA: The
chronic sequelae of non-A, non-B hepatitis. Ann Intern
Med 91: 1-6, 1979.

42. GALBREATH RM, PORTMANN B, EDDLESTON AL, WILLIAMS R, GOWER PE:
Chronic liver disease developing after outbreak of
HBsAg - negative hepatitis in hemodialysis units.
Lancet 2: 886-889, 1975.

43. SCHEUER PJH, THALER H: Acute and chronic hepatitis revisited.
Lancet 2: 914-919, 1977.

44. STEVENS CE, SZMUNESS W, HIRSCH RL: Alanine aminotransferase
levels in volunteer blood donors. In: Viral Hepatitis.
GN Vyas, SN Cohen, R Schmid (eds). Franklin Institute
Press, Philadelphia, 1978. p. 737.

45. HOLLAND PV: Gamma globulin in post-transfusion hepatitis.
In: Hepatitis and Blood Transfusion. GN Vyas, HA Perkins,
R Schmid (eds). Grune and Stratton, New York, 1972.
pp. 331-333.

46. KUHNS WJ, PRINCE AM, BROTMAN B, HAZZI C, GRADY GF: A clinical
and laboratory evaluation of immune serum globulin from
donors with a history of hepatitis: attempted prevention
of post-transfusion hepatitis. Am J Med Sci 272:
255-261, 1976.

DISCUSSION

CHAIRMAN: M.M. FISHER

FISHER: Would you comment on the woodchuck virus?

ALTER: Summers, at the Institute of Cancer Research, found in the
    woodchuck a virus-like particle very similar in appearance to
    the hepatitis B virus.   It appears now that there is a class
    of virus, similar to type B, which causes hepatitis in the wood-
    chuck and certain other animals species.   The most significant
    feature is that the woodchuck develops hepatocellular carcinoma
    at an incredible rate.   For the first time there is a model
    system to approach this problem over a relatively short period
    of time.   Studies in humans are very hard because it is such
    a slowly developing disease.

PETERS: When reports began to come out about the high frequency
    with which non A non B hepatitis progresses to chronic active
    hepatitis and cirrhosis, we analyzed all our cases of chronic
    non A non B hepatitis. We found that post-transfusion hepatitis
    frequently progressed to chronic active hepatitis or cirrhosis.
    But if the patient was a drug user there was virtually no pro-
    gression to chronic active hepatitis but persistent hepatitis
    only.   What is your experience in this regard?

ALTER: We have had no experience with an addict population and we
    don't see a lot of non A non B hepatitis in our homosexual
    community.

DIENSTAG: In Boston, probably not more than 10 of our sporadic
    cases of acute viral hepatitis in gay males are non A non B.
    We have had 7 individuals with two bouts of hepatitis in the
    last two or three years and all were either A or B.   We didn't

207

see any non A non B hepatitis in those who had two distinct bouts of hepatitis. The prevalence of sporadic non A non B hepatitis is higher in the heterosexual population, around 15-20%. In gays I think A and B are diluting out the non A non B.

KRUGMAN: B obviously is much more prevalent than non A non B in male homosexuals.

PETERS: It should be emphasized that if you have fulminant hepatitis your survival rate is far poorer with non A non B than it is with B. It also looks as though the better survival in the younger age group with fulminant hepatitis B doesn't really hold with non A non B fulminant hepatitis.

ALTER: 38% of the cases of fulminant hepatitis evaluated in the Acute Hepatic Failure Study could not be characterized as hepatitis A or hepatitis B, and were not drug associated. Patients who had hepatitis B, hepatitis A or a combination of hepatitis A and B had a 35% survival and patients with non A non B hepatitis had a 13% survival. Patients with drug hepatitis had a 12% survival. But 38% probably defines the absolute maximum contribution of non A non B hepatitis to fulminant hepatitis because what is described by exclusion as non A non B hepatitis probably includes a few other things. Some of the patients involved in the study who were originally thought to have non A non B hepatitis were later shown to have ingested a hepatotoxic drug. Similarly, some non A non B fulminant hepatitis is probably hepatitis B. There are cases of fulminant hepatitis B in which the hepatitis B surface antigen becomes undetectable about the time the SGOT drops precipitously. It is unwise now to make a concrete conclusion about the relative severity of fulminant non A non B hepatitis because the population is just too heterogeneous.

PETERS: That may well be but our own data with fulminant posttransfusion hepatitis also showed that type non A non B involves a poorer prognosis than type B.

ALTER: Is the number of cases large enough?

PETERS: Possibly not. However there were other differences. For example, the type B patients who survived tended to have high alpha-fetoproteins, whereas the non A non B patients who survived did not. This makes one wonder if there is a difference in the inducing quality of the two viruses as far as alpha-fetoprotein is concerned. This may also explain why there has been such a difference in different parts of the country concerning the prognostic value of the alpha-fetoprotein in fulminant hepatitis.

DIENSTAG: Did you notice any difference between B hepatitis and non A non B hepatitis in the occurrence of chronic liver disease after fulminant hepatitis?

PETERS: No case that we have had who survived fulminant hepatitis has developed chronic liver disease.

DIENSTAG: At least some of the patients who have survived fulminant hepatitis have undergone an enormous transfusion burden.   It would be surprising if non A non B hepatitis was not super-imposed on the fulminant acute hepatitis in some.

PETERS: Most of our cases have been drug users.   They may be less likely to have two simultaneously derived viruses or be less susceptible to non A non B.

COHEN: Will the superimposition of one type of viral hepatitis upon another, or the use of drugs or hepatotoxins during acute viral hepatitis change the clinical course, causing a more fulminant or more chronic state?

DIENSTAG: There is enough information to conclude that having one virus infection doesn't predispose to a more severe case with the second.   There are many cases of simultaneous infection in which no increase in severity or chronicity has occurred. Viruses are not metabolized the way drugs are and there is to date no evidence that viral hepatitis is more severe in individuals who are taking potentially hepatotoxic drugs or that hepatotoxic drugs are more hepatotoxic in individuals with viral hepatitis.

ROY: I would like to ask Dr. Krugman some questions on vertical transmission.   Should all expectant mothers be screened? Should Hepatitis B Immune Globulin be reserved for those babies born to mothers with e antigen or born to mothers who have had hepatitis in the last trimester? What dosage of Hepatitis B Immune Globulin do you recommend?

KRUGMAN: The decision to screen mothers depends on the particular population.   Patients from areas of the world where hepatitis B is highly endemic, patients of Chinese extraction, patients who are drug addicts, and patients with carriers in their family are high risk patients and in my opinion should be screened to see if they are carriers.   But routine screening for the population at large I think is very difficult to justify because of the cost and low yield.   That doesn't mean that you shouldn't do it.   But I think that screening of the general population should be optional.

It is clear that if a mother is a carrier and e antigen positive,

there is a very, very high likelihood that the baby is going
to be infected, shortly before, at, or even some weeks after
birth. The studies reported to date suggest that HBIG given
within 48 hours of birth may prevent the chronic carrier state
in those babies who become infected. These studies were
carried out in Taiwan. They didn't give a definite answer,
but they were suggestive. Hopefully a controlled study in
progress, to be completed by the end of this year or early
next year, will define whether multiple appropriate doses of
HBIG will be effective. In the meantime I would be inclined
to give HBIG to babies born of mothers who are carriers,
regardless of their e antigen/antibody status. I would give
0.5 - 1.0 ml HBIG as soon after birth as possible. Knowing
that the antibody persists for at least 3 months, I would wait
3 months before giving the second inoculation.

DIENSTAG: The exciting possibility is that we might soon be able
to give a combination of passive immunity and vaccinate the
baby at birth. It is also possible that the vaccine may work
rapidly enough that it alone will protect.

KRUGMAN: In preliminary studies it is clear that the presence of
antibody does not inhibit the effect of the vaccine.

SHARP: What is the evidence that in chronic active hepatitis
steroids exacerbate the disease through alteration of the
virus?

DIENSTAG: This is a very complicated area. As you are aware,
the Stanford study found that viral replication dropped
dramatically with discontinuation of steroids and the suspicion
was that the steroids had increased viral replication. But
it is hard to comment in a few words about the importance of
that study or the ways of interpreting what happened. I think
that an individual with mild chronic active hepatitis type B
probably doesn't need any intervention. On the other hand,
patients with severe chronic active hepatitis may experience
a remission initially on high dose corticosteroids, but will
deteriorate when the attempt is made to taper them to doses
which are sufficient to maintain non B chronic active hepatitis.
They will require repeated increases in corticosteroid therapy
and will still not do very well. So there is a dichotomy
between those who have mild disease and don't need any intervention and those who have severe disease and, regardless of
intervention, won't do well. Whether corticosteroids impair
virus elimination or enhance virus replication is conjectural
at this point. The question has not been approached directly.

SHARP: Dr. Alter, when you documented the fluctuating enzyme
changes in non A non B, did you recheck for all the viruses

to rule out another viral infection?

ALTER: We always recheck for B and could never implicate B. We
    don't routinely check for A and we haven't checked everything
    else.   But I am pretty confident that this is all one disease.

    I would like to comment on your previous question.   The
    question usually asked is not do steroids make it worse, but
    do steroids make it better and should they be used?   Paul Berk
    and a group at NIH reviewed three studies on steroids and
    chronic hepatitis and in particular addressed the question as to
    whether steroids should be used in asymptomatic chronic hepa-
    titis.   Although it seemed clear that steroids were beneficial
    in chronic active hepatitis of "autoimmune" origin, there was
    no evidence that steroids worked in viral induced chronic
    hepatitis and particularly in milder forms.   All the cases
    in which help was shown were the very, very severe cases and
    they proposed to do a prospective controlled trial.   The
    study was approved but not funded so I don't know if the
    answer is ever going to come.

MOROZ: I would like to ask Dr. Alter if non A non B hepatitis
    might play a role in neonatal hepatitis or biliary atresia.

ALTER: I realize that this is a pediatric meeting, but I have
    absolutely no data on non A non B in the pediatric age group.
    I suspect that whatever we can say about B we will eventually
    be able to say about non A non B and that maternal-fetal
    transmission will be documented.   I have no idea about
    biliary atresia.

KRUGMAN: The problem of hepatitis B in infants born of mothers
    with hepatitis B really wasn't recognized until the markers of
    infection became available and I think it is absolutely
    impossible to state whether there is or isn't a non A non B
    problem.   The encouraging thing is that in the high risk
    populations who can be studied, such as the male homosexuals,
    it appears that B is the big problem; non A non B is not.
    Hopefully that situation with non A non B will also be present
    in pregnancy.

SHAPERO: Is there any information on the role of steroid therapy
    in chronic active non A non B post-transfusion hepatitis?

ALTER: No study has really looked at this.   We tend not to use
    steroids because the disease is relatively mild in most cases.
    Even the few patients who have cirrhosis have none of the
    clinical stigmata of cirrhosis, are asymptomatic except for
    fatigue, and are working full-time.   It is difficult to
    evaluate treatment in a disease which has minimal symptoms

and a natural history of spontaneous regression.   But we use
steroids whenever somebody is on the sicker side and we don't
know what else to do!

TODARO: Dr. Krugman, would you comment on what to do about the
screening of medical personnel and what to do when one finds
an antigen carrier?

KRUGMAN: At the present time all medical personnel working in our
medical centre are routinely screened for both antigen and
antibody when they begin to work there.   So we know who is
antiHBs positive and who is likely HBsAg positive.   In the
event that there is an exposure, we can get in very quickly
and give the HBIG if it is indicated.

Your second question is difficult.   There are probably some
carriers in most institutions and I think that if they know
they are positive they can take the appropriate precautions.
The risk that they will transmit hepatitis is very, very low,
and there is no good indication for labelling them as "lepers".
It is only in those special circumstances where you have
someone that you can't really rely upon that you have to step
in and do something.   But that is the rare exception.   For
that person to transmit hepatitis he/she has either to inject
their blood into someone, or to get into bed with someone and
exchange secretions.   Hepatitis B is not transmitted by just
examining patients.   The epidemiology of hepatitis B encourages
us to be less and less prone to restrict the activities of
these people with very rare exceptions.

TODARO: In the nursery?

KRUGMAN: I can't see any problem in a nursery if carriers follow
the technique that they should follow.   They should be
washing their hands very carefully, and be wearing masks and
gloves when they examine the babies.   I think they really are
a negligible risk because more precautions are used in a nursery
than in other areas of the hospital.   However if something
happens to any baby in that nursery completely unrelated to
the carrier, the burden of proof will be on the administrator.
Therefore I would assign the carrier to some place other than
the nursery.

DIENSTAG: This is the hardest question to answer, even worse than
the steroid question.   There are certain groups of health
workers who, as carriers, are more likely to transmit the
disease.   Surgeons, dentists and especially oral surgeons,
obstetricians and gynecologists and members of phlebotomy
teams are examples.   What we have are occasional reports where
several cases have been traced back to a particular antigen

positive individual. There is no doubt that transmission does occur but it is rare considering the number of carriers that must exist within the medical profession. The few prospective studies that have been done with nurses and general physicians have not shown that there is a significant risk of transmission. My policy is not to change sombody's activities. But every case has to be weighed differently. I would advise not to screen all personnel until you have established a policy of what to do with the antigen positive individuals you discover. I would screen in certain areas such as dialysis units where spread can be extensive, but more as a measure of technique rather than as a means to limit occupations.

KRUGMAN: I think it is important to separate the retrospective case reports involving individuals who at the time that hepatitis B was being spread had absolutely no idea that they were carriers. That is entirely different from the situation where you begin prospectively with a carrier who, as a health professional, knows the potential risks and takes precautions.

DIENSTAG: Except in surgery or oral surgery where a cut finger cannot always be prevented. Studies are needed but are very difficult. One has to follow controls, because there is a spontaneous rate of sero-conversion in the hospital population. To follow one or two carriers means one has to follow 200-400 patients for 6-9 months. And one has to get informed consent from everybody! It is no wonder the studies are not being done.

LARK: What is the panel's view of breast-feeding by the mother who is a chronic carrier of viral hepatitis?

KRUGMAN: If you are speaking about a mother who happens to be of Chinese extraction and who is e antigen positive, the risk of the baby getting hepatitis B is very high, especially if she lives where the alternative to breast-feeding is milk that contains all kinds of enteric organisms. A study carried out in Taiwan indicated that there is no difference in the attack rate of hepatitis B in breast-fed infants as compared with infants who are not breast-fed. This is probably because the babies go into such a highly infectious environment that it makes no difference whether they are breast-fed or not. Under these circumstances it seems to me that breast-feeding should be continued. You prevent gastroenteritis and all of other things they get from the milk used in these areas. But in North America, where the risk is not 60-70% but 10% or less, it is my feeling that breast-feeding should not be recommended. Mothers can give their babies all of the necessary love and devotion without breast milk, without exchanging secretions. I think that breast-feeding might

increase the risk, who knows, from 8% up to 15 or 20%.
But I don't have the data and we will never demonstrate
this in a study.

ISSENMAN: How would you follow the infant that you have immunized
with hyperimmune globulin?

KRUGMAN: It has been shown very clearly that infants given hyperimmune globulin still get an infection and that the infection
may occur after a very long incubation period.   The incubation
period may be prolonged 5-6 months.   So an infant who has been
exposed should be followed after the inoculation of HBIG.
Most of the infants who develop antigenemia will have no
symptoms so every couple of months a sample of blood should
be taken to determine if the baby has become antigen positive,
or has developed antibody to the surface antigen.   They
should be followed in this way during the first year and
possibly during the second year.   It is also important to tell
the mother something about how hepatitis B spreads, so that she
will take precautions to prevent the horizontal spread of
infection.   But it is much more difficult for a mother to
infect a baby horizontally under the conditions that exist in
most developed areas of the world.

ISSENMAN: Are there guidelines for re-immunization?

KRUGMAN: My personal feeling about this is that re-immunization
with HBIG once you get past that first 9-10 month period, is
not really very wise.   Contacts may go for years without
getting infected under the conditions that exist in their
family and to keep giving them periodic inoculations of HBIG,
just because somebody in the family is a carrier, doesn't make
any sense to me.   Contacts of carriers would be good candidates
for hepatitis B vaccine, when it becomes available.

PETERS: The infant whose mother is an e negative chronic carrier
is perhaps constantly exposed to antigen, but not to many Dane
particles.   Does such an infant develop an immune tolerance?

KRUGMAN: After the first inoculation of the vaccine we are using
now, about 25% were immunized.   One month after the second
inoculation about 85% were immune and after the booster dose
95-100%.   Some individuals may have undetectable levels of
B antibody after the first inoculation, but on a 3-dose
schedule it is the exception that does not respond.

ALTER: Most transmission occurs around the time of delivery;
some may occur before.   The study in Hong Kong showed that a
very high proportion of neonates from antigen positive mothers

had antigen in their gastric aspirates right after delivery.
This suggested that the main route of transmission was the
swallowing of maternal blood during passage through the birth
canal and raised the possibility of preventing transmission by
doing Caesarian Sections, particularly on e antigen positive
mothers.   C-sections performed on several mothers in studies
in Taiwan did not appear to help.   We delivered two offspring
of a chronic carrier e antigen positive chimp by C-section and
both offspring became chronic carriers.

SHARP: How reliable is the current technology for Hepatitis A
testing?   We see some nonreportable types of Hepatitis A, for
example cases with IgM on the first sample and absolutely
nothing on the next.   We have also had some patients with
chronic hepatitis who are persistently IgM positive.

DIENSTAG: There are different ways to detect IgM antibody to
hepatitis A.   The test currently used by commercial laboratories involves the absorption of IgG antibody by staphylococcal
protein A.   The avidity of staph protein A for IgG is about
12 times that for IgM and if a hepatitis A antibody is absorbed
almost completely by staph A it is an IgG antibody.   But in
practice it is almost an impossible test to do in a simple
objective way and I think you are encountering false positive
tests.   I think that the staphylococcal protein A test is
unreliable for diagnosis.   Abbott's test for IgM, HABAB M,
is a reliable test and if you made your diagnosis on the basis
of that test you were probably right.

SHARP: We recently had a young child who developed hepatitis B
and became a chronic carrier, e antigen and antibody negative.
He is eligible for adoption.   What would you tell the prospective parents and the adoption agency?

KRUGMAN: I would tell them something about the epidemiology of
type B hepatitis and indicate to them that there is a potential
risk as far as other children in the family are concerned.
If he is e antigen negative the risk is a lot less, but it is
still real.

HEREDITARY FRUCTOSE INTOLERANCE

Daniel Alagille

Unité de Recherche d'Hépatologie Infantile, INSERM U 56
& Clinique de Pédiatrie, Université Paris-Sud
Hôpital d'Enfants, Bicêtre, France

INTRODUCTION

Hereditary fructose intolerance is the result of a congenital
deficiency in fructose-1-phosphate aldolase and is transmitted by
an autosomal recessive gene (1).

It is the most frequent inborn error of liver metabolism we
observe: between 1961 and 1978, 56 infants with hereditary fructose
intolerance were admitted to our department (2). The increased
incidence of this inborn error of metabolism in France is probably
due to the fact that a large number of infants are fed with a
sucrose-containing milk formula, explaining the early appearance of
symptoms in affected infants; these symptoms may appear later in
infants initially fed with non sucrose-containing milk formulas.

CLINICAL SYMPTOMS

Clinical symptoms appear as soon as fructose is introduced
into the diet (3). Among 51 infants with symptomatic hereditary
fructose intolerance, 14 were hospitalized during the first two
months of life and 37 were hospitalized 3 months or more after the
introduction of fructose in the diet. Five others, born after
an affected sibling, were put on a fructose-free diet immediately
after birth.

Before two months of age, anorexia was less frequent than
vomiting. Hepatomegaly was constant. Three infants had associated splenomegaly. Bleeding disorders were frequent. In
jaundiced infants, only three had a transitory and incomplete
stool discoloration. The eight infants with peripheral edema

217

and/or ascites also had bleeding problems.   Finally, all of these
infants were admitted to hospital critically ill, with acute liver
failure, infection, bleeding, shock or dehydration.

     In infants who were given fructose after 3 months of age,
vomiting was always present.   A distaste for sweet foods was
present even before one year of age.   One of the infants who had
clinical symptoms following food ingestion had a hypoglycemic
seizure.   Hepatomegaly was present in all; no infant had splenomegaly.   Jaundiced infants were less than 6 months of age as were
2 out of 6 infants with edema and/or ascites.   In this group,
patients were admitted to hospital with a presumptive diagnosis
of hepatitis, cirrhosis or failure to thrive.

BIOCHEMICAL SIGNS

     Biochemical signs of liver failure are more frequent in
patients under two months of age; low blood clotting factor levels,
decreased fibrinogen and sometimes signs of disseminated intra-
vascular coagulation.   Serum bilirubin, cholesterol and transaminase
levels are moderately increased.   Post-prandial hypoglycemia is
always present.   Manifestations of renal tubular dysfunction are
more frequent in patients under two months of age: proteinuria,
melituria (essentially fructosuria), aminoaciduria and hyperchlor-
emic metabolic acidosis.   Fructosuria and the increase in serum
levels of phenylalanine, methionine and tyrosine are influenced
by the amount of fructose and protein ingested.

     Because of abnormal hemostasis, liver biopsy is rarely performed
during the acute phase.   Steatosis is associated with noninflammatory
portal fibrosis.   In younger infants, intralobular fibrosis is also
seen.   Portal fibrosis progresses as long as fructose is present
in the diet and this may lead to cirrhosis.   Necrosis is especially
apparent during the acute phase.   Lobular fibrosis is associated
with disarray of the liver cell cords and pseudo-acinar formation.

DIAGNOSIS

     The diagnosis of hereditary fructose intolerance is not
always easy.   Because of pleomorphic symptoms in the younger
infants, the differential diagnosis includes pyloric stenosis,
gastroenteritis, septicemia, congenital afibrinogenemia and severe
hepatitis.   The severity of the disease at this age is also
evidenced by the early deaths of siblings from a disease compatible
with the diagnosis of hereditary fructose intolerance (4,5).   In
older infants, the clinical picture is less dramatic and the differential diagnosis is that of cirrhosis or hepatitis.

     In the differential diagnosis between hereditary fructose
intolerance and tyrosinemia or galactosemia, vomiting is a major

symptom in favour of hereditary fructose intolerance.   Therefore,
the absence of vomiting is strongly against this diagnosis.   The
onset of symptoms immediately after weaning, postprandial symptoms
and fructosuria are other helpful clues.   Finally, a positive
family history of distaste for sweet foods is also helpful (5).

After withdrawal of fructose from the diet, the diagnosis will
be supported by regression within a few hours of vomiting and
bleeding complications, and within a few days by regression of
coagulation abnormalities and renal tubular dysfunction.   It will
be later confirmed by the fructose tolerance test.   This test
should be performed 2 to 3 weeks after fructose has been excluded
from the diet and because of the risks of hypoglycemia, a strict
protocol should be followed.   After the intravenous injection of
fructose over a period of 2 to 3 minutes, there is a rapid fall in
blood glucose and phosphorus levels, concomitant with an increase
in the blood levels of fructose, non-esterified fatty acids,
magnesium and lactic acid.   The increase of fructose and lactic
acid blood levels and the fall in blood glucose level are related
to the dose of fructose injected for the test.   Therefore, at
present, if the diagnosis is suspected, we inject only 0.30 gm/Kg
fructose.   A 50% glucose solution is injected as soon as pallor
or sedation appears, and the test is stopped.

In our 50 infants, the liver fructose-1-phosphate aldolase
activity was much lower than the fructose-1,6-diphosphate aldolase
activity and the ratio of fructose-1,6-diphosphate to fructose-1-
phosphate aldolase activity was increased.

TREATMENT

Treatment is essentially dietary: fructose and sucrose are
completely excluded from the diet (6).   In acute liver failure,
emergency therapeutic measures may be instituted, according to the
following protocol: (a) immediate cessation of enteral nutrition;
(b) infusion of a glucose-electrolyte mixture; (c) blood drawing
for measurement of galactose-1-phosphate uridyl transferase activity,
when galactosemia has not been excluded; (d) exchange-transfusion
with heparinized blood (if serious bleeding tendency is present);
(e) 1 to 3 days later, progressive refeeding with a fructose-free
and low-protein diet.

PROGNOSIS

Prognosis is excellent under treatment.   The growth pattern
returns to normal.   Hepatomegaly persists for several years.
Serial liver biopsies (7) show the disappearance of intralobular
fibrosis and the stabilization or regression of portal fibrosis.
However, even if it is not as diffuse as before treatment, steatosis
persists, particularly in periportal hepatic cells, even if the

patient is under a strict fructose-free diet.   Children on such
a diet do not develop dental caries and dental examination may be
an excellent way to control the dietary treatment.

SUMMARY

Hereditary fructose intolerance (HFI) is the result of a
congenital deficiency in fructose-1-phosphate aldolase and is
transmitted by an autosomal recessive gene.   Among 51 infants
with HFI, 14 were hospitalized during the first 2 months of life
and 37 infants 3 months or more after the introduction of fructose
in the diet.   Five others, born after an affected sibling, were
put on a fructose-free diet immediately after birth.

In infants who were given fructose after 3 months of age,
vomiting was always present.   Hepatomegaly was present in all;
no infant had splenomegaly.   Biochemical signs of liver failure
and evidence of renal tubular dysfunction were more frequent in
patients under 2 months of age.   On liver biopsy, steatosis was
associated with non-inflammatory portal fibrosis.

After withdrawal of fructose from the diet, a fructose
tolerance test and evaluation of fructose-1-phosphate aldolase
activity in the liver support the diagnosis.   Treatment is
dietary: fructose and sucrose are completely excluded from the
diet.   Prognosis is excellent under treatment.

REFERENCES

1.   SCHAPIRA F, GREGORI C, HAZFELD A: Isoelectrofocusing of
        aldolase B from normal human liver and from livers with
        hereditary fructose intolerance.   Clin Chim Acta 78: 1-8,
        1977.

2.   ALAGILLE D, ODIEVRE M: Liver and Biliary Tract Disease in
        Children.   Wiley and Sons, N.Y. 1979. pp. 200-205.

3.   LEVIN B, SNODGRASS GJAI, OBERHOLZER VG, BURGESS EA, DOBBS RH:
        Fructosaemia.   Observations on seven cases.   Am J Med 45:
        826-838, 1968.

4.   CORNBLATH M, SCHWARTZ R: Disorders of Carbohydrate Metabolism
        in Infancy.   2nd ed. WB Saunders, Philadelphia. 1976.
        pp. 322-342.

5.   ODIEVRE M, GENTIL C, GAUTIER M, ALAGILLE D: Hereditary fructose
        intolerance in childhood: diagnosis, management and course
        in 55 patients.   Am J Dis Child 132:   605-608, 1978.

6. BLACK JA, SIMPSON K: Fructose intolerance.   Br Med J 4:
        138-141, 1967.

7. ODIEVRE M, GAUTIER M, RIEU D: Intolerance héréditaire au
        fructose du nourrisson: évolution des lésions histolo-
        giques hépatiques sous traitement diététique prolongé.
        Arch Fr Pediatr 26: 433-443, 1969.

DEFICIENCY OF FUMARYLACETOACETASE IN THE ACUTE FORM OF HEREDITARY TYROSINEMIA WITH REFERENCE TO PRENATAL DIAGNOSIS

S. B. Melançon, R. Gagné, A. Grenier, A. Lescault,
L. Dallaire, C. Laberge, M. Potier

Quebec Network of Medical Genetics, Centre de Recherche
Pédiatrique de l'Hôpital Sainte-Justine, Université de
Montréal and Centre Hospitalier de l'Université Laval
Québec.

The terms tyrosinemia and tyrosinosis have been widely used to describe at least seven distinct disorders of tyrosine metabolism associated with diverse clinical and biochemical consequences in infants, children and even adults (1). The only consistent bio-chemical abnormality within these syndromes has been the finding of elevated levels of plasma tyrosine, a non-essential amino acid derived from phenylalanine by the action of the enzyme phenylalanine hydroxylase. In most of the reported patients with tyrosinemia the clinical presentation resembled that of acute liver failure (acute infantile stage) while later manifestations (chronic stage) included liver cirrhosis, multiple renal tubular dysfunction, hypo-phosphatemic rickets and porphyria-like symptoms. Other less frequent modes of presentation were mental retardation, skin and corneal dystrophies and metabolic acidosis, without liver involve-ment. The major characteristics of the most common forms of tyrosinemia are outlined in Table I. For the purpose of this presentation, we will restrict our discussion to hereditary tyrosinemia.

HEREDITARY TYROSINEMIA (TYPE I)

Liver disease has been the trade mark of this familial metabolic disorder affecting infants and children from all over the world but nowhere as dramatically as in a small French Canadian isolate in the Province of Quebec (7) and with lesser frequency in the Scandinavian countries (8). Patients from other countries have showed varying degrees of severity in their clinical presentation and response to therapy, including spontaneous resolution by one

223

TABLE I

CLINICAL AND METABOLIC ABNORMALITIES IN THE TYROSINEMIAS

TRANSIENT NEONATAL TYROSINEMIA

Subjects	Prematures (30%) and full term infants (10%)
Symptoms	Lethargy, poor feeding
Signs	Late mild intellectual impairment
Biochemistry	Tyrosinemia, Tyrosyluria
Basic Defect	Delayed maturation of parahydroxyphenylpyruvic acid oxidase apoenzyme and/or relative deficiency of ascorbic acid
Therapy	Ascorbic acid supplementation and low protein diet
Genetics	Unknown

HEREDITARY TYROSINEMIA (TYPE I)

Subjects	Infants (acute stage) Children (chronic stage)
Symptoms	Vomiting, failure to thrive, fever, lethargy, irritability
Signs	Peculiar odor, jaundice, hepatomegaly, ascites, bleeding tendencies
Biochemistry	(Acute) tyrosinemia, methioninemia, hypoglycemia, hypoprothrombinemia; (Chronic) Fanconi-like syndrome with generalized aminoaciduria, phosphaturia, glycosuria, rickets, porphyria-like syndrome, cirrhosis, hepatic carcinoma
Basic Defect	Defective fumarylacetoacetate hydrolase
Therapy	Low phenylalanine, tyrosine and methionine diet; glutathione supplementation, Penicillamine therapy
Genetics	Autosomal recessive

RICHNER-HANHART SYNDROME (TYPE II)

Subjects	Infants and children
Symptoms	Photophobia, tearing, delayed milestones
Signs	Keratosis palmo-plantaris Dendritic lesions of the cornea Mental retardation
Biochemistry	Tyrosinemia, Tyrosyluria
Basic Defect	Defect in cytosol tyrosine aminotransferase
Therapy	Low phenylalanine, low tyrosine diet
Genetics	Autosomal recessive

Table 1 (continued)

OTHER LESS COMMON FORMS OF TYROSINEMIA

1) Tyrosinemia with cataracts, mental retardation, seizures, self-mutilation and growth retardation (2)

2) Tyrosinemia with mental retardation and short stature (3)

3) Tyrosinemia with metabolic acidosis, failure to thrive and spontaneous resolution by one year of age (4)

4) Tyrosinemia with glycinemia, cystinemia, generalized aminoaciduria and tyrosine crystals in the bone marrow (5)

5) Presumed tyrosinosis in myasthenia gravis patient described by Medes (6)

TABLE II

RELATIVE FREQUENCY OF PHENYLALANINE AND TYROSINE DISORDERS

IN THE PROVINCE OF QUEBEC BETWEEN 1969-1979 AS ASSESSED

BY A NEWBORN SCREENING PROGRAM [†]

DISEASE	NUMBER OF TESTS PERFORMED	NUMBER OF PATIENTS DIAGNOSED	FREQUENCY
Phenylketonuria	831,738	36	1/23,103
Hyperphenylalaninemia	831,738	40	1/20,793
Hereditary tyrosinemia	786,758	55 *	1/14,304

* 29 patients (52%) were from the Saguenay-Lac St-Jean Area

† See Reference 11

and a half years of age in two patients (4,9), while patients from
Quebec and Sweden have repeatedly demonstrated a consistent pattern
of outcome.   Most of the fifty or more patients in Quebec with
whom we have been acquainted by way of the Quebec screening
program for newborns, have died of liver failure or associated
complications before their fifth birthday.   In the Scandinavian
countries, as in other parts of the world, children tend to live
longer and develop a more chronic form of the disease ending in
complications of liver cirrhosis or hepatocarcinoma (10).

Because of the relatively high incidence of hereditary
tyrosinemia in the Province of Quebec, a compulsive neonatal
screening program was established in 1969 (Table II).   Capillary
blood specimens are obtained by heel puncture during the first
week of life or before the baby is discharged from the hospital
nursery.   Dry filter paper blood spots are analyzed for tyrosine
by an automated fluorometric method (12) and for α_1-fetoprotein by
an immunoradiometric assay (13) when tyrosine levels are above
6.0 mg/dl.   Using a discriminating value of 10 mg/dl for α_1-feto-
protein, the percentage of necessary recalls has been maintained
below 0.4%.

THE ENZYMATIC DEFECT

The abnormal tyrosine metabolism in hereditary tyrosinemia
has been attributed to a low activity of the enzyme parahydroxyphenylpyruvic acid oxidase which catalyses the formation of
homogentisic acid from parahydroxyphenylpyruvic acid (8).   The
lack of hepatic and renal involvement in infants with transient
tyrosinemia and the finding of a reduced activity of the enzymes
S-adenosylmethionine synthase (14) and porphobilinogen synthase (15)
in the liver of patients with hereditary tyrosinemia have raised
doubts as to the specificity of the parahydroxyphenylpyruvic acid
oxidase deficiency in the production of the disease.

Recent work by Linblad et al (16) has opened new avenues for
the comprehension of the pathogenesis of hereditary tyrosinemia.
These investigators have demonstrated the accumulation of succinylacetone and succinylacetoacetate in the urine of patients with the
chronic form of hereditary tyrosinemia.   These compounds would
originate from maleylacetoacetate or fumarylacetoacetate, or both,
and their increased urinary excretion indicates a block at the
fumarylacetoacetase step in the pathway of phenolic amino acid
degradation.   The investigators further suggested that the primary
enzyme defect in hereditary tyrosinemia may be a decreased activity
of fumaryl-acetoacetase (Table III).

Recently we have measured the activity of fumarylacetoacetase
in crude liver homogenates of biopsy and autopsy specimens from
patients with hereditary tyrosinemia (acute form) and control

TABLE III

DEGRADATIVE PATHWAY OF PHENYLALANINE AND TYROSINE

METABOLITE	ENZYME	DISORDERS ASSOCIATED WITH ENZYMATIC DEFECT
Phenylalanine ↓	Hydroxylase	Phenylketonuria
Tyrosine ↓	Cytosol aminotransferase	Tyrosinemia Type II
Parahydroxyphenyl-pyruvic acid ↓	Oxidase	Neonatal tyrosinemia Tyrosinemia secondary to liver damage and cirrhosis
Homogentisic acid ↓	Oxidase	Alcaptonuria
Maleylacetoacetate ↓	Isomerase	
Fumarylacetoacetate ↓	Hydrolase	Tyrosinemia Type I
Fumarate +	Fumarase	
Acetoacetate		

individuals.   Fumarylacetoacetase activity was determined according
to Hsiang et al (17).   The enzyme-catalyzed hydrolysis of aceto-
pyruvic acid was measured in 0.025 M sodium phosphate buffer at
pH 7.5 using a Unicam SP1800 ultraviolet spectrophotometer.   The
rate of decrease in absorption at 295 nm was recorded for 6 min at
22°.   Optical density units were converted to concentrations by
using a molar extinction coefficient of 7400.   One unit of enzyme
activity is defined as the amount of enzyme that catalyses the
hydrolysis of 1 millimole of substrate per minute under the above
conditions.   The rate of acetopyruvate hydrolysis was also
determined in crude homogenates of tissues by measuring the disappearance of substrate at 295 nm at one hour intervals during a
6-hour incubation.

As shown in Table IV, the activity of fumarylacetoacetase was
decreased in liver homogenates of 3 patients with hereditary tyrosinemia.   Among control livers, one patient with fructosemia
displayed the lowest fumarylacetoacetase activity.   Mixing equal
amounts of liver homogenates from patients with tyrosinemia and
controls revealed no apparent inhibition or activation.   Early in
the course of this investigation, the mother of one of our patients

with hereditary tyrosinemia became pregnant and elected to have a
therapeutic abortion.   No detectable activity of fumarylacetoacetase was recovered in the liver of the fetus "at risk" for
tyrosinemia as compared with control fetuses.

A second pregnancy "at risk" for tyrosinemia was more recently
monitored using the porphobilinogen synthase inhibition assay of
Lindblad et al (16) on maternal serum, urine and amniotic fluid
obtained at sixteen and eighteen weeks of gestation.   Control
amniotic fluids from two previous pregnancies at risk for tyrosinemia
and known to have led to the delivery of normal babies, were used
for reference.   While amniotic fluid and blood levels of tyrosine
and α_1-fetoprotein remained within normal values in all cases, the
porphobilinogen synthase inhibition assay was positive in both
amniotic fluid samples of the patient currently monitored for
tyrosinemia.   She elected to have a therapeutic abortion.   Fumarylacetoacetase activity was totally absent in the liver of her
aborted fetus as was the case for the previously presumed tyrosinemia
liver (Table IV) and no enzymatic hydrolysis of acetopyruvate was
demonstrated after prolonged incubation.   We are currently expecting
the birth of a third baby on whom all prenatal tests were normal
including the porphobilinogen inhibition assay in amniotic fluid
obtained early in the second trimester of gestation.

Although preliminary, our data support the hypothesis of
Lindblad et al (16), who implicated a deficiency of the enzyme
fumarylacetoacetase as the basic defect in hereditary tyrosinemia.
We have observed a profound deficiency of the enzyme not only in
infants with the acute form of the disease but also in fetuses at
risk for hereditary tyrosinemia.   This latter observation and the
absence of enzymatic inhibition resulting from mixing experiments
strengthen the view that fumarylacetoacetase deficiency could be
a primary inborn error of metabolism in patients with hereditary
tyrosinemia as opposed to deficiencies of other enzymes such as
parahydroxyphenylpyruvate oxidase, S-adenosylmethionine synthase
and porphobilinogen synthase.

The absence of any appreciable enzymatic hydrolysis of acetopyruvate in cultured skin fibroblasts and peripheral blood leucocytes (Figure 1) of control individuals precludes further investigation of the metabolic defect using tissue culture techniques except
from liver and possibly kidney explants.   We thus encourage
investigators who encounter patients with hereditary tyrosinemia,
to correct the blood clotting factors as early as possible in the
course of the disease and proceed to a liver biopsy for determination of fumarylacetoacetase and other appropriate enzymes (fructose
aldolase, galactose transferase and parahydroxyphenylpyruvate
oxidase) before applying a therapeutic regimen of phenolic amino
acid restriction and possibly other more dramatic procedures such
as homotransplantation of the liver (18).

TABLE IV

HEPATIC FUMARYLACETOACETASE ACTIVITY AND ACETOPYRUVATE HYDROLYSIS

IN HEREDITARY TYROSINEMIA

SOURCE OF SAMPLES	AGE	FUMARYLACETOACETASE ACTIVITY x 10^{-6}		% SUBSTRATE HYDROLYSED (6 hours)
		U/G TISSUE	U/MG PROTEIN	
REAGENT BLANK	–	0	0	7
CONTROL LIVER (AUTOPSY)				
Newborn rat	–	166 (100)*	1.94 (1.17)	88
Reye syndrome	9 months	37	1.00	93
Mucolipidosis II	2 years	112	1.74	60
Septicemia	3 months	110 (79)	1.25 (0.93)	95
(BIOPSY)				
Lactic Acidemia	6 months	115 (66)	1.62 (0.89)	79
Fructosemia	3 months	70 (52)	0.56 (0.44)	94
TYROSINEMIA LIVER (AUTOPSY)				
Acute **	6 weeks	0 (2)	0 (0.05)	10
Acute	4 weeks	14 (13)	0.30 (0.28)	17
Acute	3 months	0 (0)	0 ( )	15
FOETAL LIVER (AUTOPSY)				
Normal	18 weeks	30	0.35	56
Anencephalic	17 weeks	13 (16)	0.18 (0.21)	26
Presumed Tyrosinemia **	16 weeks	0 (0)	0 ( )	9
Confirmed Tyrosinemia ***	21 weeks	0 (0)	0 ( )	2

* Residual enzyme activity after one hour of incubation

** Same sibship

*** Increased amniotic fluid succinylacetone levels

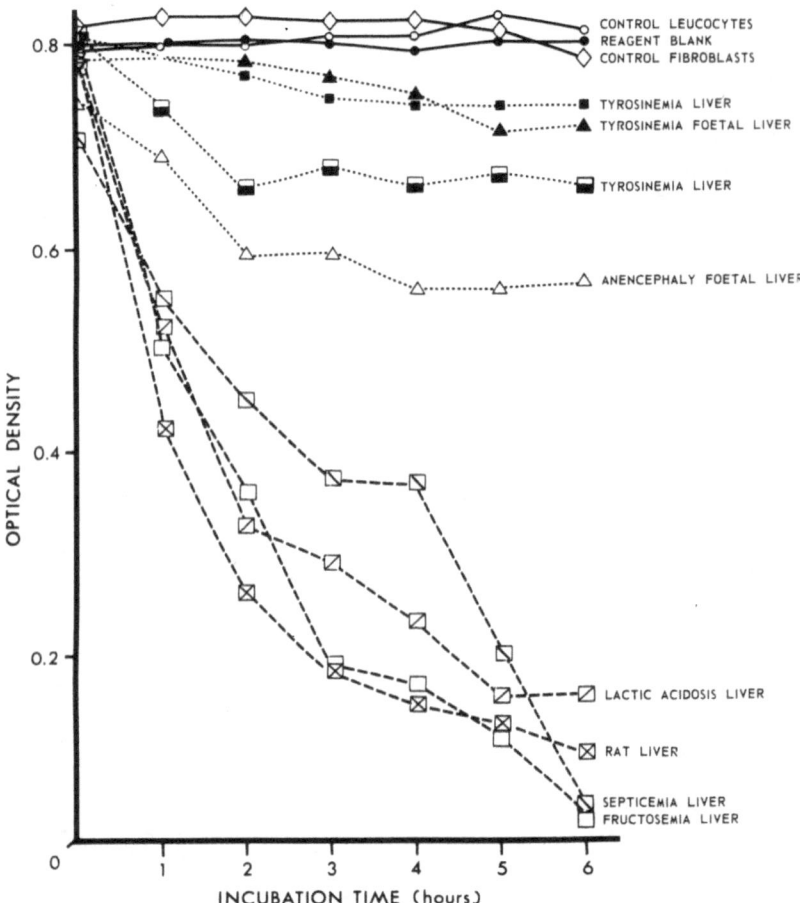

Fig. 1 *Time course of acetopyruvate hydrolysis by homogenates of*
liver, leucocytes and fibroblasts of control individuals
and by liver homogenates of patients with hereditary
tyrosinemia

SIGNIFICANCE OF THE ENZYMATIC DEFECT IN THE PATHOGENESIS OF
HEREDITARY TYROSINEMIA

        Very few investigators have accepted the view that parahydroxy-
phenylpyruvic acid (PHPPA) oxidase deficiency was the primary
defect in hereditary tyrosinemia. Retrospectively, it is obvious
that patients with the lowest PHPPA oxidase activity, early in the
course of the disease should have been protected against the
deleterious accumulation of fumarylacetoacetate and its derivatives.
This is indeed the case since Lindblad et al (16) showed that two
patients with chronic tyrosinemia, 20 and 26 years of age, had no

less than 1% detectable activity of liver PHPPA oxidase in parallel
with good clinical conditions while on a minimal dietary restriction.
Infants born with a very low level of PHPPA oxidase activity in
association with a deficiency of fumarylacetoacetase should probably
not demonstrate increased plasma values or urinary excretion of
succinylacetoacetase and succinylacetone.   The early course of the
disease should then be adequately managed with dietary restrictions
alone.   On the contrary, newborns who have normal PHPPA oxidase
activity would tend to be more severely affected by the products of
the metabolic block at the level of fumarylacetoacetase.   The
current hypothesis on the pathogenesis of liver and kidney dysfunction in hereditary tyrosinemia is outlined in Table V.   Of all
the proposed events, only a few have been so far confirmed by
experimental or human studies: 1) succinylacetone inhibits delta-
aminolevulinic acid dehydratase (porphobilinogen synthase) and
growth of malignant murine erythroleukemia cells (19),   2) the
plasma levels of tyrosine, phenylalanine and methionine are
elevated in chronic cirrhosis of the liver owing to reduced activity
of the enzymes of the tyrosine oxidative pathway (20),   and 3) high
methionine ingestion by guinea pigs leads to the production of the
hepatic, pancreatic and renal lesions seen in hereditary tyrosinemia
(21).   The prenatal origin of succinylacetone in amniotic fluid of
fetuses affected with a deficiency of fumarylacetoacetase remains
difficult to explain at the present time.   It has been clearly
demonstrated that PHPPA oxidase activity is not detectable in fetal
liver before thirty-two weeks of gestation (7).   Amniotic fluid
succinylacetone would then build up only if immediate precursors
such as homogentisic acid or maleylacetoacetate had gained access
to the fetal circulation via the maternal blood.   Such evidence
has not been obtained yet and should be further investigated.

MANAGEMENT

     Hereditary tyrosinemia is a difficult metabolic disorder to
manage.   In most instances, restriction of dietary phenylalanine
and tyrosine, using formula 3200 AB (Mead Johnson Laboratories,
Evansville, Indiana) has failed to sustain prolonged remission of
the early acute liver and kidney dysfunction.   Hypermethioninemia
is best managed by using a methionine free synthetic amino acid
mixture (22) rather than a low methionine formula (Metionaid from
Mead Johnson).   In view of the recent findings of a primary metabolic block at the level of fumarylacetoacetase, it would seem
desirable to monitor dietary measures by direct gas chromatographic
determination of circulating levels of succinylacetoacetate (16)
or by estimation of urinary succinylacetone using the porphobilinogen synthase inhibition assay (16).   If detectable amounts of the
presumed harmful metabolites of fumarylacetoacetate remain in
circulation while tyrosine and methionine concentrations are kept
within normal values, further attempts should be made to accelerate
their elimination.

TABLE   V

PROPOSED CHAIN OF BIOCHEMICAL EVENTS LEADING TO

HEREDITARY TYROSINEMIA (TYPE I)

PRENATAL: Deficient fumarylacetoacetase activity in
                   fetal liver with accumulation of succinyl-
                   acetone in amniotic fluid

POSTNATAL: Deficient fumarylacetoacetase activity in
                   newborn liver
                   ... accumulation of succinylacetoacetate
                   and immediate precursors (Maleylacetoacetate
                   and fumarylacetoacetate) in liver and body
                   fluids
                   ... increased output of succinylacetone
                   in urine

Leading to cellular damage to liver and kidney by formation
of adducts with SH-containing compounds (Glutathione)

CONSEQUENCE: Elevation of tyrosine by decreased activity
                   of parahydroxypyruvic acid oxidase

                   Elevation of methionine by decreased activity
                   of S-adenosylmethionine synthase

                   Elevation of delta-aminolevulinic acid by
                   decreased activity of porphobilinogen synthase

                   Production in kidney of a Fanconi syndrome
                   by Maleyl-derivatives

                   Induction of liver neoplasia and persistence
                   of elevated circulating α_1-fetoprotein

     A possible way to inactivate these metabolites could be the
administration of SH-containing compounds such as glutathione or
drugs like penicillamine which can form adducts with maleylacetoacetate and fumarylacetoacetate in vitro (16) and promote their
inactivation in vivo.

     Another possible approach to therapy could be the use of
enzyme inhibitors directed towards reduction of tyrosine oxidation.
Ascorbic acid deficiency would achieve this goal by decreasing
parahydroxyphenylpyruvic oxidase activity but would also lead to
scurvy (1).   Acute acetylsalicylic acid intoxication in humans is
associated with increased blood homogentisic acid levels secondary

to partial inhibition of the enzyme homogentisic acid oxidase (23). However, chronic administration of acetylsalicylic acid as in arthritis therapy does not maintain a high blood concentration of homogentisic acid and suggests that effective inhibition of homogentisic acid oxidase would not be achieved with safety owing to the bleeding tendency of hypoprothrombinemic infants with tyrosinemia.

SUMMARY

Tyrosinemia or tyrosinosis refers to a group of syndromes characterized by increased levels of tyrosine in the blood and varying clinical features. The most frequent type of tyrosinemia is a familial disorder involving the liver, pancreas and kidney with an acute presentation in infants followed by a more chronic stage in children and young adults. The primary metabolic disturbance responsible for hereditary tyrosinemia was recently identified at the level of fumarylacetoacetase, the last step in the oxidative degradation of phenylalanine and tyrosine. Defective fumarylacetoacetase activity would account for most of the secondary enzymatic defects encountered in the chronic form of the disease. Although present also in the acute infantile form of tyrosinemia, the fumarylacetoacetase deficiency does not account for the high methionine level which is a constant biochemical finding in this early form of hereditary tyrosinemia. In both acute and chronic stages, a potent inhibitor of porphobilinogen synthase, succinylacetone, derived from succinylacetoacetate, fumarylacetoacetate and maleylacetoacetate, is recovered in blood and urine. The course of both stages of the disease correlates well with the urinary output of this metabolite. Succinylacetone has also been identified in the amniotic fluid of a pregnant woman at risk for recurrence of hereditary tyrosinemia. Preliminary biochemical studies in the liver of this presumably affected fetus have revealed defective activity of the enzyme fumarylacetoacetase. The unveiling of a metabolic block at the step of fumarylacetoacetase in the tyrosine oxidative pathway further suggests new alternatives in the management of patients with tyrosinemia. These would include more effective dietary control of precursor amino acids as monitored by the level of succinylacetone in serum and urine rather than tyrosine level in blood. In addition, the usefulness of SH-containing compounds such as glutathione as supplement to the dietary measures has to be assessed.

REFERENCES

1. LA DU BN, GJESSING LR: Tyrosinosis and Tyrosinemia. In The Metabolic Basis of Inherited Disease, 4th Edition. JB Stanbury, JB Wyngaarden, DS Fredrickson (eds). McGraw Hill Co., N.Y. 1978. pp. 256-267.

2. WADMAN SK, SPRANG FJ, VAN MAAS JW, KETTING D: An exceptional
    case of tyrosinosis. J Ment Defic Res 12: 269-281, 1968.

3. LOUIS WJ, PITT DD, DAVIES H: Biochemical studies in a patient
    with tyrosinosis. Aust NZ Jl Med 4: 281-286, 1974.

4. HARRIES JT, SEAKINS JWT, ERSSER RS, LLOYD JK: Recovery after
    dietary treatment of an infant with features of tyrosinosis.
    Arch Dis Child 44: 258-267, 1969.

5. JAISWAL RB, BHAI I, NATH N, NATH MC: Tyrosinosis, clinical,
    radiological and biochemical aspects. Indian Pediat 6:
    1-17, 1969.

6. MEDES G: New error of tyrosine metabolism: tyrosinosis.
    Intermediary metabolism of tyrosine and phenylalanine.
    Biochem J 26: 917-940, 1932.

7. LABERGE C: Hereditary tyrosinemia in a French Canadian isolate.
    Am J Hum Genet 21: 36-45, 1969.

8. GENTZ J, JAGENBURG R, ZETTERSTROM R: Tyrosinemia: an inborn
    error of tyrosine metabolism with cirrhosis of the liver
    and multiple renal tubular defects. J Pediatr 66: 670-
    696, 1965.

9. GAULL GE, RASSIN DK, SOLOMON GE, HARRIS RC, STURMAN JA:
    Biochemical observations on so-called hereditary tyrosinemia.
    Pediatr Res 4: 337-344, 1970.

10. WEINBERG AG, MIZE CE, WORTHEN HG: The occurrence of hepatoma
    in the chronic form of hereditary tyrosinemia. J Pediatr
    88: 434-438, 1976.

11. GRENIER A, MORRISSETTE J, DUSSAULT JH, LABERGE C, GAGNE R:
    Les maladies métaboliques héréditaires au Québec: le
    dépistage sanguin. Union Med Can 109: 591-595, 1980.

12. GRENIER A, LABERGE C: A modified automated fluorometric method
    for tyrosine determination in blood spotted on paper: a
    mass screening procedure for tyrosinemia. Clin Chim Acta
    57: 71-75, 1974.

13. GRENIER A, MORRISSETTE J, VALET JP, BELANGER L:: Polystyrene
    tube immunoradiometric assay for human α_1-fetoprotein, and
    its use for mass screening. Clin Chem 24: 2158-2160, 1978.

14. GAULL GE, RASSIN DK, STURMAN JA: Significance of hypermethioni-
    naemia in acute tyrosinosis. Lancet 1: 1318, 1966.

15. STRIFE CF, ZUROWESTE EL, EMMETT EA, FINELLI VN, PETERING HC, BERRY HK: Tyrosinemia with acute intermittent porphyria: aminolevulinic acid dehydratase deficiency related to elevated urinary aminolevulinic acid levels. J Pediatr 90: 400-404, 1977.

16. LINDBLAD B, LINDSTEDT S, STEEN G: On the enzymic defects in hereditary tyrosinemia. Proc Natl Acad Sci USA 74: 4641-4645, 1977.

17. HSIANG HH, SIM SS, MAHURAN DJ, SCHMIDT DE: Purification and properties of a diketo acid hydrolase from beef liver. Biochemistry 11: 2098-2102, 1972.

18. FISCH RO, McCABE ERB, DOEDEN D, KOEP LJ, KOHLHOFF JG, SILVERMAN A, STARZL TC: Homotransplantation of the liver in a patient with hepatoma and hereditary tyrosinemia. J Pediatr 93: 592-596, 1978.

19. EBERT PS, HESS RA, FRYKHOLM BC, TSCHUDY DP: Succinylacetone, a potent inhibitor of heme biosynthesis: effect on cell growth, heme content and δ-aminolevulinic acid dehydratase activity of malignant murine erythroleukemia cells. Biochem Biophys Res Commun 88: 1382-1390, 1979.

20. FERNSTROM JD, WURTMAN RJ, HAMMARSTROM-WIKLUND B, RAND WM, MUNRO HN, DAVIDSON CS: Diurnal variations in plasma neutral amino acid concentrations among patients with cirrhosis: effect of dietary protein. Am J Clin Nutr 32: 1923-1933, 1979.

21. PERRY TL, HARDWICK DF, HANSEN S, POHLMAN L, WARRINGTON PD: Methionine induction of experimental tyrosinaemia. J Ment Defic Res 11: 246-253, 1967.

22. MICHALS K, MATALON R, WONG PWK: Dietary treatment of tyrosinemia type I. J Am Diet Assoc 73: 507-514, 1978.

23. MONTGOMERY JA, MAMAER OA: Profiles in altered metabolism II: accumulation of homogentisic acid in serum and urine following acetylsalicylic acid ingestion. Biomed Mass Spectrom 5: 331-333, 1978.

A METABOLIC BASIS FOR TREATMENT OF TYPE I GLYCOGEN STORAGE DISEASE

Harry L. Greene

Department of Pediatrics, Vanderbilt Medical Center
Nashville, Tennessee

Most diseases associated with excess hepatic glycogen can be traced to deficient activity of one of the enzymes involved in synthesis or degradation of glycogen (1-3). Exceptions to this are deficient activity of the glycolytic enzyme, phosphofructokinase in muscle (4), and deficient activity of the hepatic gluconeogenic enzyme glucose-6-phosphatase (G-6-Pase). The fact that glycogen synthesis and degradation can proceed unimpaired, leads to a number of clinical and chemical features unique to patients with G-6-Pase deficiency or type I glycogen storage (GSD-I).

CLINICAL AND CHEMICAL FINDINGS IN GLUCOSE-6-PHOSPHATASE DEFICIENCY

The study of mechanisms by which deficient glucose-6-phosphatase activity causes striking elevations in blood lactate, lipids, uric acid and other abnormalities has led to a better understanding of the pathogenesis and potential therapy for this form of glycogenosis. These will be discussed briefly.

Hypoglycemia

The most constant and life-threatening feature of GSD-I is the low blood glucose levels which results from relatively short periods of fasting. Fasting for as little as 2-4 hours is almost always associated with a decrease in blood glucose to less than 70 mg/dl and it is not uncommon to observe 6-8 hour fasting levels of 5-10 mg/dl. In normal individuals blood glucose levels are maintained within a relatively narrow range by hepatotrophic agents, such as glucagon, which release glucose either from stored glycogen, or from gluconeogenesis (5). In patients with GSD-I, it is possible to degrade glycogen to glucose-6-phosphate (G-6-P), but, in the

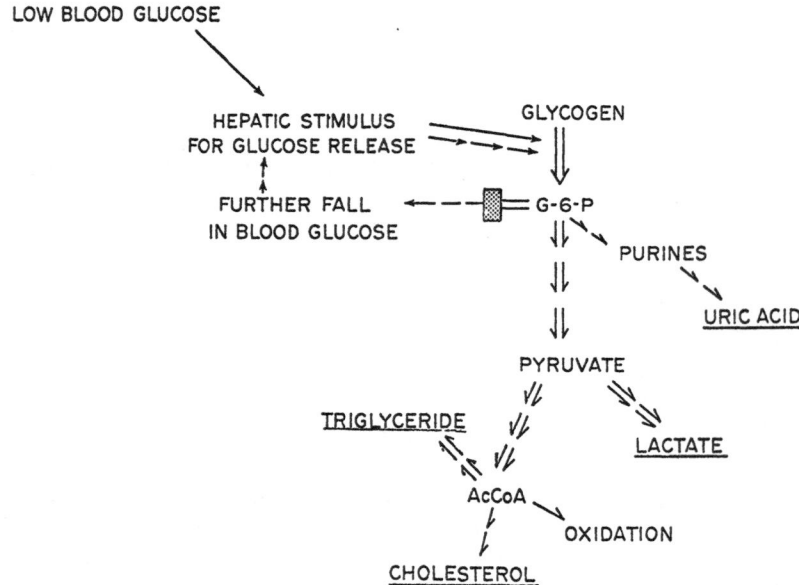

Fig. 1   *Proposed metabolic consequence of glucose-6-phosphatase
          deficiency.   The low blood glucose would promote formation
          of excess lactate, triglyceride, cholesterol and uric acid.*

absence of glucose-6-phosphatase, no glucose is released and blood
glucose levels continue to fall.   The hepatotrophic stimulus is
thus enhanced, which leads to continued glycogen degradation
resulting in secondary accumulation of lactate, urate and triglyceride as depicted in Figure 1.

Lacticemia

        Under normal circumstances, most circulating lactate is
generated from muscle glycolysis during exercise.   Removal and
metabolism of this lactate is efficiently performed by the liver (5).
By contrast, much of the circulating lactate in patients with GSD-I
is generated by hepatic glycolysis (6).   This phenomenon apparently
is the result of hepatic stimulation to release glucose from glycogen.
Excess G-6-P formed from glycogenolysis cannot be hydrolyzed because
of absent phosphatase activity and is diverted through the glycolytic pathway.   This metabolic diversion appears to be the basis
for enhanced lactate formation as well as for other chemical
abnormalities such as hypertriglyceridemia, hypercholesterolemia
and, to some extent, hyperuricemia (Figure 1).

Hyperlipidemia

Elevations in plamsa lipids are a consistent and striking
abnormality (7).   Levels of triglyceride may reach 6,000 mg/dl with
associated cholesterol levels of 400-600 mg/dl.   Free fatty acid
levels are also usually elevated.   Around puberty, xanthomas can
appear over extensor surfaces but may also appear in childhood with
involvement of the nasal septum.   These located on the septum may
contribute to the frequency of prolonged nose bleeds seen in some
patients.

As with lacticemia, elevated levels of triglyceride and
cholesterol appear to be a consequence of increased rates of glycogenolysis and glycolysis.   Observations by Sadeghi-Nejad et al (6)
suggest that excess hepatic glycolysis causes an increase in hepatic
content of NADH, NADPH, and acetyl CoA (AcCoA), 3 compounds important
in fatty acid and cholesterol synthesis.   Thus, an increase in
glycerol and AcCoA generated from the glycolytic pathway, together
with high levels of reduced cofactors, could sustain an increased
rate of triglyceride and cholesterol synthesis (8,9).   In addition
to this apparent increased rate of lipid synthesis, an event
concomitant with hypoglycemia is lipolysis from peripheral lipid
stores, which further augments the tendency for hyperlipidemia and
hepatic steatosis by increasing circulating free fatty acids (7,8,
10,11).

Hyperuricemia

Although blood levels of uric acid and the tendency to develop
gouty arthritis and nephropathy vary in different patients, those
who survive past puberty often have gouty complications (12,13).

Hyperuricemia was originally attributed to the increased level
of serum lactate and lipid which competitively inhibit urate excretion (8).   Nevertheless, the high level of urate excretion plus
the rate of incorporation of ^{14}C-1-glycine into plasma and urine
urate indicate that an increased rate of purine synthesis de novo
is probably more important in the genesis of hyperuricemia than
a decrease in urate excretion (14,15,16).   The mechanism leading
to increased purine synthesis is not yet completely understood.
There are at least two ways by which the rate of purine synthesis
may be influenced, i.e. 1) by altering the substrate concentration,
such as phosphoribosyl-pyrophosphate (PRPP) and glutamine, and
2) by altering the end product, or purine concentration (17-19).
Two substrates necessary for the first committed reaction are PRPP
and glutamine.   This reaction transfers the amine from L-glutamine
to PRPP to form 5-phosphoribosyl-1-amine.   This reaction is apparently rate limiting for the entire sequence of purine synthesis.
Although tissue levels of the two substrates have not been measured
in patients with GSD-I, blood glutamate and glutamine levels

obtained from hyperuricemic patients are 3-8 fold higher than values
obtained after urate is normalized by glucose infusion (14).   In
addition to the possibility of increased availability of glutamine,
the high levels of G-6-P produced during glycogenolysis may increase
synthesis of the second important substrate in purine synthesis,
PRPP (8,13,20).   Studies using human leukocytes indicate, however,
that an increased availability of ribose-5-phosphate does not
necessarily increase the generation of PRPP (21).   If this is
true in liver, then end product or purine concentration may be
more important in modulating the rate of purine synthesis in patients
with GSD-I.

     Low concentrations of the purines adenyl or guanyl ribonucleo-
tides or unfavorable ratios between them favor an increase in the
rate of purine biosynthesis by releasing the glutamine-PP-ribose-
P-amidotransferase from end product inhibition (22).   Although no
hepatic nucleotide levels have been determined in patients during
hypoglycemic episodes, indirect evidence suggests that hypoglycemia
in patients with GSD-I can lower adenyl ribonucleotide levels.
Such conclusions were based on an analogy with another enzyme defect,
fructose-1-phosphate aldolase deficiency (HFI).   In this disease
a substantial decrease in adenyl ribonucleotides results when large
amounts of fructose are infused into normal man or isolated rat
liver (23).   The fructose is rapidly phosphorylated and depletes
adenosine triphosphate (ATP) and inorganic phosphate (Pi) (24).
The depleted ATP and Pi then promote degradation of preformed
adenosine monophosphate (AMP) to inosine monophosphate (IMP) and
urate.   Such a sequence, therefore, not only provides a stimulus
for increased purine synthesis de novo but also increased urate
production.   An analogous situation has been proposed for patients
with GSD-I, when their blood glucose levels are sufficiently low
to cause stimulation of glycogenolysis.   Support for this proposal
can be summarized as follows:

     1) Glucagon levels are extremely high in GSD-I patients with
hyperuricemia (14,15);

     2) Glucagon infusion causes an almost immediate increase in
blood uric acid levels (within 15 minutes) without altering urinary
excretion (26);

     3) Glucagon infusion causes hepatic ATP depletion within 5
minutes in patients with GSD-I and not in other types of glycogenosis (27);

     4) Maintenance of blood glucose levels between 70 and 150 mg/dl
restores blood urate levels to normal and decreases urate excretion
(27).

Platelet dysfunction

     Patients with GSD-I usually have a prolonged bleeding time,

secondary to abnormal platelet aggregation.   Corby and co-workers
examined platelet function in 13 patients with deficient hepatic
activity of one of the following enzymes: glucose-6-phosphatase,
debrancher enzyme, phosphorylase or phosphorylase kinase (28).
Only the 7 patients with G-6-Pase deficiency showed abnormal platelet
aggregation and four of these also showed abnormal platelet adhesive-
ness.   The defect appears to be intrinsic, since crossover and
resuspension studies using patient platelets in normal plasma and
normal platelets in patient plasma did not alter in vitro platelet
function.   Two such patients had ADP content of affected platelets
measured and in both instances it was normal. Nevertheless, the
release of ADP from platelets in response to added collagen and
epinephrine was markedly impaired.   These observations suggest
that the functional defect is an impaired ability of the platelet
membrane to release ADP.   Cooper recently found a similar defect
in ADP release from platelets with elevated cholesterol content (29).
The elevated cholesterol content impaired fluidity of the membrane,
causing secondary impairment of ADP and epinephrine-induced aggregation.   Although platelet cholesterol levels have not been measured
in patients with GSD-I, the elevated serum cholesterol content might
reflect elevated platelet cholesterol content and, therefore, may
contribute to the abnormal platelet function in GSD-I patients.
If this postulate is correct, then treatment which lowers blood
and platelet cholesterol levels should also normalize platelet
function.   One of our patients recently presented with abnormal
platelet function but normal serum cholesterol and triglyceride.
This finding does not support the above hypothesis.

Growth impairment

     Children with GSD-I have short stature without disproportion
of head, limbs or trunk length.   The abdomen is usually massively
enlarged due to hepatomegaly.   Bones may be osteoporotic and some
patients show delayed bone age.   The mechanism leading to these
changes is not clear.   Growth hormone and thyroid hormone levels
are normal or increased (3,14).   Measurement of calorie-protein
intake in three patients for 2 weeks indicates adequate calorie
consumption.   Recent observations suggest that chronic lactic
acidosis with concomitant reversal of the insulin-glucagon ratio may
be more important factors in inducing a more normal growth (see
subsequent section).

Hepatic adenomata

     The development of adenomatous nodules within liver parenchyma
was an infrequent finding until recently.   In a more recent study
of eight patients, all but one had evidence of adenomata.   This is
at variance with the previously held view that they are found infre-
quently.   Adenomata develop in most patients during the 2d decade
but they may be seen in 3 year old children.   The nodules are

best demonstrated by radioisotopic scan and show decreased isotope
uptake.   At laparotomy, they appear as discrete, pale nodules
which vary in number from one to many and in size from 1 to 5 cm.
Three patients have developed hepatocellular adenocarcinoma in one
of the nodules (30,30a).   The mechanism causing the adenomata or
their malignant degeneration is unknown but treatment with portacaval shunt does not prevent their development.

Severity of illness

In spite of the fact that there is no difference in activity
of the phosphatase enzyme between patients, the expression of
symptoms and of chemical anomalies vary substantially from one
patient to another, without detectable differences in management.
Some patients may have only moderate abnormalities in blood chemistry
and decreased growth rate, whereas others may have marked alterations
in blood lipids, require frequent hospitalizations for fever and
lactic acidosis or even die in infancy or early childhood.

In addition, there appears to be some decrease in severity of
hypoglycemia after patients have reached adulthood.   In fact, a
few patients with moderately severe symptoms during childhood
improved so dramatically during adulthood as to have successful
pregnancy (15,31,32).

TREATMENT OF PATIENTS WITH GLUCOSE-6-PHOSPHATASE DEFICIENCY

Patients with some types of glycogenosis, e.g. those with
deficient hepatic phosphorylase kinase activity and some patients
with Type III (debrancher deficiency), have an excellent prognosis
without specific treatment.   In fact, with the exception of defects
in glycogen synthesis, generalized glycogenosis (acid maltase
deficiency, or Pompe's disease) and glucose-6-phosphatase deficiency,
most patients with hepatic glycogenosis have a favorable prognosis
and are successfully managed with some attention to the frequency
of feeding.   This, however, has not been true of most patients
with GSD-I.

During the past 10 years, substantial improvement in the
management of patients with GSD-I has been reported (14,25, 33-36).
The evolution of these therapeutic manoeuvers will be discussed next.

Drugs and hormones aimed primarily at improving the level of
blood glucose concentrations or the rate of growth have been used
in management of GSD-I.   Thyroid hormone, corticosteroids, cate-
cholamines, glucagon, ethanol, diazoxide and clofibrate have been
used but offer little or no benefit (37-40).   In two instances,
clofibrate showed some promise as a therapeutic agent, but because
it must be administered for an extended time and does not correct
the hypoglycemia, it is not of much practical use (14,41).   It is

possible that as the pathophysiology of GSD-I is better understood,
drug or hormone treatment will be more beneficial.

Surgical treatment of GSD-I was introduced in the late 1960's
and early 1970's.   The advent of the portacaval shunt treatment
brought about a dramatic improvement in several patients with GSD-I.

The idea was introduced in 1965, after Sexton and co-workers
observed that hepatic glycogen content decreased substantially after
portacaval transposition in dogs (42).   On this basis, Starzl and
associates proposed that a similar procedure might decrease hepatic
glycogen levels in patients with glycogenosis and also make dietary
glucose more readily available to peripheral tissues (43).   The
first of the four patients who had a portacaval transposition was
an 8-year-old girl with Type III (debrancher deficiency) glycogenosis.   She also had cirrhosis and portal hypertension and was
considered likely to benefit from decompression of the portal vein.
After the operative procedure she improved substantially;   studies
9½ years later indicated continued good health, although the predicted decrease in hepatic glycogen levels did not take place.
Two of the three other patients with GSD-I treated by this procedure
showed benefit (44), but since one patient died postoperatively with
acidosis and severe portal hypertension (43), the procedure was
abandoned for several years.

In 1972, Folkman and associates (33) showed that substantial
reduction in operative risk occurred when patients were prepared
pre-operatively with total parenteral nutrition (TPN).   In addition,
a standard end-to-side portacaval shunt resulted in continued
increase in growth and a decrease in most chemical abnormalities.

Since the portacaval shunt is technically easier and prior
treatment based on TPN diminished the risk substantially, a number
of patients in several medical centers have recently been treated
with portacaval shunts.   Assessment of long-term effects of this
treatment is not complete.   In spite of initial improvement in
most patients, two major problems have emerged, namely premature
closure of the shunt and persistence of hypoglycemia.

Hypoglycemia is by far the more serious complication.   Before
surgical intervention, extremely low levels of blood glucose were
generally tolerated without serious consequences.   After portacaval
shunt, however, the same level of hypoglycemia induced acidosis
and prolonged seizure activity, which may be lethal.   Thus,
intensive medical management is even more critical to prevent
symptomatic hypoglycemia after the portacaval shunt (25).

Although metabolic results of portacaval shunting provided a
better understanding of the pathophysiology of the illness and
appeared to offer an almost "magical cure" for several patients

with GSD-I, much of the initial enthusiasm has been replaced by
caution since some patients have exchanged one set of problems
for another.

   Dietary manipulation has evolved as the preferred method of
management.   Most authors recommend frequent feedings that should
at least provide for the energy-protein needs of a normal child of
comparable age.   Qualitatively, the diet restricts fat, purines,
fructose and galactose and therefore sucrose and lactose.   The
fact that a number of patients have reached adulthood suggests
that this type of dietary management is sufficient for some patients,
although most have recurrent bouts of acidosis, growth failure and
complications resulting from persistent hyperuricemia.

Theoretical considerations

   Present recommendations for treatment of GSD-I stem primarily
from the studies of Folkman and associates (33), who first illustrated the reversal of most biochemical abnormalities after TPN.
Their observation that both TPN and portacaval shunt delivered
nutrients primarily into the systemic circulation suggested that
hepatic exposure to nutrients was important in the pathogenesis of
many biochemical abnormalities.   Nevertheless, it was later demonstrated that the same beneficial effect seen with TPN or portacaval
anastomosis could be achieved with an intragastric infusion of a
nutrient solution similar in content to that used during TPN (34,35).
This suggested that bypassing the liver with nutrients was not the
most important factor in reversing the abnormalities.   The similarity in these three types of treatment (e.g. portacaval shunt,
TPN and continuous intragastric infusion of glucose) was that a
hormonal stimulus to the liver to produce glucose was decreased
or averted.   Specifically, TPN and continuous intragastric feeding
both prevented a hepatic stimulus glucose release by maintaining
blood glucose levels in the range of 90-150 mg/dl, whereas the
portacaval shunt prevented such a stimulus by diverting pancreatic
and enteric blood into the systemic circulation.   On this basis,
the hypothesis for treatment illustrated in Figure 2 was formulated.

   The hypothesis states that, as blood glucose falls below a
critical level, compensatory mechanisms cause glycogen degradation
to glucose-6-P.   In the absence of glucose-6-phosphatase, G-6-P
is not hydrolyzed to release free glucose and the hepatic stimulus
for glycogenolysis results in formation of other intermediates such
as lactate, triglycerides and possibly uric acid.   To interrupt
the stimulus, treatment with an exogenous source of glucose should
inhibit the release of hepatotrophic stimuli and therefore the
excess glycogenolysis.   If this postulate is correct, any method
of treatment which maintains blood glucose above this critical level
should also prevent or at least improve biochemical manifestations
of the illness.   In addition, the hypothesis suggests that portal

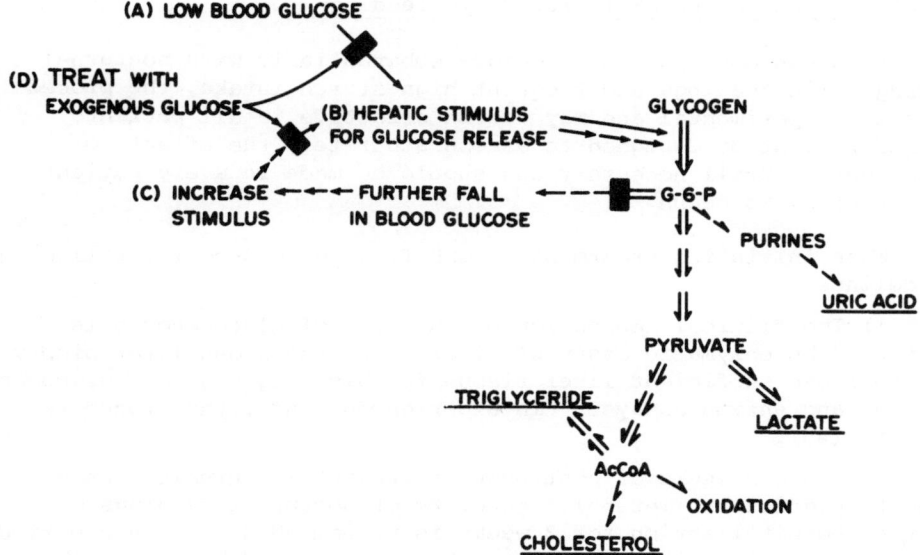

Fig. 2 *Proposed mechanism whereby exogenous glucose should*
decrease the hepatic stimulus for glycogenolysis and
thereby form the basis for treatment.

diversion should dilute hepatotrophic agents in the systemic circulation.   This dilution would therefore result in less hepatic
stimulation for glycogenolysis.

Thus, theoretically, either portacaval shunt or continuous
infusion of a high glucose diet should be effective in reversing
most manifestations of the illness, with the exception that portacaval shunt should have little or no beneficial effect on hypoglycemia.   Thus, portacaval shunt is not recommended as a sole
form of treatment for those patients who are expected to have frequent episodes of very low blood glucose levels or for small children
whose shunt may be more likely to close spontaneously.

Although TPN and continuous intragastric infusion of glucose
are effective treatment modalities for GSD-I, they are impractical
on a long-term basis.   A more practical method was devised to
maintain blood glucose concentrations at a level that would prevent
stimulation of excess glycogenolysis.   This treatment consisted
of a high-glucose diet given enterally during night-time sleep and
consumption of a high-starch diet at frequent intervals while awake.
Such a regimen has successfully maintained a number of patients
relatively symptom-free for almost 5 years and provided normal or
near-normal growth and development.

Studies using nocturnal intragastric feedings

    Although most patients improve substantially with nocturnal·
intragastric feedings and frequent high-starch intake, the procedure
is still experimental and may not be effective in all patients.
Therefore a study designed to assess accurately the effects of
treatment is still necessary and should be made in every patient
when therapy is begun.

    When initiating treatment of GSD-I, we have used the following
guidelines:

    1) The clinical impression of the type of glycogenosis is
confirmed by enzymatic assay of liver.   Percutaneous liver biopsy
can retrieve sufficient liver tissue for histologic study, glycogen
content and enzyme assays.   In experienced hands, the procedure
is safe (45).

    2) Since 2 weeks of continuous intragastric infusion can be
used to predict the metabolic benefits of nocturnal feedings,
initial hospitalization for 3 weeks is recommended.   Such a period
has been essential in determining the clinical and biochemical
responses of treatment.   It is also optimal for counseling the
parents and patients for future outpatient care.

    3) Although treatment is based on the maintenance of blood
glucose levels above 70 mg/dl, during at least the first 3 months
we recommend a solution containing glucose oligosaccharides as well
as a nitrogen source with added vitamins and minerals.   We prefer
Vivonex or Vivonex High Nitrogen (Eaton) because of ease in mixing
but have used less expensive solutions, such as Precision LR (Doyl)
or Polycose (Ross) plus added casein.   With these preparations
there have been fewer problems with hypoglycemia and better growth
rates than with glucose alone.

Protocol for treatment

    The treatment protocol is illustrated in Figure 3.   Patients
with prior hepatic enzyme measurements may not require repeat
liver biopsy.   Patients with normal bleeding time at admission
have a liver biopsy performed within the first 3 days of hospitalization (none of these patients had G-6-Pase deficiency).   If
bleeding time is abnormal, it is corrected within 7 days by continuous intragastric infusion and then liver biopsy is performed.

    Initial blood, radiographic and anthropometric measurements
are made on day 1 and the diet prescribed before admission (e.g.
frequent high-starch feedings at 3-4 hour intervals) is continued
for 4 days.   Blood samples are taken at 4-hour intervals for
blood glucose, lactate, insulin, glucagon and growth hormone levels
on day 2.   In small children, only glucose and lactate levels are

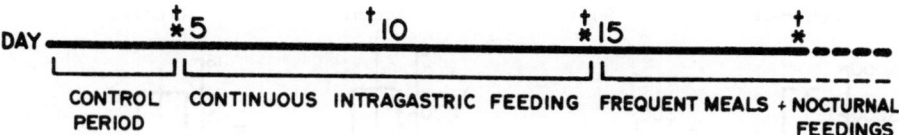

DAY

CONTROL PERIOD
CONTINUOUS INTRAGASTRIC FEEDING
FREQUENT MEALS + NOCTURNAL FEEDINGS

*Blood for liver function, lipids, urate, lactate, glucose, platelet function.

†Blood glucose, lactate, glucagon, insulin every 4 hours for 24 hours.

Fig. 3   Protocol for treatment

measured and in infants, only blood glucose is measured, using 20 µl samples from each fingerstick.

By day 3, baseline measurements are completed and continuous intragastric feedings are begun at the same daily caloric intake as during the first 3 days of admission.   In infants and small children, infusion is better tolerated by the intestinal tract if it is mixed at a concentration of 20 calories/oz.   If it can be tolerated at 30 cal/oz, however, there is less urinary frequency.   A small nasogastric tube (No. 5 or 8-French, 14 gauge or O.D.=0.067 in.) is inserted.   The first few times the tube is inserted, the nares are sprayed with a 1:1 mixture of 0.5% Neo-Synephrine and 2% Xylocaine.

After 11-14 days of continuous infusion, blood measurements are repeated to determine the potential benefit of long-term treatment. If there is no substantial improvement during this period, it is doubtful that nocturnal feedings will offer further chemical benefit.

The aim of continuous nocturnal feedings, along with frequent high-carbohydrate feedings during the day, is to maintain blood glucose levels above 70 mg/dl.   This usually can be done by giving 1/3-2/5 of the daily caloric needs as the nocturnal infusion and the remainder as oral feedings during the day.   To ensure that this blood glucose level is maintained, blood is obtained at 4-hour intervals for 24 hours soon after beginning the infusion, again some months later and annually thereafter.   Adjustments in diet or nocturnal feedings are made accordingly.

The first four patients treated were readmitted for studies at 3 months, 6 months, 1 and 2 years.   Subsequent evaluations of these and other patients (as outpatients) have been made annually.

The diet is modified to meet the individual idiosyncrasies of patients and general guidelines with emphasis on maintenance of glucose levels at 70-150 mg/dl have been more effective than specific

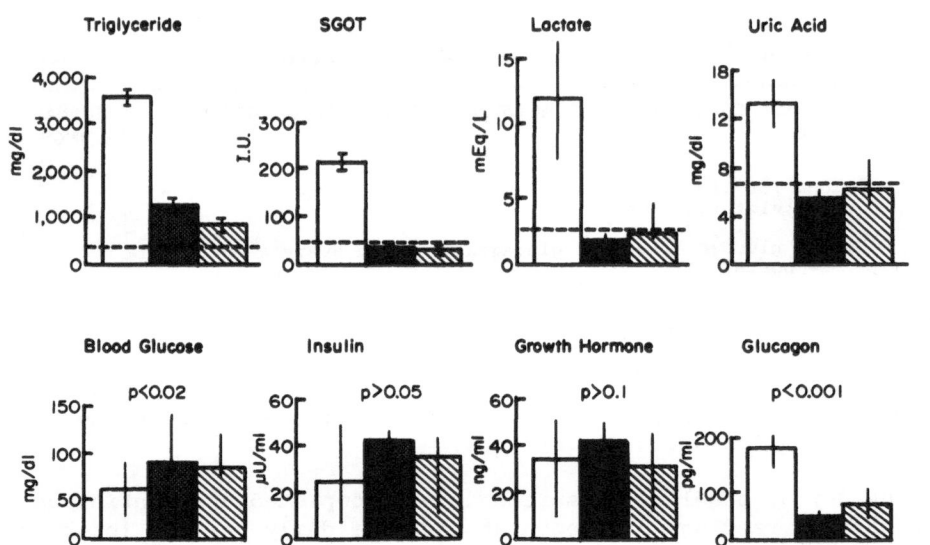

Fig. 4   *Treatment-induced changes in patients with GSD-I.*
Open bars = control period. Cross-hatched bars = two weeks
after treatment with continuous intragastric infusion.
Single-hatched bars = 4-5 years after frequent daytime
feeding and continuous nocturnal feeding.

do's and don'ts.   Caloric proportions approximate 60-70% as
carbohydrate (almost exclusively starch), 10-15% as protein and
the remainder as fat.   Daily intake is divided into equal proportions and given at 3-hour intervals.   Fructose (sucrose) and
lactose (galactose) intake is discouraged but allowed if the
restricted diet is refused or not taken appropriately.

RESULTS OF TREATMENT

Figure 4 compares blood profiles in seven patients before
treatment, after two weeks of continuous intragastric infusion,
and after five years of treatment with frequent daytime feedings
plus continuous nocturnal intragastric feedings.   After two weeks
of continuous feeding the mean blood glucose levels increased from
62 (range 28 to 96) to 97 (range 71 to 151 mg/dl).   There was
also a significant decrease in SGOT, lactate, urate, and bleeding
time values.   Triglyceride concentrations also decreased significantly from 3,612 ± 123 to 1,181 ± 110 mg/dl.   There was also a
demonstrable decrease in palpable hepatic size.   Hepatic biopsy
in two patients indicated that the change in size was accountable
more by a decrease in triglyceride (from 124 to 44 and from 108 to

27 mg/gm liver) than by glycogen content (from 9.5 to 9.8 and
from 9.2 to 7.8%) (14).

Hormone values were quite variable between patients.   Some
patients showed initial insulin levels as high as 35 µU/l with
concomitant blood glucose values less than 70 mg/dl.   This suggested
some degree of insulin resistance prior to treatment.   Treatment
caused an increase in circulating insulin from a mean of 25 (range
7 to 50) to 44 (range 26 to 53) µU/l but this increase was not
significant (P > 0.05).   Similarly the change in growth hormone
levels from 36 (range 10 to 51) to 41 (range 8 to 49) ng/ml was
not significant.   By contrast, the markedly elevated glucagon
levels with a mean of 190 (range 171 to 308) decreased significantly
(P < 0.01) to a mean of 44 (range 26 to 53) pg/ml following treatment.

Treatment with nocturnal intragastric infusion and frequent
meals maintained most blood chemical values within normal limits
after the initial corrections with continuous infusion.   Six of
seven patients maintained normal blood uric acid and transaminase
levels;   four maintained normal blood lactate, and three a normal
bleeding time.   Although triglyceride levels were lowered substantially, they remained elevated to varying degrees in all but
two patients.   Those with highest triglyceride levels also showed
elevated blood cholesterol levels and concomitant prolonged bleeding
time.   Glucagon levels, which decreased to normal during continuous
infusion, remained normal during the period of nocturnal infusion.

The most striking change caused by treatment was an accelerated
rate of growth.   Before treatment all patients were considerably
less than the third percentile for age.   After five years of
therapy all were greater than the tenth percentile.

Complications

There were no complications resulting from repeated tube
placement (aspiration, nasal irritation, etc.).   Symptomatic
hypoglycemia was the only complication noted in seven patients
followed in our hospital (46).   Three to five hours of no dietary
glucose or starch usually resulted in symptomatic hypoglycemia and
lactic acidosis.   Attention to this possibility provided some
margin of safety for most children.   One patient, age 4½ years
(follow-up data not included), apparently developed an acute gastroenteritis followed by several episodes of vomiting which led to
hypoglycemia and severe acidosis.   The symptoms continued for
several hours before seeking medical attention.   In spite of
attempts at resuscitation and correction of his intractable acidosis,
he died in a community hospital.   This unfortunate complication
illustrates the importance of early correction of symptomatic
hypoglycemia and acidosis.

SUMMARY

Studies suggest that the clinical and biochemical abnormalities
present in GSD-I result from an excess rate of glycogenolysis
secondary to a decrease in blood glucose concentrations below
70 mg/dl.   The lack of glucose-6-phosphatase activity prevents
hepatic release of glycogen to glucose and continued stimulation of
glycogenolysis causes excessive formation of glucose-6-phosphate
and secondarily increases lactate, triglyceride and uric acid.
In addition, abnormal platelet function, prolonged bleeding time and
impaired growth are prominent features of the illness.

Biochemical and clinical aberrations in GSD-I can be substantially improved by treatment aimed at decreasing the hepatic stimulus
for glycogenolysis by maintaining the blood glucose concentration
between 70 and 150 mg/dl.   This is most effectively done by total
parenteral nutrition or continuous intragastric infusion of a
high-glucose diet (i.e. Vivonex High Nitrogen or Precision LR).
The equally effective, more practical and most acceptable method of
maintaining blood glucose levels is continuous infusion of the diet
at night for 8-12 hours, followed by high-starch feedings every
3 hours while awake.   This treatment has been very effective in
providing the necessary milieu for normal growth and development
in 7 patients for 4 years (46).

REFERENCES

1. HUG G: Glycogen storage diseases. Birth Defects XII: 145,1976.

2. SENIOR B: The glycogenoses. Clin Perinatol 3: 79, 1976.

3. HOWELL RR: The Glycogen Storage Diseases. In The Metabolic
        Basis of Inherited Disease, Stanbury JB, Wyngaarden JB,
        Fredrickson DS (eds) (4th Edition). McGraw-Hill Co.,
        New York, 1977. p. 137.

4. TARUI S, OKUNO G, IKUKA Y, TANAKA T, SUDA M, NISHIKAWA J:
        Phosphofructokinase deficiency in skeletal muscle: a new
        type of glycogenosis. Biochem Biophys Res Commun 19:
        517, 1965.

5. COLEMAN JE: Metabolic interrelationships between carbohydrates,
        lipids and proteins. In Diseases of Metabolism, Bondy PK,
        Rosenberg LE (eds). (7th Edition) WB Saunders Co.,
        Philadelphia, 1974. p. 107.

6. SADEGHI-NEJAD A, PRESENTE E, BINKIEWIEZ A, SENIOR B: Studies
        in type I glycogenosis of the liver. The genesis and
        deposition of lactate. J Pediatr 85: 49, 1974.

7. JAKOVCIC S, KHACHADURIAN AK, HSIA DYY: The hyperlipidemia in
    glycogen storage disease. J Lab Clin Med 68: 769, 1966.

8. HOWELL RR, ASHTON DM, WYNGAARDEN JB: Glucose-6-phosphatase
    deficiency glycogen storage disease. Studies on the inter-
    relationships of carbohydrate, lipid and purine abnormali-
    ties. Pediatrics 29: 553, 1962.

9. OCKERMAN PA: Glucose, glycerol and free fatty acids in glycogen
    storage disease type I: blood levels in the fasting and
    non-fasting state: effects of glucose and adrenalin admini-
    stration. Clin Chim Acta 12: 370, 1965.

10. FORGET PP, FERNANDES J, BEGEMANN PH: Triglyceride clearing in
    glycogen storage disease. Pediatr Res 8: 114, 1974.

11. HULSMANN WD, EIJENBOOM WHM, KOSTER JF, FERNANDES J: Glucose-
    6-phosphatase deficiency and hyperlipaemia. Clin Chim
    Acta 30: 775, 1970.

12. FINE RN, STRAUSS J, CONNEL GN: Hyperuricemia in glycogen
    storage disease type I. Am J Dis Child 112: 572, 1966.

13. HOWELL RR: The interrelationship of glycogen storage disease
    and gout. Arthritis Rheum 8: 780, 1965.

14. GREENE HL, SLONIM AE, O'NEILL JA,Jr, BURR IM: Continuous
    nocturnal intragastric feeding for management of type I
    glycogen storage disease. N Engl J Med 294: 423, 1976.

15. ALEPA FP, HOWELL RR, KLINEBERG JR, SEEGMILLER JE: Relation-
    ships between glycogen storage disease and tophaceous gout.
    Am J Med 42: 58, 1967.

16. JAKOVCIC S, SORENSEN LB: Studies of uric acid metabolism in
    glycogen storage disease associated with gouty arthritis.
    Arthritis Rheum 10: 129, 1967.

17. HENDERSON JF, KHOO KY: Synthesis of 5-phosphoribosyl-1-pyro-
    phosphate from glucose in Ehrlich ascites tumor cells in
    vitro. J Biol Chem 240: 2349, 1965.

18. GREENE HL, SEEGMILLER JE: Elevated erythrocyte phosphoribosyl-
    pyrophosphate in x-linked uric aciduria: importance of
    PRPP concentration in regulation of human purine biosynthe-
    sis. J Clin Invest 48: 32a, 1969.

19. RAIVIO KO, SEEGMILLER JE: Role of glutamine in purine synthesis
    and in guanine nucleotide formation in normal fibroblasts
    and in fibroblasts deficient in hypoxanthine phospho-

ribosyltransferase activity. Biochim Biophys Acta 299: 282, 1973.

20. HOWELL RR: Hyperuricemia in childhood. Fed Proc 27: 1078, 1968.

21. BROSH S, BOER P, JUPFER J, DEVRIES A, SPERLING O: De novo synthesis of purine nucleotides in human peripheral blood leukocytes: excessive activity of the pathway in hypo-xanthine-guanine phosphoribosyl-transferase deficiency. J Clin Invest 58: 289, 1976.

22. HOLMES EW, McDONALD JA, McCORD JM, WYNGAARDEN JB, KELLY WN: Human glutamine phosphoribosyl-purophosphate amidotrans-ferase: kinetic and regulatory properties. J Biol Chem 248: 143, 1973.

23. BODE JC, ZELDER O, RUMPELT HJ, WITTKAMP U: Depletion of liver adenosine phosphates and metabolic effects of intravenous infusion of fructose or sorbitol in man and in the rat. Eur J Clin Invest 3: 436, 1973.

24. WOODS HF, EGGLESTON LV, KREBS HA: The cause of hepatic accumu-lation of fructose-1-phosphate on fructose loading. Biochem J 119: 501, 1970.

25. CRIGLER JR, Jr, FOLKMAN J: Glycogen storage disease: new approaches to therapy. In Hepatotrophic Factors, Porter R, Whelan J (eds), Ciba Foundation Symposium, Amsterdam, 1978. p. 331.

26. ROE TF, KOGUT MD: The pathogenesis of hyperuricemia in glycogen storage disease type I. Pediatr Res 11: 664, 1977.

27. GREENE HL, WILSON FA, HEFFERAN P, TERRY AB, MORAN JR, SLONIM AE, CLAUS TH, BURR IM: ATP depletion, a possible role in the pathogenesis of hyperuricemia in glycogen storage disease type I. J Clin Invest 62: 321, 1978.

28. CORBY DG, PUTNAM CW, GREENE HL: Impaired platelet function in glucose-6-phosphate deficiency. J Pediatr 85: 71, 1974.

29. COOPER RA: Abnormalities of cell-membrane fluidity in the pathogenesis of disease. N Eng J Med 297: 371, 1977.

30. HOWELL RR, STEVENSON RE, BEN-MENACHEM Y, PHYLIKY RL, BERRY DH: Hepatic adenomata with type I glycogen-storage disease. J Am Med Assoc 236: 1481, 1976.

30a. ROE TF, KOGUT MD, BUCKINGHAM BA, MILLER JH, GATES GF, LANDING BH:

Hepatic tumors in glycogen-storage disease type I.
Pediatr Res 13: 931, 1979.

31. SIDBURY JB: The genetics of the glycogen storage disease.
Prog Med Genet 4: 32, 1965.

32. FARBER M, KNUPPEL RA, BINKIEWICA A, KENNISON RD: Pregnancy
and von Gierke's disease. Obstet Gynecol 47: 226, 1976.

33. FOLKMAN J, PHILIPPART A, TZE WJ, CRIGLER J,Jr: Portacaval
shunt for glycogen storage disease: value of prolonged
intravenous hyperalimentation before surgery. Surgery
72: 306, 1972.

34. BURR IM, O'NEILL JA, KARZON DT, HOWARD LJ, GREENE HL:
Comparison of the effects of total parenteral nutrition
continuous intragastric feeding and portacaval shunt on a
patient with type I glycogen storage disease. J Pediatr
85: 792, 1974.

35. ROE TF, KOGUT MD: Chronic effects of oral glucose alimentation and portacaval shunt in patients with glycogen storage
disease type I. Pediatr Res 10: 414, 1976 (abs).

36. BAKER L, MILLS JL: Long-term treatment of glycogen storage
disease type I: clinical improvement but persistent
abnormalities of lactate and triglyceride concentration.
Pediatr Res 12: 502, 1978 (abs).

37. KOULISCHER N, PICKERING DE: Glycogen-storage disease: a
study on the effect of sodium l-thyroxine and glucagon.
Am J Dis Child 91: 103, 1956.

38. LOWE CU, SOKAL JE, DORAY BH, SARCIONE EJ: Biochemical studies
and specific therapy in hepatic glycogen storage disease.
J Clin Invest 38: 1021, 1959 (abs).

39. LOWE CU, MOSCOVICH LL: The paradoxical effects of alcohol on
carbohydrate metabolism in four patients with liver
glycogen disease. Pediatrics 35: 1005, 1965.

40. RENNERT OM, MUKHOPADHYAY D: Diazoxide in von Gierke's disease.
Arch Dis Child 43: 358, 1968.

41. GREENE HL, HERMAN RH, STIFEL FB: Glycogen storage disease due
to glucose-6-phosphatase deficiency: treatment with
clofibrate. Pediatr Res 6: 398, 1972 (abs).

42. SEXTON AW, MARCHIORO TL, WADDELL WR, STARZL TE: Liver deglyco-
genation after portacaval transposition. Surg Forum 15:
120, 1964.

43. STARZL TE, MARCHIORO TL, SEXTON AW, ILLINGWORTH B, WADDELL WR,
     FARIS TD, HERMANN RJ: The effect of portacaval trans-
     position on carbohydrate metabolism: experimental and
     clinical observations. Surgery 57: 687, 1965.

44. RIDDELL RG, DAVIES RP, CLARK AD: Portacaval transposition
     in the treatment of glycogen storage disease. Lancet 2:
     1205, 1966.

45. HONG R, SCHUBERT WK: Menghini needle biopsy of the liver.
     Am J Dis Child 100: 42, 1960.

46. GREENE HL, SLONIM AE, BURRIM: Type I glycogen storage disease:
     advances in treatment. In Advances in Pediatrics,
     Barness L (ed) vol. 26: 63-92, 1979.

DISCUSSION

CHAIRMAN: C.C. ROY

COX: I would like to ask Dr. Greene about those very high triglyceride levels merely from excess production. Might there
also be some effect on the lipoprotein lipase degradation
system?

GREENE: Yes. I didn't really have time to go into all the
mechanisms, but there clearly are two or three sources of
the elevated triglycerides: dietary intake, lipolysis and
synthesis in the liver.

WONG: We have seen four patients with tyrosinemia in the past
three years. All died and all had marked hypoglycemia.
All had high insulin secretion during the time they had hypoglycemia and at autopsy all had pancreatic islet hyperplasia.
Does Dr. Melancon have any explanation for these phenomena?

MELANÇON: I agree but I don't know what comes first. It is
reasonable that with hypoglycemia one has excess insulin
secretion and eventually islet cell hyperplasia. But chronic
tyrosinemics end up with diabetes mellitus and no secretion of
insulin. My assumption is that the hypoglycemia comes first.
It might be that they are feeding less and less tricarboxylic
acids into the cycle but I don't know if this would be enough
to create hypoglycemia.

ISSENMAN: Patients with Type I glycogen storage disease seem to
have their homeostasis severely disturbed by intercurrent
infections. Has Dr. Greene had an opportunity to study any
patients in this regard?

GREENE: Since we started treatment we haven't had any of these
     problems and I am not sure that every patient that gets fever
     has an infection.   One of the most severe patients that I
     have ever seen had intermittent fevers for which we were never
     able to show any intercurrent infection.   But every time her
     blood glucose dropped below 40 or 50 mg% she produced lactate
     at astronomical levels as if she were generating energy that
     was dissipated in the form of heat rather than stored as
     ATP.   I think some patients during acidosis and hypoglycemia
     will develop fever.   Following manipulation to normalize their
     triglyceride and uric acid concentrations we have not had any
     more "infectious" complications than in a normal group of
     children.   In patients with elevated serum uric acid we have
     found abnormalities in leucocyte cell migration.   This disease
     may in fact alter the patient's immune response.

SHARP: The liver disease that you examined in regard to fumaryl-
     acetacetase activity was not particularly severe.   With
     severe liver disease do you see low activity and do hetero-
     zygotes have intermediate activity?

MELANÇON: We haven't looked at many liver diseases and at no
     heterozygotes.   We have another way to look at heterozygotes,
     by loading with homogentisic acid and measuring the amount of
     urinary succinyl acetone.

SHARP: Could you elaborate on the neurologic complications that
     you see and have you investigated pancreatic function on an
     intraluminal basis?

MELANÇON: We have not done any other pancreatic studies.   The
     group in Quebec City has demonstrated that the actual inhibitor
     of glucagon is not tyrosine.   We have been able to show that
     the acetoacetate derivatives can reduce the activity of PHPP
     oxidase.   I cannot tell you much about the brain damage except
     that we found inclusions in the brain of one of our patients
     that looked very much like something that was reported as
     sudanophilic leucodystrophy.   We are now looking back at some
     of the brains of tyrosinemics, mostly in the Chicoutimi area,
     to find out if these inclusions were present also.   Obviously
     any ketone body can eventually damage brain cells and leave
     microscopic lesions.

DE BELLE: How many patients have been picked up during the ten
     years that the screening program for tyrosinemia has been in
     effect?   In what clinical status were these babies found and
     what has been their follow-up?

MELANÇON: We have picked up 55 patients during the last ten years,
     29 from the Chicoutimi area.   About 50 were actually sick at

the time the diagnosis was made.

DE BELLE: In other words, none of the children was picked up
   before he or she became ill?

MELANÇON: I am not familiar enough with all the patients to
   answer that question.

DE BELLE: I have a child with "congenital" fructosemia who was
   picked up in early infancy but who now, at over 2 years of age,
   has improved fructose aldolase levels. The levels are still
   not normal but they are above what they were at birth, and the
   liver biopsy is now normal. Must such children still be on
   a diet?

ALAGILLE: The absence of aldolase activity is not transitory.

DE BELLE: Do improved levels go against the diagnosis of
   congenital fructosemia?

ALAGILLE: Yes. The problem is to exclude first galactosemia and
   then hereditary fructosemia. If these diagnoses have been
   excluded it is possible to wait. The three or four patients
   we have studied in this condition had a final diagnosis of
   hereditary tyrosinemia.

THALER: In a relatively asymptomatic child with hereditary fructose
   intolerance, one often diagnosed because another sibling is
   picked up, we usually find only growth retardation. And when
   fructose is taken out of the diet a significant growth spurt
   occurs. Have you found this to be true and if so, what do
   you think the mechanism of growth retardation is?

ALAGILLE: We haven't seen this.

THALER: Dr. Greene's results may be explained if patients with
   glycogen storage disease prefer to use calories from ethanol
   in comparison with normal. Does anyone know what the utilization of nonalcoholic calories is during ethanol administration?

GREENE: To my knowledge no studies have been done to look at
   substrate utilization during alcohol infusion in glycogen
   storage disease. We do know that in normal men who have been
   given alcohol, several of the glycolytic enzymes are decreased.
   I think that the paradoxical response of lactate, the paradoxical response of glucose and the rapid metabolism of
   ethanol may point toward the microsomal ethanol-metabolizing
   system (MEOS) pathway demonstrated by Lieber and his group.
   In patients who take alcohol over a prolonged period of time
   the MEOS pathway, normally not utilized, is activated. A

similar mechanism may occur in patients with chronic lactic acidosis, who have to find another mechanism to oxidize their DPNH.

SHARP: How do the three treatments for Type I glycogen storage disease compare and are there any differences in response to treatment between Type IA and Type IB?

GREENE: I assume by the three modalities of therapy that you mean total parenteral nutrition, portacaval shunt and intragastric or enteral feedings?   I don't think there is any place for total parenteral nutrition at home in the management of patients with Type I glycogenosis.   It is an impractical form of therapy.   Secondly, in spite of the almost magical cure rate reported initially, patients with a portacaval shunt still have episodes of hypoglycemia.   In fact, two of our patients who had portacaval shunts elsewhere are now on nocturnal feedings to prevent this problem.   With intragastric feedings at night you are at least able to maintain normal blood glucose concentrations.   So of the three treatment programs for those patients who require more than simple frequent feedings 24 hours a day, the most practical is some form of enteral feeding so that they can sleep through the night.

The Type IB patients are those who have normal glucose-6-phosphatase activity but all the signs and symptoms of Type IA. They seem to respond just as well except for the persistence of their neutropenia, abnormalities in leucocyte migration and frequent infections.

ALAGILLE: We perform portacaval shunt in severe cases of Type I or Type III Glycogen Storage Disease.   In 16 cases we have observed a dramatic fall of hyperlipidemia and hyperuricemia. Growth retardation has been corrected, and the general condition of the children and their tolerance for hypoglycemia have improved.   We know very well your results and our present difficulty is to decide whether or not we should stop performing portacaval shunts and try your nocturnal gastric feeding treatment.

ROY: Have you had any patients who had attacks of pancreatitis?

GREENE: No. We have had two patients with recurrent abdominal pain but it wasn't pancreatitis.   I know of one patient who died from hemorrhagic pancreatitis which remained undiagnosed until the time of postmortem.

ROY: We have had two who had pancreatitis.   They are now on nocturnal feedings and doing very well.   Do you come down so hard on TPN because of the complication rate?

GREENE: It is very difficult to do it at home, it is not necessary, it is expensive and you don't get that much advantage from it.

GORESKY: A fructose load in adults will double or triple the rate of disappearance of ethanol from the circulation. Therefore I would be very surprised if what you see in the children is due to a MEOS phenomenon. I would guess that it is probably related to loading the intermediate substrates in the glycolytic chain.

GREENE: I think that you are absolutely right. If you first normalize the lactate, triglyceride and uric acid concentrations for one week prior to the alcohol, they will react normally.

WILSON'S DISEASE - HEPATOLENTICULAR DEGENERATION

THE IMPORTANCE OF EARLY DIAGNOSIS

Andrew Sass-Kortsak

Department of Paediatrics, Faculty of Medicine
University of Toronto, and the Research Institute
The Hospital for Sick Children, Toronto

Wilson's disease is a genetically determined disease, due to
a defect in a single gene (1).   Both parents are heterozygous
carriers of this abnormal gene and never develop any signs or
symptoms of Wilson's disease.   However, their children have a
1:4 chance of being homozygous and thus having Wilson's disease.
They also have a 1:2 chance of being heterozygous carriers like
their parents and a 1:4 chance of being homozygous normal (2).
All this is characteristic of an autosomal recessive form of
inheritance.

The pedigree of a large family with Wilson's disease is shown
in Figure 1.   The parents in generation II were heterozygous
carriers and had 18 children (generation III).   Five of them had
Wilson's disease; the others were either heterozygous carriers or
homozygous normal.   The first patient had 4 children and then died
with cirrhosis of the liver.   The other four patients are alive.
Two (No. 6 and 14) had chronic liver disease when diagnosed but the
others (No. 12 and 18) were diagnosed before they developed manifestations of their disease.   All four of these patients are being
treated with D-penicillamine and have done very well.   These five
patients have had 12 children, all of whom are heterozygous carriers
of Wilson's disease (generation IV).

Patients with Wilson's disease usually do not present with
typical symptoms and signs until they are between 10-30 years of
age and rarely even later than 30 years of age.

The earlier they present the more likely do they present with
symptoms of liver disease.   Later presentation is often with
neurological disease.   The third obvious sign of this disease is

261

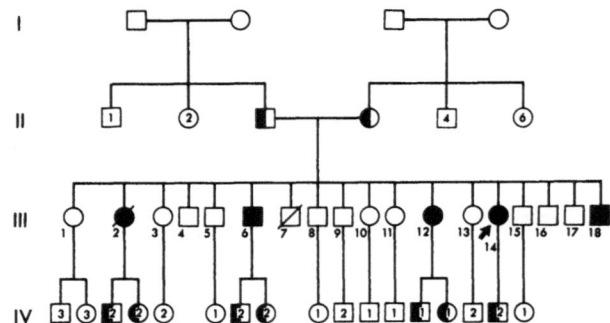

Fig. 1 Pedigree of a family with Wilson's disease.
        The propositus (III.14) developed liver disease at 17 years
        of age. Survey of his sibship (generation III) revealed
        4 additional homozygous abnormals: III.2, presumed, died
        earlier of liver disease; III.6 and III.18 presymptomatic,
        with evidence of latent liver disease; III.12, presymptom-
        atic, with no evidence of disease. Parents in generation
        II and the children of patients in generation IV are
        obligate heterozygotes. The genotypes of the others are
        not known. Note that homozygous abnormal patients are not
        found in generation I, in generation II, among 13 sibs of
        the parents, and in generation IV, among 29 children of
        the propositus and his sibs.

the presence of Kayser-Fleischer rings of the corneae. However,
these rings can be absent, especially in the teenager. Thus the
absence of Kayser-Fleischer rings in a young individual does not
exclude Wilson's disease. Finally, patients have kidney involvement but this is functional and not clinically obvious.

     The typical patient with Wilson's disease has: (a) liver
disease, cirrhosis of the liver, (b) neurological disease, tremors,
incoordination, spasticity, dystonia, etc., (c) Kayser-Fleischer
rings of the corneae, (d) mild but definite functional renal involvement. However, the diagnosis of this disease must be made much
before this full-blown picture has developed.because an effective
form of treatment is available. Orally administered D-penicillamine
(3-7) or triethylene-tetramine (8,9) is most effective provided
treatment is started early, before permanent, irreversible damage
has occurred in vital organs like the liver, brain or kidneys.

     We still do not know the exact genetic defect in Wilson's
disease. However, we do know that it involves a serious problem
with the handling of copper (1). It is estimated that we take
3,000 - 5,000 micrograms of copper daily in our food (1). Approximately 2/3 of this daily oral intake of copper is absorbed from

the bowel (2,000-3,500 µg per day).   Copper that has been absorbed
from the bowel is carried in the blood attached to a specific site
on serum albumin.   It disappears from the blood very rapidly and
is taken up mainly by the liver.   Most of this copper is promptly
excreted by the liver via the bile so that the copper content of
the liver is maintained at 5-15 µg/g wet weight, or approximately
10 mg copper in the liver of a human adult.

In Wilson's disease there is no problem with the absorption
of copper from the bowel or with the uptake of copper by the liver.
However the hepatic excretion of copper is defective.   Thus copper
accumulates, primarily in the liver but also in certain other organs,
notably the brain, kidneys, and corneae of the eyes.

Treatment with D-penicillamine or triethylene-tetramine is
effective because these agents cause excretion of copper through
the kidneys.   Normally, in spite of the absorption of 2,000-3,500 µg
of copper per 24 hours, the urine contains only a trace amount of
copper, less than 40 µg per 24 hours.   After ingesting 1 g D-penicillamine per day, a normal individual will excrete 10-20 times more
copper via the urine, that is 400-800 µg copper per 24 hours.
Patients with Wilson's disease have 50-100 times the normal amount
of hepatic copper and excrete increased amounts of urinary copper,
150-300 µg per 24 hours.   Patients ingesting 1.0g D-penicillamine
daily will excrete 2,000-5,000 µg copper per 24 hours.

The urinary copper excretion of a patient undergoing treatment
with D-penicillamine decreases slowly and approaches normal.   When
treatment is stopped after 2-3 years a patient will excrete < 40 µg
copper per 24 hours and will excrete only 400-800 µg copper per
24 hours in response to 1 g D-penicillamine.

Patients slowly improve during the first 2-3 years of treatment.
Signs and symptoms of liver disease disappear and kidney function
normalizes.   Neurological problems also improve but more slowly.
After 3-5 years of constant treatment, the Kayser-Fleisher rings
fade and with more time will completely disappear.

The important question of how much improvement will occur can
be answered only with uncertainty.   The patient whose diagnosis is
made early will probably return to normal, but not before 1-2 years
time.   One can expect this when liver disease is the primary manifestation.   But when the patient presents with neurological symptoma-
tology the prognosis must be more guarded, especially with the
dystonic, spastic form of the disease.

During the past 30 years I have seen over 80 patients with
Wilson's disease.   Approximately 10-15 of these have died, some
before treatment was available, some because they could not take
the treatment, and some because treatment was started too late.

Thirty to thirty-five patients have improved markedly, but the normal
state was not re-established in all.   A few of the latter have liver
problems, but most have neurological symptoms.   Less than half the
total number of patients that I am seeing regularly are living a
normal life.   This is the case because the diagnosis was made too
late.

      The diagnosis must be made early, before symptoms of the disease
are present.   Is this possible?   The answer is very definitely
yes.

      Generally speaking there are three approaches to the early
diagnosis of Wilson's disease:

   1) Paying attention to the unusual presentations of Wilson's
      disease.

   2) Recognition of Wilson's disease when the signs of liver
      and/or neurological disease are minimal.

   3) Screening the total population between 5-7 years of age.

Unusual presentations of Wilson's disease

      a) Hemolytic crises.   Rarely a severe acute hemolytic crisis
is the first sign of Wilson's disease (10-13).   Anaemia, hemolytic
jaundice and splenomegaly are the typical signs.

      The hemolysis is associated with the sudden release of a large
amount of copper from the liver.   How and why this occurs we do not
know.   A great deal of the increased copper in the liver is bound
to a low molecular weight protein, metallothionein.   This protein
has a very rapid turnover rate and if its rate of production is
suddenly and markedly decreased the copper which is bound to it may
be released into the plasma and lead to massive hemolysis.   This
of course remains to be proven.   We have measured in a patient with
Wilson's disease and a severe hemolytic crisis a plasma copper level
of 650 µg/100 ml with a low normal serum ceruloplasmin level.   We
calculated that the non-ceruloplasmin bound copper level in this
patient was close to 600 µg/100 ml of plasma.   The increase of
non-ceruloplasmin bound copper from the normal level of 10 µg/100 ml
to 600 µg/100 ml may have been the reason for the massive hemolysis.

      We have since made the diagnosis of Wilson's disease in two
young girls (8 and 11 years of age) who presented with an acute
hemolytic crisis, and without obvious signs of liver or neurological
disease.   They had anaemia, hemolytic jaundice and splenomegaly.
Careful examination revealed that their livers were slightly enlarged
and firmer than normal.   Search for the usual factors causing hemolytic disease revealed no etiology.   Their serum ceruloplasmin
levels were low, their serum total copper reduced, and their urinary

excretion of copper increased.   Kayser-Fleischer rings were present
in both.   Studies with radioactive copper confirmed the diagnosis
of Wilson's disease.   A 3-year-old sister of one of these girls was
also found to have Wilson's disease.   In all three of these cases
treatment was started within weeks of the diagnosis and before the
onset of manifest liver or neurological disease.   All three are
perfectly well and leading normal lives 7-10 years after diagnosis.

        b) <u>Kidney disease</u>.   Patients may present with renal problems
before the usual signs and symptoms of Wilson's disease develop (14).

        A 15-year-old girl was admitted to our hospital with a urinary
tract stone which had to be removed surgically.   One and a half
years later, she presented with neurological symptoms and the diagnosis of Wilson's disease was made.   This diagnosis should have
been made at the time of her admission with the renal stone.

        In patients with Wilson's disease the serum uric acid levels are
low because there is reduced reabsorption of uric acid by the kidneys.
This increased renal uric acid excretion can lead to stone formation.
There are other renal reabsorption deficiencies in patients with
Wilson's disease.   For this reason, children who present with
nephrolithiasis should be suspected of having Wilson's disease.

        Another patient, a 9-year-old girl, was referred to our renal
service with moderate proteinuria and episodic hematuria.   We found
a firm liver edge at the costal margin.   Slit lamp examination
revealed Kayser-Fleisher rings.   Serum ceruloplasmin was very low,
serum total copper was reduced and urinary copper excretion was
markedly increased.   The diagnosis of Wilson's disease was made,
and treatment with D-penicillamine initiated.   She is now 24 years
old and perfectly well.   She has never developed the typical signs
of Wilson's disease and she never will develop liver or neurological
disease provided she continues the D-penicillamine treatment.

        c) <u>Vitamin D-resistant rickets - Fanconi's syndrome</u>.   The
diagnosis of Wilson's disease has been made in several young children
presenting with Vitamin D-resistant rickets or with Fanconi's
syndrome (15-17).   This has been reported mainly from India.

        We have diagnosed Wilson's disease in two Indian children.
One was a 2-year-old boy with very low serum ceruloplasmin levels,
low total serum copper and a slowly increasing urinary copper excretion.   The other, a girl born in Canada, is 7½ years old.   She
was admitted with early chronic liver disease, very low serum
ceruloplasmin and copper, increased urinary copper excretion and
marked aminoaciduria.

        d) <u>Kayser-Fleischer rings</u>.   Among the 80-90 patients with
Wilson's disease that I have seen there was only one in whom the

diagnosis was made by an ophthalmologist.   This patient, a 17-year-old boy, was perfectly well and was sent to an ophthalmologist to have his presbyopia checked.   A routine slit lamp examination was done and Kayser-Fleischer rings of the corneae were discovered. It would seem advisable for ophthalmologists always to use the slit lamp when examining children over 6 years of age.

       e) Psychiatric involvement.   I have not seen children with Wilson's disease present with psychiatric involvement.   This, however, can be a rare form of presentation at a later age, during the third and fourth decades of life.

Early recognition of Wilson's disease when signs of liver and/or neurological disease are minimal

       Most of our patients with Wilson's disease were diagnosed when the disease was so advanced that proper and effective treatment could not reverse the disease completely.

       During the early stages of Wilson's disease the history and clinical examination are of little help in making the diagnosis. There is nothing specific about the liver and/or neurological disease.   Even later in the disease process, there are no clinical findings that are only present in Wilson's disease.   Therefore, one must look for the specific manifestations of Wilson's disease if the diagnosis is to be made early.

       First, one must look for Kayser-Fleischer rings by slit lamp examination.   In order to do this one must have an experienced ophthalmologist.   Then one should measure the serum ceruloplasmin and total copper levels.   One must take the blood with a plastic syringe, place it in a copper-free tube and handle the specimen in such a way that contamination with copper is avoided.   Finally, one must measure the copper content of at least two 24-hour urine collections.   These collections must be directly into plastic containers which have been carefully washed with deionized or double-distilled water.

       A patient who has liver and/or neurological symptomatology will most likely have Kayser-Fleischer rings, low serum ceruloplasmin and total copper levels and increased copper excretion in the urine. Conversely, the diagnosis of Wilson's disease can be excluded if Kayser-Fleischer rings are absent, the serum ceruloplasmin and copper levels are normal or raised and the urinary copper excretion is normal (< 40 µg/24 h) or only minimally increased (< 100 µg/24 h) (1).

       Very rarely the patient may have Wilson's disease and yet Kayser-Fleischer rings cannot be found even by careful slit lamp examination.   This can happen when a young patient presents with

liver disease.   When Wilson's disease presents with neurological
symptoms Kayser-Fleischer rings are always present.   Rarely the
serum ceruloplasmin levels are normal, perhaps "low normal", and
the serum total copper levels quite increased.   Ceruloplasmin
contains 0.315% copper, and this ceruloplasmin-bound copper can be
calculated using an enzymatic (oxidase) method.   In normals the
non-ceruloplasmin bound copper is less than 10 or 15 μg/100 ml
serum.   In Wilson's disease the amount of non-ceruloplasmin bound
copper is increased quite markedly, often to 30-40 μg/100 ml.   For
reliable measurements one must resort to several testings.   The
urinary excretion of copper is always increased in Wilson's disease,
and when a patient is found to have increased urinary copper excretion, it is worth while to continue the collection for an additional
3-5 days while the patient (who is close to adult size) receives
0.5 g D-penicillamine, q 12 h.   Under these circumstances normal
adults excrete 400-800 μg of copper per 24 hours, whereas the
patient with Wilson's disease excretes 1,500-5,000 μg/24 hours or
even more.

By these methods, the diagnosis of Wilson's disease can almost
always be made in a patient who has presented with liver and/or
neurological disease.   But rarely one may have to go further.

Kidney function tests may be helpful.   There is usually no
obvious renal disease but there may be proteinuria, not severe,
and the urinary sediment may contain some red blood cells.   Uric
acid excretion is increased and the serum uric acid level is quite
low.   Aminoaciduria may be present and quite marked in some
instances.   There may be other failures of tubular reabsorption.

If one is still in doubt about the diagnosis, one may carry
out studies with radioactive copper (^{64}Cu or ^{67}Cu).   Following
the intravenous administration of a single tracer dose of radioactive copper attached to human serum albumin, one measures
repeatedly total plasma and ceruloplasmin bound activity and the
urinary and fecal excretion of radioactivity for a 3-4 day period.
^{67}Cu has a half-life of 60.3 hours and when it is used one may also
measure the decrease in total body radioactivity over 2-3 weeks.
Obviously these copper studies have to be done in institutions
where such studies can be performed.

Screening of the total population for Wilson's disease

Screening before symptoms of Wilson's disease appear could be
carried out at the time children enter school, between 5-7 years
of age, and this could be the ideal way to make the diagnosis.

Measurement of the serum ceruloplasmin level, by an immuno-
chemical method, only requires a capillary blood sample.   The
serum could be separated by centrifugation, then frozen and shipped

to a central laboratory.   There could be one problem.   Serum
ceruloplasmin levels may be normal (usually "low normal") at the
time the diagnosis of Wilson's disease is made.   This may occur
in 3-5% of patients.   However I believe that the serum ceruloplasmin levels are always below the normal range during the presymptomatic phase of Wilson's disease.

We have seen 8-10 patients with Wilson's disease whose serum
ceruloplasmin levels at the time of diagnosis were within the normal
range, greater than 20 mg/100 ml.   During the first 2-3 years of
D-penicillamine treatment their serum ceruloplasmin levels decreased.
In many of these individuals the levels became very low, 5-10 mg/
100 ml or even lower.

There is a second observation that suggests that the serum
ceruloplasmin levels are low before the symptoms of Wilson's disease
appear and specifically before liver involvement becomes marked.
In the sibships of patients with symptomatic Wilson's disease and
normal serum ceruloplasmin levels we have found four younger presymptomatic sibs with Wilson's disease and low serum ceruloplasmin
levels.

A second problem is that heterozygous carriers of Wilson's
disease may have lower than normal serum ceruloplasmin levels.
However, only 7% of heterozygous carriers will have this abnormality
and further studies will identify these individuals.

For these reasons, I believe that there will not be many
"false positive" results when measuring serum ceruloplasmin levels
between 5-7 years of age during the presymptomatic phase of the
disease.   Unfortunately, this condition is thought to be so rare
that total population screening for this one single condition
will probably be considered prohibitively expensive.   Therefore
we may have to wait until screening at this age is introduced for
other diseases in which early diagnosis and treatment may be of
benefit.

SUMMARY

1)   Wilson's disease is based on an abnormality of a single
gene.   The mode of inheritance is autosomal recessive.

2)   Treatment for this condition is available and is most
effective, provided it is instituted early and carried on for the
rest of the patient's life.   Early diagnosis is the key to successful treatment.

3)   When patients present with liver and/or neurological
disease Wilson's disease should be ruled in or out as soon as
possible.

4) Unusual presentations of Wilson's disease include acute hemolysis, renal disease, vitamin D resistant rickets, Fanconi's syndrome, Kayser-Fleischer rings, and psychiatric problems.

5) Screening the total population at the age of 5-7 years could be the ideal solution to the problem of making the diagnosis of Wilson's disease before symtoms arise.

REFERENCES

1. SASS-KORTSAK A, BEARN AG: Disorders of copper metabolism (Wilson's Disease (hepatolenticular degeneration) Menkes' Disease (Kinky-hair or steely-hair syndrome)). In The Metabolic Basis of Inherited Disease, 4th Edition, JB Stanbury JB Wyngaarden, DS Fredrickson (eds). McGraw-Hill Book Co. N.Y. 1978. pp. 1098-1126.

2. BEARN, AG: A genetical analysis of thirty families with Wilson's disease (hepatolenticular degeneration). Am J Hum Genet 24: 33-43, 1960.

3. WALSHE JM: Penicillamine, a new oral therapy for Wilson's disease. Am J Med 21: 487-495, 1956.

4. STERNLIEB I, SCHEINBERG IH: Penicillamine therapy for hepatolenticular degeneration. J Am Med Assoc 189: 748-754, 1964.

5. RICHMOND J, ROSENOER VM, TOMPSETT SL, DRAPER I, SIMPSON JA: Hepato-lenticular degeneration (Wilson's disease) treated by penicillamine. Brain 87: 619-638, 1964.

6. MILNE MD, LEWIS AAG, LYLE WH (eds): Penicillamine. Proceedings of Conference, The Royal Society of Medicine, London, Nov. 27, 1967. Postgrad Med J Suppl, Oct. 1968.

7. WALSHE JM: The physiology of copper in man and its relation to Wilson's disease. Brain 90: 149-176, 1967.

8. DIXON HBF, GIBBS K, WALSHE JM: Preparation of triethylenetetramine dihydrochloride for the treatment of Wilson's disease. Lancet 1: 853, 1972.

9. WALSHE JM: Copper chelation in patients with Wilson's disease; a comparison of penicillamine and triethylenetetramine dihydrochloride. Quart J Med, N.S. 42: 441-452, 1973.

10. WALSHE JM: Wilson's Disease: The presenting symptoms. Arch Dis Child 37: 253-256, 1962.

11. McINTYRE N, CLINK HM, LEVI AJ: Hemolytic anemia in Wilson's
     disease. N Eng J Med 276: 439-444, 1967.

12. WILLMS B, BLUME KG, LÖHR GW: Hämolytische Anämie bei Morbus
     Wilson (Hepatolentikuläre Degeneration). Klin Wschr 50:
     995-1002, 1972.

13. ISER JH, STEVENS BJ, STENNING JF: Hemolytic anemia of Wilson's
     disease. Gastroenterology 67: 290-293, 1974.

14. WIEBERS DO, WILSON DM, McLEOD RA, GOLSTEIN NP: Renal stones
     in Wilson's disease. Am J Med 67: 249-254, 1979.

15. CAVALLINO R, GROSSMAN H: Wilson's disease presenting with
     rickets. Radiology 90: 493-494, 1968.

16. JOSHUA GE: Hepatolenticular degeneration (Wilson's disease)
     and rickets in children. Indian J Med Res 61: 1876-1884,
     1973.

17. DESTUR DK, MANGHANI DK, WADIA NH: Wilson's disease in India.
     I. Geographic, genetic and clinical aspects in 16 families.
     Neurology 18: 21-31, 1968.

ALPHA-1-ANTITRYPSIN DEFICIENCY

Diane Wilson Cox

Research Institute, The Hospital for Sick Children
and the Departments of Paediatrics, Medical Genetics
and Medical Biophysics, University of Toronto, Ontario

INTRODUCTION

Alpha-1-antitrypsin (α_1AT) is one of several protease
inhibitors in serum which together control proteases involved in
such vital processes as activation of the clotting system, activation and control of the complement system, removal of dead cells
and tissues, and possibly control of the immune response. α_1AT
is the most abundant of the serum protease inhibitors on a molar
basis and inhibits a wide spectrum of proteases including leukocyte
proteases, thrombin, and bacterial proteases. This serum protein
is particularly interesting from a genetic viewpoint in that it
illustrates how a genetic predisposition can interact with other
factors (genetic or environmental), to produce disease.

A deficiency of the α_1 band on agarose electrophoresis
occurring in patients with emphysema was the first recognition,
in 1963, of a disease association for this protease inhibitor (1).
Individuals with the deficiency were susceptible to early onset
emphysema (2). In 1969, α_1AT deficiency was reported to be
associated with cirrhosis in children by Sharp et al (3). Individuals with α_1AT deficiency have a different type of α_1AT with a
different electrophoretic mobility from the normal. The deficient
type is named Pi (protease inhibitor) type Z (genotype ZZ); the
normal is Pi type M (genotype MM).

CLINICAL MANIFESTATIONS

Among children with liver disease, α_1AT deficiency is not a
rare problem. In a study at the Hospital for Sick Children of
104 patients with liver disease of unknown etiology, we found that

271

TABLE I

α_1AT DEFICIENCY: CLINICAL ONSET

35 PATIENTS AT HSC

Presentation	No.
Neonatal obstructive jaundice	22
Hepatomegaly	6
Failure to thrive	3*
Other: non-liver	4
TOTAL	35

(*includes 1 SCID)

10 children (9.6%) had α_1AT deficiency, Pi type ZZ. A further two children (1.9%) were of Pi type SZ, another Pi type associated with a low concentration of α_1AT.

During the past 10 years, 35 patients with α_1AT deficiency (including two sibs) have been identified at The Hospital for Sick Children.   The mode of clinical onset is indicated in Table I. Of the four patients not ascertained because of the presence of liver disease, one each had the following conditions: ulcerative colitis, nephrotic syndrome, anomalous pulmonary drainage, and emphysema.   The majority (71%) of patients with clinically recognized abnormalities of the liver had neonatal obstructive jaundice. One child with failure to thrive had severe combined immune deficiency (SCID)   (4).   Frequently, infants with α_1AT deficiency have features typical of 'neonatal hepatitis syndrome'.   In a series of HSC patients with neonatal hepatitis, five of 17 patients (29.4%) had α_1AT deficiency, Pi type ZZ (5).   This is similar to the frequency obtained in a study in England (6).   A minority of individuals with α_1AT deficiency develop clinical evidence of liver disease.   A study of 120 deficient individuals, obtained from a newborn screening of more than 20,000 infants in Sweden, has shown that approximately 17% develop clinical manifestations of liver disease (7).

BIOCHEMICAL MANIFESTATIONS

Liver function tests in affected children indicate typical cholestatic jaundice, with an increase in direct bilirubin. Liver enzymes indicative of liver disease such as SGOT are moderately increased. Rose Bengal results typically show 10 to 15% excretion, indicating some impairment of biliary excretion. In several respects then, this condition might be mistaken for biliary atresia although biliary excretion is not totally impaired. It is not clear whether α_1AT is involved in some way in the metabolism of bile acids or bilirubin, or if the failure in biliary excretion is merely an indication of the damaged liver. The concentration of α-fetoprotein in serum has been reported to be normal in patients with α_1AT deficiency, although levels are somewhat elevated in infants with neonatal hepatitis not associated with α_1AT deficiency (8).

Protein electrophoresis on a cellulose acetate strip is unreliable for the detection of α_1AT deficiency. This routine semi-quantitative assay for serum proteins usually includes a densitometer scanning of the strip, with the results converted into quantities of protein classes. Typically the figures for the small α_1 peak, which is predominantly α_1AT, are normal even in individuals who have α_1AT deficiency. However direct examination of the strip, not using the densitometer figures, will indicate in most cases, a definite flattening of the α_1 peak. A more reliable method to detect α_1AT deficiency is by an immunological method, specifically for the quantitation of α_1AT. This can be done by radial immunodiffusion, a method available in a number of commercial kits, or by electroimmune assay (9). It is important that each laboratory knows its normal values as the normal values reported with commercial kits are sometimes not appropriate. The point at which a value is considered normal is also of prime importance. Children with α_1AT deficiency and evidence of liver disease generally have concentrations of α_1AT about 20 to 45% of normal. Adults with α_1AT deficiency and lung disease frequently have levels in the range of 10 to 15% of normal. For the screening of children with liver disease, it is therefore important to carry out further testing for any children having a serum α_1AT concentration of 50% or lower. Pi typing of such sera is necessary for confirmation of α_1AT deficiency, as a secondary reduction in α_1AT can result from advanced liver disease, from inflammatory conditions of the gut, or from loss of α_1AT into the urine in kidney disease.

GENETIC ASPECTS

More than 30 genetic variants of α_1AT have been described. These genetic variants or Pi (protease inhibitor) types were first identified by electrophoresis in starch gel, followed by a second electrophoresis into specific α_1AT antibody in agarose (10). The

TABLE II

PI TYPES

IN NORMAL POPULATION

(TORONTO, CANADA)

Phenotype	Number	Percent
M	910	88.6
MS	82	8.0
MZ	23	2.2
SS	3	0.3
FM, lM	4	0.4
Other	5	0.5
TOTAL	1027	100.0

method most commonly used at present is isoelectric focusing in polyacrylamide gels. Even more genetic variants have been recognized using this method. In the Canadian population, the most common Pi types have the frequencies indicated in Table II. The genetic type cannot be assumed by quantitation of α_1AT since α_1AT is an acute phase reactant susceptible to increase even in slight infections. Usually a deficiency of α_1AT is associated with Pi type Z (genotype ZZ). The approximate concentrations of α_1AT for the most common Pi types are as follows: MM - 100%; MS - 86%; MZ - 64% (11). Rare deficient alleles include Pi Mmalton, Pi Mduarte and null. In the latter, no α_1AT is produced.

The inheritance of the specific type of α_1AT is said to be codominant because each genetic type is expressed in the heterozygote. For example, the heterozygote type MZ is an individual who produces both M and Z types of α_1AT. However, the appearance of liver or lung disease appears to be recessive, as it occurs only in those with a deficiency (Pi ZZ), while heterozygotes (Pi MZ) are usually normal. The implications of this recessive disease risk are that 1 in 4 sibs of a patient with α_1AT deficiency will also have the deficiency. The testing of sibs is therefore important.

PATHOLOGY

A complete review of the pathology of the liver and lungs in α_1AT deficiency has recently been published (12). In general, the liver shows evidence of intrahepatic cholestasis, evidence of hepatocellular injury of varying degrees and giant cells particularly in the periportal regions. Fibrosis can be observed even in livers of patients who have not shown evidence of liver disease. In some livers, cirrhosis, both macro and micro nodular, is observed. Occasionally the liver shows paucity of bile ducts. The bile ducts may have disintegrated to such a degree that the pathological picture appears similar to that of extrahepatic cholestasis.

As first reported by Sharp (13), the liver of patients of Pi type ZZ shows typical inclusions which stain bright pink with PAS stain after diastase treatment. Typically, these inclusions are in the rough endoplasmic reticulum. Larger inclusions generally occur in the periportal regions. In children, dust-like particles can be seen in other areas of the hepatocytes. This positive stain with PAS indicates that the inclusions contain carbohydrate. A more specific identification of the inclusions of α_1AT can be obtained by immunofluorescence, using fluoroscein conjugated monospecific α_1AT antibodies. Fluorescence is positive even in very young infants in whom PAS inclusions may not yet be visible. Immunofluorescence can be carried out on formalin-fixed material, although better results are obtained with fresh frozen samples (14). Immunoperoxidase is an even more sensitive stain that can identify small amounts of α_1AT even in individuals of Pi type MM (15).

The storage of α_1AT in inclusions is particularly apparent in the rough endoplasmic reticulum. The normal Z protein is therefore accumulating at the site of synthesis, perhaps due to aggregation or insolubility. These inclusions have been purified from the liver, and have been shown to lack sialic acid, as would be expected from their position in the rough endoplasmic reticulum (16). The addition of sialic acid occurs in the Golgi apparatus, a position not reached by the majority of the abnormal Z molecules. Studies of purified Z α_1AT indicate an amino acid substitution of glutamic acid for lysine in the normal protein (17,18). It is still not known how the amino acid substitution leads to adherence of the α_1AT within the hepatocytes.

α_1AT inclusions occur with other deficient alleles (Mmalton and Mduarte) but not with Pi null, a truly deficient type of α_1AT in which no product is detectable.

An increased risk for hepatoma has been reported in adults with α_1AT deficiency (19). Cirrhosis occurs at a low frequency among adults with α_1AT deficiency, probably in only a few percent (20). We have observed a patient, a 55-year-old female, with hepatoma and no other abnormalities of the liver.

TABLE   III

PROGNOSIS IN α_1AT DEFICIENCY

WITH LIVER SYMPTOMS

Present Status	No.
Deceased (2-16 years)	10*
Abnormal liver function	1
Minor signs	6
Normal	6
TOTAL	23

(*includes 2 non-liver)

PROGNOSIS

The earliest reports of liver disease associated with α_1AT deficiency indicated a poor prognosis, with progressive cirrhosis and early death.   A report of 18 patients of Pi type ZZ at The Hospital for Sick Children has indicated that some children, perhaps as many as two-thirds, recover from their liver abnormalities and become virtually normal (5).   Of the 35 patients from H.S.C., listed in Table I, 31 (including two sibs) were first ascertained because of their clinically apparent liver disease.   The status of those who have been followed to at least two years of age is given in Table III.   The cause of death for two of the ten patients was not related to their liver disease: sudden infant death at four months in a child with a very mild liver abnormality, and death from severe combined immune deficiency at two years of age. Seven of the ten deaths occurred between five and 16 years of age. One of the 23 has definitely abnormal liver function tests, with an SGOT elevated to three times normal.   Six children have shown steady improvement and have only minor signs of liver impairment: hepatomegaly with normal tests of liver function, or a slight increase in SGOT to about 1½ times normal as the only abnormal findings.   Excluding the two children who died of disease not related to their liver abnormality, nine children have had an unfavourable prognosis and 15 appear to be normal or almost normal. Among the earlier cases followed from our hospital, most of those were ascertained because of a continual history of liver disease.

TABLE IV

PROGNOSIS IN α_1AT DEFICIENCY

FOLLOWED TO AT LEAST 2 YEARS

Present Status	SGOT at 2-3 years		
	Increased >100 IU	Normal <100 IU	Unknown
Deceased	3	-	5
Liver Abnormalities	1	-	-
"Normal" (minor signs)	4	2	0
Normal	-	4	2

Among the more recent patients, not yet followed to two years of age, many appear to be recovering from their liver disease. There has probably been a tendency for our figures to show a worse prognosis than the true one because of the bias of the early cases. Longer follow-up periods are required.

In our earlier publication, the data indicated that the concentration of SGOT appeared to be the only possible indicator of outcome (5). Patients with a favourable course tended to have a steady decrease in SGOT while those with a less favourable prognosis tended to have a steady increase in SGOT. In Table IV the prognosis is indicated in relation to an increased SGOT, considered to be greater than 100 IU/l (approximately three times normal). This bears out our previous impression that the SGOT at two to three years of age can give some indication of the outcome. However as cirrhosis proceeds, SGOT may show only a small elevation, but hepatomegaly and jaundice are also usually present.

With the majority of patients showing a favourable prognosis, it is important to be positive, although guarded, in giving information to parents during the neonatal period about the prognosis of their child.

OTHER CLINICAL ABNORMALITIES

There is a well-established association between early onset emphysema and α_1AT deficiency. Seven of our patients have had tests of lung function at six years of age or older. At six years of age, two patients of two tested showed normal tests of

lung function.   By 12 years of age, four of five children tested
showed abnormalities of lung function.   In a study in progress
to follow the sibs of adults with α_1AT deficiency and obstructive
lung disease, we find that non-smokers frequently have normal
tests of lung function up to 25 years of age.   The frequency of
abnormal lung function in children ascertained through their
liver disease appears to be excessively high, although the numbers
are too small at present for drawing conclusions.

Membranoproliferative glomerulonephritis (MPGN) has been
reported previously in three of our patients with liver disease (21).
Of six children with liver disease who have now been examined,
four have had MPGN.   Clinical signs of kidney disease have not
necessarily been present.   There appears to be deposition of α_1AT
on the glomerulus.   Subendothelial deposits have been noted by
electron microscopy.   These deposits of α_1AT may be part of
immune complexes.

STATUS OF SIBS

The 30 probands with clinical evidence of liver disease have
a total of 35 sibs.   Their Pi types are as follows: 7 MM, 15 MZ,
and 13 ZZ, compared with the expectations of a 1:2:1 ratio.   Of
the 13 Pi ZZ sibs, one had definite evidence of cirrhosis.   Two
of 13 have minor signs, as described for our follow-up studies.
Based on the Swedish data, we expect 17% of infants of Pi type ZZ
to show some clinically apparent evidence of liver disease.   If
one third of these have a poor outcome, then we would expect 6% of
the sibs to have liver disease and poor prognosis.   This is compatible with the 1 in 13 we have found.   There does not therefore
appear to be evidence for a marked increase in risk for developing
childhood liver disease among the sibs of probands with clinically
apparent liver disease.   This may not be true in all centres and
will depend to a great extent on whether only the most severely
affected patients are admitted to the centre.   We feel we have a
broad range of patients under study, including those children who
have a transitory hyperbilirubinemia.

VALUE OF DIAGNOSIS

In spite of the fact that there is no known direct therapy for
α_1AT deficiency at the present time, there are several important
reasons for diagnosing the deficiency in children with liver disease:

(1) Some information is available regarding the prognosis,
which appears to be favourable in a high percentage of cases.

(2) Genetic counselling can be offered to the parents.   They
can be told they have a 25% or 1 in 4 risk for having a child with
α_1AT deficiency, Pi type ZZ (assuming they are each of Pi type MZ).

Their chance of having a child who is Pi type ZZ and develops
clinical evidence of liver disease is 25% x 17% = 4%.   If 1/3
of these have a poor prognosis, their overall risk for having a
child with severe liver disease is 1 to 2%.   Amniocentesis, using
a sample of foetal blood, has been reported to be successful in
detecting the Pi type of the fetus (22).   However, against this
must be balanced a relatively low risk for having a child with
severe liver disease.

(3) Prevention: Smokers are known to have considerable
increase in risk for developing emphysema of early onset.   It has
been estimated that smokers develop their first evidence of obstructive lung disease at least 13 years earlier than non smokers with
this deficiency (23).   Early knowledge of the condition may then
help make possible an appropriate lifestyle for the affected child
in the future.   Recommending that parents (Pi MZ) avoid smoking
is useful in two respects: the susceptible child is not exposed
to the harmful effects of smoke and secondly may be less inclined
to develop smoking habits him or herself.

(4)   Treatment may become available in the future.   Replace-
ment of α_1AT is a real possibility.   This may be more helpful for
patients with obstructive lung disease than for those with liver
disease since we do not yet have a reasonable hypothesis for the
cause of the liver disease.   Albumin lysosomes containing a synthetic inhibitor have been tested in animals (24).   Low molecular
weight inhibitors have been found useful in animal models in
preventing emphysema (25).

CONCLUSION

There are still several major unanswered questions regarding
α_1AT deficiency.   We do not know the basic cause for storage of
α_1AT in the liver.   The mechanism of liver damage is not known.
Damage does not appear to be due to the storage of α_1AT itself,
as all individuals of Pi type ZZ accumulate α_1AT in the liver but
only a small percentage of these develop liver disease.   We know
there is considerable variability in the clinical course but we
do not yet know how to alter the course of the disease.

It is important to consider α_1AT deficiency in the differential
diagnosis of liver disease of unknown etiology.   The biochemical
methods used to test for the deficiency must be adequate.   Sibs
of patients with α_1AT deficiency should be tested.   Finally, it
is important to keep in mind that the prognosis in this condition
can be favourable.

SUMMARY

Alpha$_1$-antitrypsin (α_1AT) deficiency is now recognized as a frequent cause of obstructive jaundice in the neonatal period. Approximately one third of infants with the clinical features of the neonatal hepatitis syndrome have α_1AT deficiency. This deficiency can also first manifest as hepatosplenomegaly or failure to thrive.

There is a large number of genetic variants of α_1AT, most of which are associated with a normal concentration of α_1AT and are differentiated only by their electrophoretic mobility. A deficiency of α_1AT is usually associated with the Pi (protease inhibitor) type ZZ. The abnormal Z α_1AT is not secreted normally from the liver, and forms PAS positive globules in the rough endoplasmic reticulum, particularly in periportal areas. Because of the increased retention of α_1AT, serum concentration is reduced, usually to 10 to 20% of the normal amount. However, in children with liver disease the amount of α_1AT in an individual of Pi type ZZ can rise to 40% of normal. Because of the relatively increased concentration of α_1AT, cellulose acetate electrophoresis is not necessarily reliable in identifying α_1AT deficiency.

The prognosis for this disease appears to be better than was originally reported. From our studies of 31 infants and children of Pi type ZZ who have had evidence of liver disease, the majority, about two-thirds, appears to have recovered normal liver function and they are in good health.

REFERENCES

1.   LAURELL CB, ERIKSSON S: The electrophoretic α_1-globulin pattern of serum in α_1-antitrypsin deficiency. Scand J Clin Lab Invest 15: 132-140, 1963.

2.   ERIKSSON S: Studies in α_1-antitrypsin deficiency. Acta Med Scand 177: suppl. 432: 5-85, 1965.

3.   SHARP HL, BRIDGES RA, KRIVIT W, PREIER EF: Cirrhosis associated with alpha-1-antitrypsin deficiency: a previously unrecognized inherited disorder. J Lab Clin Med 73: 934-939, 1969.

4.   GELFAND EW, COX DW, LIN MT, DOSCH HM: Severe combined immune-deficiency disease in patient with α_1-antitrypsin deficiency. Lancet 2: 202, 1979.

5.   MOROZ SP, CUTZ E, COX DW, SASS-KORTSAK A: Liver disease associated with alpha$_1$-antitrypsin deficiency in childhood. J Pediat 88: 19-25, 1976.

6. PORTER CA, MOWAT AP, COOK PJL, HAYNES DWG, SHILKIN KB, WILLIAMS R: α_1-antitrypsin deficiency and neonatal hepatitis. Br Med J 3: 435-439, 1972.

7. SVEGER T: Liver disease in alpha$_1$-antitrypsin deficiency detected by screening of 200,000 infants. N Eng J Med 294: 1316-1321, 1976.

8. JOHNSTON DI, MOWAT AP, ORR H, KOHN J: Serum alpha-fetoprotein levels in extrahepatic biliary atresia, idiopathic neo-natal hepatitis and alpha-1-antitrypsin deficiency (Pi Z). Acta Paediat Scand 65: 623-629, 1976.

9. LAURELL CB: Quantitative estimation of proteins by electro-phoresis in agarose-gel containing antibodies. Anal Biochem 15: 45-49, 1966.

10. FAGERHOL M: The Pi-system. Genetic variants of serum α_1-antitrypsin. Ser Haematol 1: 153-161, 1968.

11. COX DW, HOEPPNER VH, LEVISON H: Protease inhibitors in patients with chronic obstructive pulmonary disease: the alpha$_1$-antitrypsin heterozygote controversy. Am Rev Resp Dis 113: 601-606, 1976.

12. CUTZ E, COX DW: α_1-antitrypsin deficiency: The spectrum of pathology and pathophysiology. In Perspectives in Pediatric Pathology. HS Rosenberg, RP Bolande (eds). Masson, New York, 1979. pp. 1-39.

13. SHARP HL: Alpha-1-antitrypsin deficiency. Hospital Practice 5: 83-96, 1971.

14. HUANG SN, MINASSIAN H, MORE JD: Application of immunofluores-cent staining on paraffin sections improved by trypsin digestion. Lab Invest 35: 383-390, 1976.

15. FELDMANN G, GUILLONZO A, MAURICE M, GUESNON J: Depressed secretion of plasma proteins synthesized by the liver: An ultrastructural investigation based on immunoperoxidase. In First International Symposium on Immunocytochemical Techniques. INSERM. G. Feldman et al (eds). North-Holland Publishing Co., Amsterdam. 1976. pp. 378-394.

16. JEPPSSON JO, LARSSON G, ERIKSSON S: Characterization of α_1-antitrypsin in the inclusion bodies from the liver in α_1-antitrypsin deficiency. N Eng J Med 293: 576-579, 1975.

17. JEPPSSON JO: Amino acid substitution Gly-Lys in α_1-antitrypsin
    PiZ. FEBS Lett 65: 197-197, 1976.

18. YOSHIDA L, LIEBERMAN J, GAIDULIS L, EWING C: Molecular
    abnormality of human α_1-antitrypsin variant (Pi Z) assoc-
    iated with plasma activity deficiency. Proc Natl Acad
    Sci USA 73: 1324-1328, 1976.

19. ERIKSSON S, HAGERSTRAND I: Cirrhosis and malignant hepatoma
    in α_1-antitrypsin deficiency. Acta Med Scand 195:
    451-458, 1974.

20. LARSSON C: Natural history and life expectancy in severe
    $alpha_1$-antitrypsin deficiency, Pi Z. Acta Med Scand 204:
    345-351, 1978.

21. MOROZ SP, CUTZ E, BALFE JW, SASS-KORTSAK A: Membranoprolifera-
    tive glomerulonephritis in childhood cirrhosis associated
    with $alpha_1$-antitrypsin deficiency. Pediatr 57: 232-238,
    1976.

22. JEPPSSON JO, FRANZEN B, SVEGER T, CORDESIUS E, STROMBER P,
    GUSTAVII B: Prenatal exclusion of α_1-antitrypsin
    deficiency in a high risk fetus. N Eng J Med 300:
    1441-1442, 1979.

23. BLACK LF, KUEPPERS F: $Alpha_1$-antitrypsin deficiency in non-
    smokers. Am Rev Resp Dis 117: 421-428, 1978.

24. MARTODAM RR, TWUMASI DY, LIENER IE, POWERS JC, NISHINO N,
    KREJCAREK G: Albumin microspheres as carrier of an
    inhibitor of leukocyte elastase: Potential therapeutic
    agent for emphysema. Proc Natl Acad Sci USA 76: 2128-
    2132, 1979.

25. KLEINERMAN J, RANGA V, RYNBRANDT D, IP MC, SORENSEN J,
    POWERS JC: The effect of the specific elastase inhibitor
    alanyl alanyl prolyl alanine chloromethylketone, on
    elastase-induced emphysema. Am Rev Resp Dis 121: 381-
    387, 1980.

DISCUSSION

CHAIRMAN: H. SHARP

GORESKY: What is the incidence of problems with penicillamine in
    the treatment of patients with Wilson's disease?

SASS-KORTSAK: In only one of 80 patients have we had to discontinue
    treatment with penicillamine.   But we work very hard to make
    patients tolerate penicillamine when problems develop.   The
    patient may develop, 6-7 days after the start of treatment,
    an acute sensitivity reaction with skin rash, fever etc.
    One discontinues the penicillamine for 4-7 days, and then
    re-start with 5 mg and the next day 10 mg and the day after
    20 mg and so on.   Eventually the patient tolerates 1 g
    penicillamine.   If this does not work, then we discontinue
    again, wait until the reaction is gone, put the patient on
    a medium dose of prednisone, and re-start the penicillamine
    using the dose schedule I just mentioned.   Our one failure
    developed severe proteinuria, 5-8 g protein/24 hours, after
    3 or 4 months of treatment.   This is a different type of
    reaction and one must discontinue the penicillamine, death
    from nephrotic syndrome having been reported in this situation.

SHARP: We have allowed these patients to continue on penicillamine
    but have weaned them down to a very low dose.   We have not
    had problems.   But we do fear the Goodpasture type of reaction
    and do not generally recommend this alternative approach.

WONG: What is your experience in using a penicillamine load for
    identifying heterozygotes?

SASS-KORTSAK: Not very good, because the individual who is
    heterozygote for Wilson's disease has anywhere from two to

283

five times the normal amount of copper in the liver and will, in response to a penicillamine load, excrete more copper in the urine than a normal individual.   So you can't use the penicillamine loading test to separate homozygotes from heterozygotes.

PERRAULT: Two of our seven MZ children had neonatal hepatitis and one has hepatomegaly.   Does that fit with the incidence of liver disease in your MZ patients?

COX: What was your source of MZ children?

PERRAULT: They were relatives of subjects with alpha-1-antitrypsin deficiency.

COX: None of our 15 MZ sibs has had liver abnormalities.

SHARP: We haven't seen liver abnormalities in the MZ siblings either but we see a much higher incidence than the Toronto group in ZZ siblings.

COX: We have studied 60 patients with alpha-1-antitrypsin deficiency and lung disease and only one of these has liver disease.   One of the MZ subjects had severe hepatitis and I wonder whether MZ people do worse if they get hepatitis of whatever type.

PERRAULT: Our patients with neonatal hepatitis recovered.

COX: That agrees with our general finding.

PETERS: I want to interject one word of caution about testing. We do a lot of the ceruloplasmin and alpha-1-antitrypsin testing in our area and find that the commercial plates are not very good.   In fact if one takes a standard from one kit and tests it on another one gets very different values. We also find that the commercial laboratories in the Los Angeles area make Wilson's Disease almost epidemic.   They regularly get levels of 5 when it is really 20.   Although the test is simple, the commercial laboratories do it very badly.

COX: The immunological kits for alpha-1-antitrypsin do vary tremendously in their normal values because until recently there had been no standard purification technique.   This is why we express it as a percentage of a normal pool.   For transportation purposes, sodium azide is often added to the serum because it preserves the protein pattern for electro-phoresis.   However sodium azide inhibits ceruloplasmin and if you use such sera in an enzymatic assay you certainly will come up with a lot of patients with Wilson's disease. If you test for ceruloplasmin immunologically, it will be normal.

PETERS: There had been a lot of conjecture that liver cell carcinoma and alpha-1-antitrypsin have a relationship. We have found no ZZ's in 120 cases of liver cell carcinoma. We have found perhaps an insignificant increase in MZ. What has been your experience along these lines?

COX: We have been looking for hepatoma in alpha-1-antitrypsin patients with lung disease and in alpha-1-antitrypsin adults with liver disease. One adult patient with liver disease developed a hepatoma. We also had one very interesting alpha-1-antitrypsin deficient patient with lung disease who had no evidence at all of liver disease but who at autopsy was found to have a hepatoma. Perhaps there is a relationship.

SHARP: The answer is not in and the problem is really that no group has enough patients to find out whether individuals with abnormalities in alpha-1-antitrypsin are predisposed to certain diseases.

CLOSING COMMENTS

CLAUDE C. ROY

Three books have been published during the past year on
Pediatric Liver Disease: Alexander Mowat from King's College
Hospital in London, a second one edited by Ranjit Chandra, who is
at St. John's, Newfoundland, and one by Daniel Alagille and Michel
Odièvre from l'hôpital des enfants de Bicètre in Paris. This
Fifth International Symposium of the Canadian Liver Foundation has
further alerted us to the importance of Pediatric Hepatology as a
rapidly developing field.

This two-day symposium has been quite an experience for all
of us through the exchange of ideas and the fraternization. It
has provided a very good update on current clinical problems while
attracting special attention to those clinical and research areas
where answers are urgently needed. Some of the data presented
was new information; although some of it still appears quite
fragile and vulnerable, it has given us some sense of direction in
the field. The program was drawn up so that the differences
between pediatric and adult hepatology would become evident. I
think the meeting has been successful in that sense.

Before closing I would like to express very special thanks to
Valerie Price, Executive Director of the Foundation, who has
played a key role in organizing this meeting, to Woody Fisher and
to Jim Weber who have been essential components of the Program
Committee to put this Symposium together. I am grateful to the
Session Chairmen for their skilful direction, to the speakers who
have been extremely good at reporting their work in such a scholarly
fashion, and to all of you. We should all thank the Canadian
Liver Foundation for giving us this unique opportunity in such
pleasant surroundings.

CONTRIBUTORS

D. Alagille,
        Clinique de Pédiatrie
        Université Paris-Sud
        Hôpital de Bicêtre
        Bicêtre, France

H. J. Alter,
        Immunology Section, Blood Bank Department
        Clinical Center, National Institutes of Health
        Bethesda, Maryland

D. H. Carver,
        Department of Paediatrics
        University of Toronto
        Hospital for Sick Children
        Toronto, Ontario

D. W. Cox,
        Departments of Paediatrics and Genetics
        University of Toronto
        The Hospital for Sick Children
        Toronto, Ontario

E. Cutz,
        Department of Pathology
        University of Toronto
        Hospital for Sick Children
        Toronto, Ontario

R. C. de Belle,
        Department of Paediatrics
        McGill University
        Montreal Children's Hospital
        Montreal, Quebec

J. L. Dienstag,
        Department of Medicine
        Harvard Medical School
        Massachusetts General Hospital
        Boston, Massachusetts

M. M. Fisher,
        Department of Medicine
        University of Toronto
        Sunnybrook Medical Centre
        Toronto, Ontario

L. M. Gartner,
        Department of Pediatrics
        University of Chicago
        Chicago, Illinois

H. L. Greene,
        Department of Pediatrics
        Vanderbilt University Hospital
        Nashville, Tennessee

S. Krugman,
        Department of Pediatrics
        New York University Medical Center
        New York, New York

J. R. Lilly,
        Department of Surgery
        University of Colorado Medical Center
        Denver, Colorado

S. B. Melançon,
        Centre de Recherche Pediatrique
        Hôpital Sainte-Justine
        Université de Montréal
        Montréal, Québec

A. B. Okey,
        Department of Paediatrics
        University of Toronto
        The Hospital for Sick Children
        Toronto, Ontario

R. L. Peters,
        Department of Pathology
        University of Southern California School of Medicine
        Los Angeles, California

C. C. Roy,
          Département de Pédiatrie
          Université de Montréal
          Hôpital Sainte-Justine
          Montréal, Québec

A. Sass-Kortsak,
          Department of Paediatrics
          University of Toronto
          Hospital for Sick Children
          Toronto, Ontario

B. Shandling,
          Department of Surgery
          University of Toronto
          Hospital for Sick Children
          Toronto, Ontario

H. L. Sharp,
          Departments of Pediatrics and Medicine
          University of Minnesota Health Sciences Center
          Minneapolis, Minnesota

I. M. Taylor,
          Department of Anatomy
          Faculty of Medicine
          University of Toronto
          Toronto, Ontario

M. M. Thaler,
          Department of Pediatrics
          University of California
          San Francisco, California

J. B. Watkins,
          Department of Pediatrics
          University of Pennsylvania School of Medicine
          The Children's Hospital of Philadelphia
          Philadelphia, Pennsylvania

A. M. Weber,
          Département de Pédiatrie
          Université de Montréal
          Hôpital Sainte-Justine
          Montréal, Québec

J. L. Weber,
        Department of Paediatrics
        University of Toronto
        Hospital for Sick Children
        Toronto, Ontario

C. L. Witzleben,
        Department of Pathology
        University of Pennsylvania School of Medicine
        Children's Hospital of Philadelphia
        Philadelphia, Pennsylvania